A Handbook of TCM Pediatrics

A Handbook of TCM Pediatrics

Bob Flaws

Blue Poppy Press

Published by:
BLUE POPPY PRESS
A Division of Blue Poppy Enterprises, Inc.
5441 Western Ave. #2
BOULDER, CO 80301

FIRST EDITION, JANUARY 1997
SECOND PRINTING, JUNE 2002
SECOND EDITION, MARCH 2006

ISBN 0-936185-72-4
LC 96-86028

COPYRIGHT 2006 © BLUE POPPY PRESS

All rights reserved. No part of this book may be reproduced, stored in a retrieval system, transcribed in any form or by any means, electronic, mechanical, photocopy, recording, or any other means, or translated into any language without the prior written permission of the publisher.

Disclaimer: The information in this book is given in good faith. However, the translators and the publishers cannot be held responsible for any error or omission. Nor can they be held in any way responsible for treatment given on the basis of information contained in this book. The publishers make this information available to English language readers for scholarly and research purposes only.

The publishers do not advocate nor endorse self-medication by laypersons. Chinese medicine is a professional medicine. Laypersons interested in availing themselves of the treatments described in this book should seek out a qualified professional practitioner of Chinese medicine.

COMP Designation: Original work using a standard translational terminology

Text & Cover design by Eric Brearton

Printed at National Hirschfeld, Denver, CO

10 9 8 7 6 5 4 3 2 1

Contents

Preface vii

Book One

1	Introduction	3
2	The Unique Characteristics of Children	7
3	The Main Cause of Most Children's Diseases	13
4	Key Points in Diagnosing Children	17
5	Key Points in Treating Children	29
6	Chinese Dietary Therapy & Pediatrics	33
7	Chinese Herbal Medicine	43
8	Acupuncture & Moxibustion	49
9	Antibiotics & Immunizations	51

Book Two

1	The Diagnosis & Treatment of Commonly Encountered Pediatric Diseases	63
2	Emergency Formulas	305
3	Case Histories	315

Appendix 1: Developmental Mileposts — 321
Appendix 2: Resources for Going Further — 325
Bibliography — 331
General Index — 331
Formula Index — 343

Preface

In 1985 I published a book on Oriental pediatrics titled *Turtle Tail and Tender Mercies*. It was based on my research of the English language literature available at that time and my study of and clinical experience in pediatric *tui na* in China. That book sold well and undoubtedly helped many practitioners and patients alike. Blue Poppy Press still gets orders for that book even though it has been out of print for some years. However, although *Turtle Tail* filled a need in its time, after several years it became apparent to me that, as a clinical manual of TCM pediatrics, it was seriously flawed. As publisher of Blue Poppy Press, I have tried several times to commission a really good TCM pediatric text to meet the needs of Western practitioners and their patients. Unfortunately, no one has submitted a completed manuscript though more than one Chinese practitioner has promised. In the intervening years, I have taught myself to read medical Chinese. Thus I have taken it upon myself to create a new English language clinical manual on the TCM treatment of pediatric diseases.

As my practice has developed over the years, I have more and more concentrated on the prescription of internally administered Chinese herbal medicines. *Turtle Tail* gave herbal, acupuncture, and *tui na* treatments for most of the diseases it covered. In this book and consistent with the majority of Chinese TCM pediatric books, except for a short chapter on pediatric acupuncture in general and a short section on acupuncture under most of the diseases discussed, I have primarily focused on the herbal treatment of pediatric diseases. Acupuncture can be an effective modality for the treatment of certain pediatric diseases. However, I find the prescription of Chinese herbal medicines mostly sufficient, quite convenient to administer, and I prefer, if possible, not to make my little friends cry. For more detailed information on pediatric acupuncture, the reader is referred to Julian Scott's *Acupuncture in the Treatment of Children* published by Eastland Press of Seattle, WA. As for pediatric *tui na*, Blue Poppy Press has published a treatment manual on pediatric *tui na* written by Dr. Fan Ya-li formerly of the Shandong

College of TCM. Therefore, I have left it to that book to discuss that treatment modality.

In reviewing the Chinese literature on pediatrics, it is clear that most Chinese pediatric manuals discuss a number of diseases that Western children do not commonly suffer from, such as malnutrition, epidemic dysentery, and epidemic encephalitis B. Other conditions discussed in Chinese manuals, such as polio, tetanus, and leukemia, are better and more appropriately treated by modern Western medicine. Therefore, I have kept the topics discussed in this book solely to the diseases and conditions which typically present in a TCM outpatient clinic in the West. These diseases, other than seasonal epidemics such as measles and mumps, have been presented in a roughly longitudinal manner, meaning that they have been introduced more or less chronologically in terms of their likelihood of appearance. For additional information on the treatment of common skin diseases in children, the reader is referred to Liang Jian-hui's *Handbook of Traditional Chinese Dermatology*, also published by Blue Poppy Press, and to *Manual of Dermatology in Chinese Medicine* by Shen De-hui, Wu Xiu-fen, and Nissi Wang published by Eastland Press.

The material in this book is taken from a number of Chinese sources. These are listed in the bibliography. I have used Nigel Wiseman's terminology as it appears in *A Practical Dictionary of Chinese Medicine*, Paradigm Publications, 1998, as consistently as possible. Medicinals are identified in Pinyin followed by Latin pharmacological nomenclature in parentheses. These identifications are primarily based on Bensky *et al. Chinese Herbal Medicine: Materia Medica.* In a very few cases, they are based on Hong-yen Hsu's *Oriental Materia Medica: A Concise Guide,* or the Shanghai Science & Technology Press's *Zhong Yao Da Ci Dian (Dictionary of Chinese Medicinals)*.

This book is meant for students and professional practitioners of Traditional Chinese Medicine. It is not intended as a parent's guide. For parents and lay readers, I have specifically written *Keeping Your Child Healthy with Chinese Medicine: A Parent's Guide to the Care and Prevention of Common Childhood Diseases.* That book is meant as a companion volume to this one, explaining traditional Chinese theories on diet and child care. Although that book does give a number of simple home remedies for common pediatric complaints, parents of children who are ill are advised to seek out professional TCM care for their charges. The full benefit of TCM pediatrics is only made manifest when treatment is based on a professional pattern discrimination which is beyond the means of most Western parents.

Many readers know that my first specialty is TCM gynecology. However, because

I treat so many women, when they see how much good Chinese medicine has done for them, they frequently ask me to also treat their children. Therefore, it is not uncommon for me to see in my clinic as many or even more infants and toddlers in a day than adult women. As a father myself, I love babies and children of all ages, and it is one of my joys in life to be able to relieve the suffering of what in Chinese are called 'our little friends.' Some Western TCM practitioners are hesitant to or simply do not treat babies and children in their practices. However, it is my experience that Chinese medicine offers quick and effective treatment for the majority of common childhood complaints. Once one knows the key essentials of TCM pediatric diagnosis and treatment, TCM pediatrics is a relatively simple specialty and one which deserves much more attention in the Western world. Hopefully this book will help to show how easy it is to diagnosis and treat our little friends with Chinese medicine.

Bob Flaws
Boulder, CO

BOOK ONE

1
Introduction

Pediatrics is one of the oldest specialties within Chinese medicine. Zhang Zhong-jing's *Jin Gui Yao Lue (Essentials of the Golden Cabinet)* and Wang Shu-he's *Mai Jing (Pulse Classic)* both date from the late Han dynasty (*i.e.*, the late 200s CE) and both contain chapters specifically on pediatrics. Wang Dao's *Wai Tai Mi Yao (Secret Essentials of an Outer [i.e., Frontier] Official)*, Sun Si-maio's *Bei Ji Qian Jin Yao Fang (Emergency Formulas [Worth] a Thousand [Pieces of] Gold)*, and Chao Yuan-fang's *Zhu Bing Yuan Hou Lun (Treatise on the Origins & Symptoms of Various Diseases)* all contain chapters specifically about pediatrics. Qian Yi, also known as Qian Zhong-yang, was one of the earliest and most famous Chinese pediatric specialists. Living in the Song dynasty from 1032-1113 CE, he was the author of the first book devoted solely to pediatrics in Chinese medical literature, the *Xiao Er Yao Zheng Zhi Jue (A Collection of Essential Pediatric Patterns & Treatments)*. He was also the first Chinese pediatrician to detail the different patterns in measles, scarlet fever, chicken pox, and smallpox. Qian pointed out the unique characteristics of infants and young children and he introduced new methods of diagnosis and treatment based on those unique characteristics. Also in the Song dynasty, Liu Fang wrote a book on pediatrics titled *You You Xin Shu (The Heart Book of Pediatrics)* which sits on the shelf in front of me as I write this introduction.

In the Ming dynasty (1368-1644 CE), a number of influential pediatricians summarized their experiences and theories in various books on TCM pediatrics. Xue Liang-wu, a distinguished imperial physician, wrote the *Bao Ying Cuo Yao (Essentials for the Care & Protection of Infants)* in 1556 in which he stressed the importance of the correct adjustment of herbal formulas for children depending on their age and size. In 1534, Wang Luan wrote the *You Ke Lei Cui (A Collection of Pediatric Cases)*. This is a comprehensive text which lists the pulse, treatment principles, acupuncture protocols, and herbal formulas under each pediatric disease.

Wan Quan, also know as Wan Mi-zhai, was one of the most famous Ming dynasty pediatricians. He was the third generation in his family to practice medicine and he, therefore, inherited his father and grandfather's lifelong experience in pediatrics. Wan Quan advocated that children should be frequently exposed to sunlight and fresh air, trained to resist cold, protected from being frightened, and should not be overfed or given too much medicine. Wan's most famous works on pediatrics include *Dou Zhen Shi Yi Xin Fa (Heart Methods Handed Through the Generations for Poxes & Rashes)*, *You Ke Fa Hui (An Exposition on Pediatrics)*, and *Yu Ying Jia Mi (Family Secrets in Pediatrics)*.

In the Qing dynasty (1644-1911 CE), He Meng-yao wrote *You Ke Liang Fang (Fine Formulas in Pediatrics)* and *Dou Zhen Liang Fang (Fine Formulas for Poxes & Rashes)*. And besides entire books devoted to pediatrics, numerous premodern Chinese doctors included sections on pediatrics in their collected life's works. One Qing dynasty example is Shen Jin-ao's *Shen Shi Zan Sheng Su (Master Shen On the Importance of Preserving Life)*. In addition to chapters on materia medica, pulse examination, febrile and miscellaneous diseases, and gynecology, Shen included a section on pediatrics. This book, because of its rich content, is still a popular book in TCM circles in China.

Today, every TCM college in China teaches undergraduate and postgraduate courses in pediatrics, and every TCM hospital has a pediatric department. In addition, hundreds of books on TCM pediatrics have been published in China in this century. When one visits such a department in a Chinese TCM hospital or if one looks at a modern Chinese TCM pediatric textbook, one will see that the primary modality employed is the prescription of Chinese herbal medicine. This is because, traditionally, pediatrics (*er ke*) was seen as a subdivision (along with gynecology [*fu ke*]) or was at least connected with internal medicine (*nei ke*), and *nei ke* in China means the administration of internal herbal medicine. This means that, although many Chinese acupuncture books contain sections on pediatric diseases and although one can see some children receiving treatment in Chinese acupuncture clinics, the specialty of pediatrics in TCM implies, at least to the Chinese, the use of Chinese herbal medicine.

However, there is one other place where pediatrics is also practiced and written about as a specialty within Chinese medicine, and that is in *tui na*. *Tui na* is Chinese medical massage, and within *tui na* there is the very healthy and robust specialty of *xiao er tui na* or pediatric massage. Chinese pediatric massage developed in the Jin (265-420 CE), Northern & Southern (420-589 CE), Sui (589-618 CE), and Tang (618-907 CE) dynasties. However, its real blossoming occurred in the Ming dynasty. For instance, there is a chapter on pediatric massage in Yang Ji-zhou's *Zhen Jiu Da Cheng (Great Compendium of Acupuncture & Moxibustion)*. During the Ming and Qing dynasties, numerous books were published on pediatric massage and now every Chinese TCM college and hospital have their pediatric massage departments. Readers interested in Chinese pediatric massage should see the bibliography at the back of this book for English language titles and videotapes.

As mentioned above, in Chinese medicine, infants and young children are not just miniature adults. Children's anatomy and physiology are intrinsically different from an adult's. The child is immature, and this immaturity is reflected in their immature anatomy and physiology just as much as their immature mental and emotional capacities. This means that, in TCM pediatrics, young children are prone to certain disease causes and disease mechanisms, certain methods are used specifically for diagnosing young children, and that children even have their own treatment principles and treatment modalities. Therefore, in TCM, pediatrics is really very much a specialty. The good news is that, if one keeps these basic differences in mind and understands their implications, then the rest of TCM pediatrics is relatively easy to understand and practice.

2
The Unique Characteristics of Children

The Two Main Characteristics of Pediatric Physiology

There are two main characteristics to pediatric physiology according to TCM theory.

1. The viscera and bowels are tender and delicate and the form qi is not full.

In the Warring States period, approximately 200 BCE, the *Ling Shu (Spiritual Pivot)* stated: "Children's flesh is fragile, their blood is scanty, and their qi is weak." Eight hundred years later, Chao Yuan-fang, in his *Zhu Bing Yuan Hou Lun (Treatise on the Origins & Symptoms of Various Diseases)* reiterated this point when he said, "Children's viscera and bowel qi is soft and weak." Qian Yi, in his Song dynasty *Xiao Er Yao Zheng Zhi Jue (A Collection of Essential Pediatric & Patterns & Treatments)*, says, "The five viscera and six bowels are made but not complete . . . are complete but not strong." And finally, the *Xiao Er Bing Yuan Fang Lun (Treatise on the Origins of Pediatric Diseases & Their Treatments)* says, "The skin and hair, muscles and flesh, sinews and bones, brain and marrow, the five viscera and six bowels, the constructive and defensive, and the qi and blood of children as a whole are not hard and secure." All these quotes from the earliest written TCM records to modern books on Chinese pediatrics agree that all the physical and physiological constitutions of children are weak and immature.

2. Children have a pure yang constitution.

This means that yin and yang within young children's bodies are not well integrated. Because yin is not capable of checking and controlling yang, yang easily becomes hyperactive. When yang becomes hyperactive, it may easily manifest as evil heat.

The Two Main Characteristics of Pediatric Pathophysiology

There are two main characteristics of pediatric pathophysiology according to TCM theory.

1. Children are easily susceptible to disease which then transmits and changes rapidly.

This means that children are prone to getting sick more easily than adults. Every parent and pediatrician is well aware of this fact. However, when children do get ill, their diseases progress more rapidly through the various divisions or stages described by Chinese medical theory than in adults. According to TCM theory, there are three main viscera responsible for the majority of pediatric diseases. These are the lungs, spleen, and liver.

A. The lungs

It says in the *Zhong Yi Er Ke Xue (A Study of Chinese Medicine Pediatrics)* that:

> Children's exterior defensive is not secure. Therefore, external evils easily enter the exterior and assail the lungs.

The exterior defensive refers to the exterior of the body guarded and controlled by the defensive qi. The defensive qi is, in turn, controlled by the lungs. If evils enter the exterior of the body, they hinder and obstruct the free flow of the defensive qi which then accumulates in the exterior producing symptoms of muscular aches and pains as well as fever. This accumulation of defensive qi in the exterior hinders the lungs' control over downward depuration or perfusion and depuration. Thus the lung qi counterflows upward, resulting in sneezing and coughing. In addition, because fluids are not sent down to the bladder, fluids may accumulate in the lungs, transforming or congealing into phlegm. Once evils enter the body, they may also enter the lungs internally due to the lungs being the "tender viscus." This all explains why children are prone to catching cold and developing coughs, asthma, bronchitis, allergies, etc.

B. The spleen

It also says in the *Zhong Yi Er Ke Xue (A Study of Chinese Medicine Pediatrics)*:

> Children's transportation and transformation is not fortified and complete. Therefore, they are easily damaged by food.

The terms transportation and transformation refer to the spleen's transportation and transformation of water and grains or foods and liquids. In addition, the word fortify also technically implies the spleen in Chinese medicine. When one specifically wants to supplement the spleen, we say that the spleen should be fortified. This means that spleen function *vis a vis* digestion is weak and immature in children. If the spleen's function of the transportation and transformation of foods and liquids is weak, then stagnant food may easily accumulate in the stomach.

When this happens, it may result in several possible diseases or disease mechanisms. First, it may give rise to indigestion and other digestive tract complaints, such as vomiting and/or diarrhea, with the signs and symptoms of food stagnation. Secondly, it may give rise to symptoms of evil heat. This is because food depression is a yin evil which obstructs the flow of yang qi. When yang qi is not allowed to flow freely, it becomes stagnant or depressed and accumulates. Because it is yang, when it accumulates, it may manifest as heat, since warmth is one of the inherent characteristics of yang qi. Third, food stagnation implies that the clear and the turbid are not separated as they should be. The clear is not upborne and the turbid is not downborne. Thus turbid fluids accumulate and these may transform and congeal into phlegm. And fourth, because stagnant food hinders and obstructs the upbearing of the clear qi, the spleen is not fortified by this qi. Thus the spleen becomes damaged and vacuous, and this spleen qi vacuity only results in the spleen's further loss of control over transportation and transformation. This then becomes a vicious circle about which we will have plenty more to say.

C. The liver

Zhu Dan-xi, one of the four great masters of internal medicine of the Jin-Yuan dynasties, in his *Dan Xi Xin Fa (Dan-xi's Heart Methods)* says that, in children, "The liver commonly has a surplus." The clinical implication of this is that children may easily develop internal stirring of liver wind. This is due to several reasons. First, we have already seen that children's blood is inherently scanty. It is the liver which stores the blood and the sinews are controlled by the liver. Thus children's blood may not always nourish their sinews adequately. If the sinews do not receive adequate nourishment and moistening from the blood, then they contract, causing spasms. Secondly, if food, dampness, or phlegm become depressed due to impeded lung and/or spleen function, the qi will not flow easily and uninhibitedly but rather it will also tend to become stagnant and depressed. Stagnant qi results in the liver losing its control over coursing and discharge. Thus the liver becomes replete (at least in terms of qi). This liver qi repletion and depression may easily lead to liver yang hyperactivity due to children's inherent pure yang constitution. And liver yang hyperactivity may, in turn, give rise to liver fire and/or internal stirring of wind. Third, if evil heat accumulates in the body for any reason, again due to children's inherently pure yang constitution, this heat may transform into fire which then may become internal stirring of wind. Since the liver is the wind wood viscus, internal stirring of wind is typically associated at least in some way with the liver in TCM, if not causally, at least in terms of treatment.

2. Children's visceral qi is clear and effective; therefore, they easily and quickly return to health.

Because children are young and new, their viscera and bowels have not yet accumulated a lifetime of evil qi. The types of evil qi we accumulate with age are dampness and turbidity, stagnant qi and static blood, and deep-lying or hidden evils. The famous TCM geriatrics specialist, Yan De-xin, in his book *Aging & Blood Stasis*, says that aging is due to blood stasis which impedes the functioning of the viscera and bowels. This blood stasis may be due to enduring disease, traumatic injury, long-term qi stagnation, or any evil qi, such as dampness, phlegm, or food stagnation which hinder and obstruct the free flow of qi. Secondarily then, the viscera and bowels do not engender and transform the same amounts of qi and blood. Consequently, the body does not receive adequate nourishment and prenatal or former heaven essence is used up.

In children, this has not yet happened to any appreciable degree. Therefore, when they do get ill, they tend to recuperate very rapidly. This also means that they tend to respond to light treatment and small doses.

Other key statements of fact about the unique pathophysiological characteristics of children

In addition, there are a number of other traditional sayings about the unique pathophysiological characteristics of children. First of all, "Because of immature yang body, evils easily enter." The yang referred to here is the defensive yang. Because the defensive yang is inherently weak, external evils may easily enter a child's body and cause disease.

Secondly, "Because of delicate and tender flesh and muscles, they transmit changes easily." This means that if external evils enter the body, they are easily transmitted or work their way from one division of the body to another. Division here refers to the six divisions of the *Shang Han Lun (Treatise on Damage [Due to] Cold)* and the four divisions of *wen bing xue* or warm disease theory. This means that external evils may easily and relatively quickly go from the *tai yang* to the *shao yang* or from the *wei* to the *ying* or *xue fen*.

Third, "Because of sensitive stomachs, they spit up food and milk easily." This is simply a restatement that children's spleens are inherently weak and immature and they easily suffer from food damage.

Fourth, "Because of immature essence qi, they gain and lose weight easily." This essence qi refers to the postnatal or latter heaven essence. The spleen is the root of latter heaven essence manufactured from the excess of qi and blood engendered and transformed by the spleen from food and liquids. When one goes to sleep, this excess or superabundant qi and blood are transformed into acquired or postnatal essence. Because children's spleens are inherently immature and weak, they do not manufacture much in the way of excess qi and blood. Therefore, they do not store as much acquired essence as a more mature person does. Consequently, because they do not have this backup reserve of acquired essence which can be turned back into qi and blood, they easily lose weight if anything damages their spleen function.

Fifth, "Because of cowardly spirit qi, they easily become emotionally upset." Li Dong-yuan, another of the four great masters of internal medicine of the Jin-Yuan dynasties, in his monumentally important *Pi Wei Lun (Treatise on the Spleen & Stomach)* has this to say about the production of spirit in the human body:

> Qi is the forefather of spirit and essence is the child of qi. Thus qi is the root of essence and spirit. Great is qi! When qi accumulates, it produces essence. When essence accumulates, it renders essence wholesome.

This means that spirit is nothing other than an accumulation of qi and essence in the heart. However, since essence is nothing other than an accumulation of qi, spirit is really nothing other than an accumulation of qi. As we have already seen, the spleen is the postnatal root of engenderment and transformation of qi and, in young children, the spleen is inherently vacuous and weak. Thus it is easy to see why the spirit would be so restless and easily upset in infants and young children. The spirit is quiet or calm only if it is nourished by sufficient qi and blood. Since these tend to be scanty and weak, the spirit likewise is easily upset.

Sixth, "Because of fetal toxins accumulated, they are more susceptible to pox." It is believed in Chinese medicine that toxins can be inherited from the parents at the moment of conception or may be engendered during gestation due to the mother's faulty diet and lifestyle. Such congenital toxins are called fetal toxins in TCM, and they are a species of deep-lying or hidden warm evils. Deep-lying or hidden evils are evils which remain latent in the body until some later circumstance allows them to become active. If children have inherited or developed fetal toxins *in utero*, certain types of invading seasonal or pestilential qi can combine with these fetal toxins and result in rather virulent epidemic pox diseases. These include rubella, rubeola, and chicken pox as specifically pediatric pox diseases.

And seventh, "Because of soft, weak viscera and bowels, they easily become cold and hot, hungry and full." Once again this goes back to children's inherent scanty and weak qi and blood which, in turn, have to do with their inherently weak spleen qi. It is qi which keeps the body warm. Therefore, if qi becomes weak, there is cold. If qi becomes inhibited and depressed, then there is depressive or transformative heat. Because children's bodies lack reserves (*i.e.*, acquired essence), they easily become hungry, but, because their spleen qi is weak, they easily also become full. In the latter case, the spleen is not strong enough to transport and transform a lot of food at one time. Thus infants and young children have to eat many small meals throughout the day.

3
The Main Cause of Most Children's Diseases

In theory, pediatric diseases may be due to either external, internal, or neither external nor internal causes. External causes refers to the six environmental excesses and pestilential qi. Internal causes refers to damage by the seven affects or emotions. And neither external nor internal causes refers to a miscellaneous collection of disease causes, such as diet, lifestyle, sex, trauma, poisoning, drowning, etc. Although pediatric diseases may be due to any of these three groups of disease causes, in children under six years of age, diet is, by far in my experience, the leading cause of the commonly encountered pediatric complaints with external and internal causes aggravating the ill effects of a faulty diet.

Diet as the key cause of most children's diseases

In particular, children under the age of five or six are believed to have immature or weak digestion and it is this fact which accounts for most of the commonly encountered pediatric diseases, including colic, earache, cough, swollen glands, allergies, and pediatric asthma and eczema. In Chinese medicine, the digestion is spoken of as the spleen and stomach and it is a statement of fact that, "In children the spleen is insufficient."

The Chinese medical conception of digestion

According to TCM, the process of digestion is likened to the process of the distillation of alcohol. The stomach is likened to a fermentation vat. It receives the food and drink which are "rottened and ripened" in the stomach. However, this pot of the stomach sits on a stove. That stove is the spleen which provides the heat which drives off the essence of the food and drink the same way that fire under a still drives off the alcohol from the mash. This means that it is the warmth of the spleen which provides the force for the transformation of food and liquids. This warmth of the spleen is called the spleen yang when describing its warming function, while it is referred to as spleen qi when describing its transforming and transporting function.

Thus the spleen yang qi transforms the finest essence of food and liquids and sends this upward to the heart and lungs. This finest essence of food and liquids becomes qi in the lungs, while it becomes blood in the heart. The lungs then send the qi out to the rest of the body just as the heart sends the blood out to the rest of the body. The qi provides the motivating force for all other transformations and transportations in the body, while the blood provides the moistening and nourishment for all the tissues of the body. If the qi and blood are sufficient and flow freely and without impediment to the entire body, then there is power to function and nourishment to build and repair the body and also to fuel that function. If, however, there is insufficient qi and blood, then function and nourishment are weak and deficient and there is the possibility of disease.

The finest essence which becomes the qi and blood is like the essence of alcohol that is driven off to collect in the cooling coils of a still. In Chinese medicine, this finest essence is often simply referred to as the clear. In contradistinction, the dregs or what is left behind are called the turbid. Hence the creation of qi and blood out of the finest essence of food and drink is also described as the separation of clear and turbid. The clear is sent upward to become the qi and blood, while the turbid is sent downward to be excreted as waste from the body through urination and defecation.

As stated above, Chinese doctors believe that the baby's spleen and stomach or digestion is inherently weak and immature. This means that the baby's digestion has a hard time separating clear and turbid efficiently and completely. On the one hand, this means that, although the baby eats and drinks, they do not make the same amount of qi and blood an adult would. Thus the baby spends much more time sleeping than the adult. On the other hand, this means that turbid qi is not always excreted as efficiently as possible. Instead, this turbid material may collect internally and "gum up the works."

Food, phlegm & dampness

In Chinese medicine, this turbid material may collect in the stomach and intestines where it obstructs the free flow of the stomach and intestinal qi and depresses their function. This then causes abdominal distention, stomachache, constipation, diarrhea, and/or vomiting. This turbid material may also overflow from the middle burner or middle section of the body, the home of the spleen and stomach. Typically, this turbid residue is seen as damp in nature. Thus this turbid dampness may cause all sorts of symptoms associated with excess dampness, such as diarrhea and vomiting as well as damp skin lesions. If this dampness congeals, it may form phlegm.

According to Chinese medicine, phlegm is nothing other than congealed dampness resulting from incompletely digested food and drink. Because it is the spleen which is the motivating force for the separation of clear and turbid, *i.e.*, the digestion of food and drink, it is said, "The spleen is the source of phlegm production." However, phlegm, once it is produced, tends to accumulate in the lungs. This is supported by the saying, "The lungs are the place where phlegm is stored." If phlegm gathers in the lungs, it obstructs and inhibits the flow of lung qi and this results in stuffy nose, runny nose, sneezing, coughing, and even asthmatic wheezing.

The most commonly encountered pediatric diseases are either upper respiratory tract complaints, such as cough, cold, asthma, and allergies, or are digestive tract complaints, such as colic, diarrhea, stomachache, and vomiting. The first group of diseases all have to do with phlegm accumulating in the lungs, while the second group have to do with poor digestion. However, since according to the Chinese medical theory, phlegm is a by-product of poor digestion, one can say that all these complaints are, in children, at root all due to their immature and, therefore, faulty digestion. This is why my first teacher of Chinese medicine, Dr. (Eric) Tao Xi-yu of Denver, was fond of saying that all pediatric diseases are due to indigestion.

Inflammation & upward counterflow

In Chinese medicine, qi is inherently warm. Qi is also what transports and transforms food and liquids. If qi fails to transport and transform these foods and liquids and a turbid residue gathers and accumulates, this may obstruct the free and normal flow of the qi. The qi builds or backs up. Since it is inherently warm, if the qi backs up abnormally, there will be an abnormal accumulation of heat in that part of the body and this pathological accumulation may manifest as inflammation. Thus dampness may become damp heat, stagnant food may become stagnant food and stomach heat, and phlegm may become phlegm heat.

If this qi builds up to a certain point, eventually it must go somewhere. If turbid dampness, food, and phlegm keep the qi from flowing normally and it builds up like gas in a balloon, eventually it must find some avenue of escape. Because qi is yang, it also has an inherent tendency to move upward. That means that if it builds up past a certain point, qi will tend to counterflow abnormally upwards. This may then produce hiccup, burping and belching, vomiting, and/or coughing.

Therefore, one can see that the poor digestion associated with young infants and children under the age of five or six canot only produce excessive dampness and phlegm inside the body but can also indirectly be associated with counterflowing qi and inflammatory heat. When one adds these two disease mechanisms to the list, one can see that weak digestion may play a part in even more of the diseases and symptoms associated with infants and children.

And further, it is the qi which protects the body from invasion by various pathogens in the external environment. In Chinese medicine, various pathological bacteria, viruses, and fungi existing outside the body are called external evils. If the spleen and stomach promote good, efficient digestion, sufficient qi and blood are manufactured and this sufficient qi defends the exterior of the body by these external evils or pathogens. If this qi is not manufactured in sufficient quantities, then the exterior of the body may be abnormally susceptible to invasion. Thus because babies have weak stomachs and spleens, they are also more easily invaded by external pathogens than adults. In layperson's terms, this means that they "catch" germs more easily.

The implications of the above theory

The fact that weak or immature digestion is the root of most common pediatric diseases has three main implications. First and very obviously, if digestion plays such a pivotal role in the health and well-being of infants and young children, then diet is extremely important both in terms of preventing disease as well as treating it. The following chapter is devoted to a discussion of diet and children's health. Secondly, treatment for most children's disease should also pivot around regulating and strengthening digestion. As we will see below, when it comes to the TCM treatment of the most commonly encountered children's diseases, attention to regulating and improving digestion is central. And third, because the spleen and stomach automatically mature around the age of six or so, most common pediatric diseases are self-limiting. This means that children automatically tend to outgrow them. This is an important point which laboring parents should keep in mind when they have lost sleep for the third night in a row due to a coughing son or a feverish, crying daughter with an earache.

4
Key Points in Diagnosing Children

Sun Si-miao, the most famous Chinese doctor of the Tang dynasty (618-907 CE) said, "Better to treat 10 men than 1 woman; better to treat 10 women than 1 baby." What he meant by this was that, because women have menstrual cycles, there is more to take into account when diagnosing and treating them. Therefore, Sun felt it was harder to diagnose and treat women than men. Further, babies cannot talk. Therefore they cannot explain what they are feeling. Because of this, pediatrics has sometimes been jokingly referred to in Chinese medicine as specialization in mutes. Because he could not question his young patients the way he would adults, Sun felt that they were even more difficult to diagnose than women.

Happily, TCM gynecology and pediatrics has made great progress since the Tang dynasty, and I feel just the reverse of Sun Si-miao. If one understands the pivotal role of diet and indigestion in pediatrics, babies are actually much easier to diagnose and, therefore, treat than women. (And if one understands how to read the monthly report card of a woman's monthly cycle, women are much easier to diagnose than men who never tell you what is really going on anyway.) Therefore, I love to treat babies and do not find them all that difficult to diagnose. Essentially, what the Chinese doctor is trying to determine in most pediatric illnesses is whether the baby is abnormally hot or cold, whether their righteous qi is sufficient or insufficient, and whether there is some evil or unhealthy qi or substance which needs to be eliminated from the body. In order to make those determinations, the TCM practitioner uses four basic methods called the four examinations. These consist of looking, listening/smelling, feeling, and questioning.

Looking

In 1575, Zhou You-fan compiled a list of 15 steps in a pediatric diagnosis. Eleven out of those 15 steps all have to do with looking or inspection. In general, what the TCM practitioner looks at is the baby's eyes and facial color, the color of their hands and nails, the color, size, and shape of the vein at the base of the index finger, and at any particular area which is painful or diseased.

Inspecting the spirit

Looking at the eyes tells the practitioner how serious the disease is. This is called inspecting the baby's spirit. If the eyes are clear and shining and the baby is aware and intelligent, then the disease is not all that serious and should respond to treatment without too much worry. If on the other hand, the baby's eyes are dull, filmy, and lack awareness or consciousness, then the disease has become serious and great care needs to be taken, possibly including seeing a Western MD.

Inspecting the facial complexion

Next the practitioner looks at the color of the baby's skin. This includes the baby's nails and lips in particular.

1. A red facial complexion

A healthy child should have a pink facial complexion which is lustrous or shiny. If the baby is redder than normal, this suggests that there is some abnormal heat within the baby's body. The deeper or darker the shade of red, the more intense the heat. If there are habitually redder than normal cheeks, this typically suggests food accumulation or stagnation with transformation of heat. If the cheeks are only redder than normal in the afternoon, this suggests either damp heat or vacuity heat. If both cheeks are bright red while the rest of the face is a bright white, and if there is accompanying cold limbs and a chilly sweat, this indicates that vacuous yang has lost its root and is counterflowing upward. If the facial complexion is red with a white forehead, this suggests internal heat combined with lung vacuity. Traditionally, the right cheek was indicative of the lungs and the left cheek was indicative of the liver. However, in modern TCM, if only one cheek is redder than normal, local inflammation due to teething should be suspected.

2. A pale facial complexion

A paler than normal face usually indicates qi or yang vacuity. If the face is a somber white, this suggests qi vacuity, while if it is a bright white, this indicates a yang vacuity. If the facial complexion is bright white with chilled limbs, this may indicate yang desertion, while a white, edematous face suggests qi or yang vacuity with dampness.

3. A yellow facial complexion

If the baby's facial complexion is a withered or sallow yellow, this indicates qi and blood vacuity usually due to spleen vacuity. If there is a bright yellow facial complexion, then dampness is mixed with heat. If this yellow color is dull, then dampness is associated with spleen qi vacuity. If there is a dull yellow facial complexion with white, powdery patches on the cheeks lateral to the corners of the mouth, then intestinal parasites should be suspected.

4. A green-blue facial complexion

A green-blue facial complexion indicates either cold or considerable pain. If there is a green-blue, purplish color, this indicates blood stasis. If there is a green-blue complexion with purplish, *i.e.*, cyanotic, lips, this suggests obstruction of the lung qi resulting in blood stasis as in pneumonia.

In particular, the practitioner should look at the vein at the root of the bridge of the nose between the two eyes. This area is called *shan gen* in Chinese. This translates as the root of the mountain, the nose being the mountain of the face. If a blue vein is visible here, this suggests that the baby's spleen, *i.e.*, their digestion, is weak, and the more prominent and visible this vein is, the weaker the spleen. This is a very reliable diagnostic sign and one which is easy to determine.

Inspecting the bodily form

Inspecting the bodily form means visually assessing the child's muscles and bones. Are they appropriately developed for the child's age? It also means looking at the child's head hair. Is the hair on the child's head healthy looking and lustrous or does it look withered and brittle or sparse? Are there any bald spots on the head? Withered, dry, brittle hair suggests extreme qi and blood vacuity for some reason, while underdeveloped muscles and bones also suggests visceral weakness and insufficiency. The practitioner should also look to see if the child's backbone and legs are straight. Further, if the belly is distended with prominent blue veins, this may suggest chronic indigestion and, therefore, malnutrition associated with parasites. In addition, the practitioner should look to see whether the child moves about normally, if they are limping, guarding, or protecting some body part, or if they are holding some body part as if in pain.

If the child is asleep or unconscious when the practitioner inspects them, sleeping on the abdomen may be a sign of food stagnation or intestinal parasites, while sleeping on the back suggests a prolonged or serious disease. Sleeping with many covers and the body curled up in a ball suggests cold, while sleeping with the arms and legs thrown outward and the covers and bedclothes thrown off suggests heat. Arched back rigidity of the neck and spasms and contracture of the four limbs suggest infantile convulsions as do frequent, occasional startled reactions.

Inspecting the tongue, eyes, nose, mouth, ears & two yin

1. Inspecting the tongue

It is usually impossible to inspect the tongue of a very young child. But, in those children who are a little older and who can understand and comply with the request to "Stick out your tongue", looking at the tongue is just as important a part of TCM pattern discrimination as it is in adults. Basically, tongue signs in children mean the same things they do in adults. For instance, a paler than normal tongue means qi and blood vacuity. A red tongue indicates heat. A deep red tongue in the case of a warm disease suggests that heat has entered the constructive and blood divisions. And a thorny red tongue like a red bayberry indicates toxic heat in the blood division with consumption and exhaustion of yin fluids. A purplish tongue indicates stasis and stagnation.

As for the fur or coating, a white, slimy coating indicates dampness and phlegm internally. If the coating is yellow and slimy, then there is damp heat or turbid dampness in the middle burner. If the tongue coating is yellow, slimy, and dirty looking, there is food stagnation with depression transforming heat. A dry, scanty, or peeled tongue coating suggests yin fluid vacuity and consumption, while a geographic or patchy tongue coating which comes and goes from time to time indicates spleen and stomach vacuity weakness. However, when it comes to a tongue coating in very young children and infants, any tongue coating which is thicker than normal usually indicates food stagnation and the presence of internal heat due to depression. This is due to babies' viscera being clearer or cleaner than adults and also to their pure yang constitution.

2. Inspecting the eyes

We have already discussed inspecting the eyes for the presence of spirit. Here we are looking more closely for particular pathological signs in the eyes. If the sclera are red, this often suggests wind heat. Watering eyes are an early sign of measles or a severe common cold. A yellow sclera indicates the presence of damp heat internally, while black or dark bluish spots in the sclera point to the presence of intestinal parasites. Abnormally dilated or contracted pupils suggest kidney qi exhaustion and vacuity. Slight corneal opacity in infants and young children may be a sign of malnutrition. And staring straight ahead with fixed eyes and a dull expression indicates infantile convulsions.

3. Inspecting the nose

A stuffy nose or runny nose with a clear, watery discharge indicates either a common cold, respiratory allergies, or chronic spleen vacuity with dampness. A thicker nasal discharge indicates the presence of some heat. The thicker this discharge becomes and if it turns from white to yellow to green, this indicates more severe heat affecting the lungs. However, the practitioner should be careful at this point. Yellow, thick, or even green mucus indicate heat affecting the lungs, but the site of engenderment of this heat may be the spleen, stomach, and/or liver. If the wings of the nose tremble or move with breathing, this is characteristic of pneumonia. Dry, yellow nasal mucus or crusting around the nose of dry mucus suggests dryness and heat. And nosebleeding suggests heat in the lung channel if it accompanies an obvious upper respiratory disease but heat in the stomach if it occurs after eating and particularly after eating greasy, fatty, and/or spicy, hot food.

4. Inspecting the mouth

Red, swollen gums with erosion indicate upward counterflow of stomach fire, while canker sores typically indicate spleen damp heat. Sores on the tongue are mostly due to heat in the heart and spleen, while a patchy white covering on the tongue indicates thrush and is usually associated with damp heat. However, this damp heat may typically be associated with concomitant spleen vacuity. Dental caries also usually indicate stomach fire and/or spleen damp heat. If the teeth fail to grow on time, this is due to kidney qi vacuity since, "The teeth are the surplus of the kidneys."

If the throat is red and inflamed, this indicates a wind heat invasion. If the tonsils are swollen and red, then there is wind heat with heat toxins or heat retained in the lungs and stomach. If the tonsils are swollen and inflamed and are covered with a white or yellowish white membrane which can be wiped away, then there are definitely heat toxins causing tonsillitis. If there is a greyish white membrane covering the back wall of the throat which cannot be wiped away, this suggests diphtheria.

5. Inspecting the ears

Swelling and pain of the auditory duct of the ear with a greenish yellow, purulent discharge from the ear canal indicates heat counterflowing and upwardly harassing. Most often, this heat is due to food stagnation transforming into depressive heat. Locally, this heat is in the gallbladder and triple burner channels, but the site of its engenderment is in the stomach and intestines. If there is a watery, slightly turbid, whitish discharge from the ear, this is due to enduring spleen qi vacuity not containing fluids. It is seen in cases where the eardrum has ruptured and then fails to heal. If there is marked swelling and pain in the glands under the ears, this suggests epidemic parotitis or mumps due to wind heat toxins invading the foot *shao yang*.

6. Inspecting the two yin

In Chinese medicine, the two yin refer to the anus and urethra in males and to the anus and vaginal meatus including the urethra in females. The urethra and vaginal meatus are the front or anterior yin, while the anus is the rear, back, or posterior yin. If the external genitalia are red and moist in little girls, this indicates the presence of damp heat in the lower burner. Itching of the anterior yin indicates pinworms or trichomoniasis of the vagina. If the scrotum is unusually flaccid in little boys, this suggests kidney qi vacuity, while one-sided enlargement and downward drooping of the scrotum indicates hernia due to spleen qi vacuity.

Dampness and itching of the anus with white, thread-like worms crawling out from inside the anus at night indicates a pinworm infestation, while redness, inflammation, chapping and cracking of the skin, and possible oozing of turbid fluids suggests diaper rash due to damp heat.

Inspecting skin rashes & eruptions

1. Small, papular eruptions

Small, fine papular eruptions or rashes are characteristic of measles, rubella, and scarlet fever.

2. Vesicular eruptions

Raised vesicles which are red colored at their base and which may occur on the head, face, and four limbs are characteristic of chicken pox and impetigo. Chicken pox begins as fine, raised papules which then become water blisters the size of soybeans. After the eruptions break, they dry up, crust, and scab. The water blisters of chicken pox can cover the enter body. Impetigo, on the other hand, is characterized by turbid, pus-filled lesions with red bases or roots which typically affect only a localized area. These lesions may then spread if the pus filling the lesions touches the surrounding skin.

3. Macular eruptions

Bright red macular eruptions which are not noticeably raised, thorny, or papular on palpation and which do not lose their color when pressed are characteristic of heat toxins having entered the constructive and blood divisions. If macular eruptions are indistinct or dark purplish in color accompanied by a pale complexion, cold limbs, and a fine pulse, then qi is too vacuous to contain and restrain the blood within its vessels. These are called yin eruptions as compared to the yang eruptions above and indicate a serious pathological condition.

Inspecting the stools & urine

1. The stools

Newborns and nursing infants usually have soft stools frequently throughout the day. These are yellow in color and neither too dry nor too wet. This is normal. If the stools of a newborn or infant change from this norm in any way, this is a very important indicator of the presence of disease. Small, hard, round, dry stools with several days between movements indicate replete heat in the *yang ming* or consumption of yin fluids due to warm disease. Loose stools containing white milk curds or brightish yellow in color and smelling like rotten eggs indicate food stagnation due to unregulated feeding. Blood and pus or mucus in the stools suggest the presence of damp heat in the intestines. If there is more blood, there is more heat. If there is more pus or mucus, there is more dampness. If the stools are bloody like the color of soy sauce in a nursing infant accompanied by crying from time to time, this indicates intestinal obstruction and intussusception.

2. The urine

Normal urine is clear and light yellow in color. If the urine becomes scanty and dark yellow during very hot weather and profuse perspiration, this is also normal. If the urine is dark yellow, frequent, and painful or burning, this suggests the presence of damp heat percolating downward. Turbid urine like rice washing water is due to turbid dampness in turn due to unregulated feeding. Deep brown or reddish urine suggests hematuria. In order to determine the cause of this hematuria, one must check other signs and symptoms.

Inspecting the vessel of the three bars at the tiger's mouth

Next the practitioner will look at the vein at the base of the palmar side of the index finger. This is a special diagnostic method developed in the Tang dynasty specially for children under 2-3 years of age. This vein is called the *hu kou san guan zhi mai* or vessel of the three bars at the tiger's mouth. The tiger's mouth is the angle between the thumb and index finger when both are fully extended. The three bars are the three joints of the index finger. The metacarpal-phalangeal joint is called the wind bar. The first interphalangeal joint is called the qi bar. And the second or distal most interphalangeal joint is called the life bar. Inspection of the vein at these three anatomical positions on the index finger is both a method of "pulse examination" and a method of inspection. Why this can be called a pediatric method of pulse examination is that the word in Chinese for pulse, *mai*, also means vessel and any visible vein is a type of vessel in Chinese medicine. This type of pulse examination was developed to take the place of palpation of the pulse in infants which is much harder to do accurately and efficiently than in adults.

Traditionally, it was the left index finger which was inspected in little boys and the right index finger in little girls. Nowadays in China, the right index finger is examined in both boys and girls. Depending upon the size, color, prominence, location, and shape of the vein on the palmar surface of the index finger, the practitioner can tell whether the disease is hot or cold, vacuous or replete, how far it has progressed, and how dangerous the condition is.

One begins by moistening the palmar surface of the index finger in order to see this vein more clearly. This is the same as moistening a piece of wood or a stone in order to reveal the grain more clearly. Next, one gently stretches the index finger backwards in order to also make the vein more visible. In general, observation of this vessel is divided into four basic criteria: 1) the depth of the vessel, 2) its color, 3) its size, and 4) its location in terms of the three joints of the index finger.

1. Depth

In a normally healthy child, this vein should only be dimly visible. If the vein is easily seen and looks close to the surface of the skin, this indicates an exterior pattern. If the vein looks indistinct and deeper under the skin, this indicates an interior pattern.

2. Color

In a healthy child, the vein is a pale purple color or reddish brown in color. If the color changes from this norm, then this suggests pathology. A light red vein suggests vacuity cold or qi and blood dual vacuity, while a red vein indicates replete heat. If the vein is dark red or purplish red, this suggests accumulation and/or depression of heat. Whereas, a bluish purple vein indicates spasms and tremors, painful conditions, and blood stasis.

3. Size

A thicker than normal vein indicates repletion, while a thinner than normal vein indicates vacuity.

4. Location

In a healthy child, this vein should only be seen at the wind bar. If there is an easily seen vein at the metacarpal-phalangeal joint but no easily seen vein at the other two more distal joints of the index finger, this traditionally shows that any externally invading evil qi is in the exterior. This is why this is called the wind gate. However, in modern clinical practice, a visible vein here more often simply means the disease is not severe. In my experience, an engorged, slightly purplish or red purplish vein at the wind bar indicates food stagnation with depressive heat due to unregulated feeding. If one changes the child's diet, this vein's size and visibility will recede even without other professional treatment. Typically, the symptoms which go along with a visible vein at the wind bar are headache, bodily heaviness, loss of appetite, and a slight fever.

If the vein is visible and unusually prominent at the wind bar *and* the first or proximal interphalangeal joint, then disease has either entered the channels or is more serious. Therefore, this section is called the qi bar. The symptoms which commonly go along with this sign are high fever, no appetite, fatigue and somnolence, and diarrhea. The child should be treated professionally, but the disease should respond to treatment without difficulty.

If the vein is visible at all three joints or bars or is prominently visible at the third or life bar, then the disease has entered the viscera. In this case, the symptoms are more severe and include possible vomiting, continued or even higher fever, nightmares, delirium, and convulsions. This disease most definitely requires speedy professional treatment and, if left untreated, the consequences may be permanent or life-threatening. This is why the third joint is called the life bar.

In addition, the TCM practitioner will also want to look at any place the child or the parent says they hurt or any location which is diseased. For instance, if there is a diaper rash, the practitioner will want to see that rash to determine what color red it is, how extensive it is, whether it is wet or dry, and whether the skin is broken or intact. Likewise, any other skin rash would be inspected in the same way. If a rash was very red, then this suggests pathological heat. If its reddish purple, then the TCM practitioner may be thinking about TCM concepts such as toxins and/or blood stasis. If the rash is wet and weeping, this suggests pathologic dampness, while if there is pus production, this also suggests toxins.

Listening/smelling

In Chinese medicine, there is a single verb which translates as listening and smelling together. What the Chinese medical practitioner is listening for is the sound of any cough. Is it strong or weak? A strong cough typically goes along with a replete pattern, while a weak cough goes along with a vacuity pattern. Is it wet or dry? A wet cough indicates profuse phlegm, while a dry cough indicates insufficient lung fluids. Is the cough spasmodic? In modern TCM, this question helps determine not so much the pattern of the cough but the necessity of using certain wind medicinals which have a pronounced antispasmodic ability. The practitioner listens to the sound of breathing. Is it asthmatic and wheezing? Does it sound phlegmy and obstructed? If there is either the sound of phlegm obstructing the nose or phlegm in the throat, then the practitioner knows there is the presence of phlegm. Further, the practitioner listens to the sound of the voice and the speech. Is the voice hoarse or raspy? A hoarse or raspy voice indicates either a wind heat invasion or yin vacuity. Is the voice a normal loudness or very faint and weak? Normal volume suggests that the righteous qi is sufficient, whereas disinclination to speak and/or a weak voice suggests vacuity weakness. Can the child speak normally for their age? This tells us about their development which in turn tells us about their spleen and kidneys. Are they delirious? Delirium in a warm disease suggests that heat has affected the pericardium and thus given rise to disquietude and, therefore, chaos and confusion of the heart spirit.

As for smelling, the practitioner smells the breath. This is very important for finding out if there is stagnant food in the stomach. If there is, the breath will tend to be sour and bad-smelling. If the breath is fresh and clean, then food stagnation is probably not the issue. Further, the practitioner will want to at least know from the parents how the stools smell. If they are very foul-smelling, then there is probably heat and possibly food stagnation. If they are odorless, this suggests that the spleen is weak. Is the urine strong smelling? If it is, this again suggests heat. In actual practice, it is mostly the parents doing the smelling of the urine and stools and the practitioner questions the parents about this.

Feeling

When the child first comes in, the practitioner will usually pat the child's head and the side of their face. The parent may not know this, but the practitioner has already begun their diagnosis. By patting or stroking the head gently, the practitioner is seeing if the fontanelle has closed properly for the baby's age. By patting or stroking the baby's cheek, they can tell if the baby is hot or cold. They may then take the child's hands to play with, but while playing, they are also assessing whether the child is hot or cold. At some point in the examination, the practitioner will probably lie the child on their back and feel their abdomen. Is it too hot or cold? Is it too firm and distended or too slack and infirm? The practitioner may or may not feel the baby's pulse at their wrist depending upon how old the child is, but the practitioner will want to feel any place the child or the parent says is affected by the complaint. For instance, if there is a sore throat (or even if there is not), the practitioner will want to feel the glands to see if they are swollen, hard, and/or tender to the touch.

Pulse examination

If the child is more than 2-3 years old, then the practitioner should at least try to examine the child's pulse at the *cun* opening on the wrists. Since the child's three positions are smaller than an adult's, the practitioner will have to hold their three palpating fingers more closely together. Even still, their fingers may not be able to distinguish adequately these three positions. In that case, one can feel the entire pulse with only one or two fingers, attempting to get an overall impression of whether the pulse is floating or deep, fast or slow, weak or forceful, large or fine, slippery or wiry. Li Shi-zhen says that when feeling the pulse on infants, one need only use a single finger to check all three positions and it is enough to check for strong or weak, slow or rapid pulses.

When attempting to examine a child's pulse, the practitioner should keep in mind that a child's pulse is normally faster than an adult's. If one does not remember this, then one may mistake a cold for a hot disease. According to Li Shi-zhen, the normal pulse rate for children between the ages of 3-5 years old is seven beats per respiration. Eight or nine beats per respiration cycle indicates heat, while four or five beats per respiration cycle indicates cold. A more modern interpretation is that:

120-140 beats per minute is a normal pulse rate in newborns
110-120 beats per minute is normal in a one-year-old
110 beats per minute is normal in a four-year-old
90 beats per minute is normal in an eight-year-old
75-80 beats per minute is normal in a 14-year-old.

Questioning

Although questioning the child itself is often not possible due to youngness of age, the practitioner will question the parent. They will want to know how the disease began, how long it has been going on, what are the symptoms, how is the appetite, the stools, urination, energy, mood, and sleep. What color is any phlegm? What treatments have already been tried and with what result? What does the child eat? What were they eating when they got ill? What else was happening when they got ill? Has the child had any fever? Do they seem to be running hot or cold, etc., etc.?

The exact questions which the practitioner will ask very much depend on the major complaint. For instance, if the major complaint is vomiting of milk in a child which is still breast-feeding, then some of the questions will include: How long ago did the vomiting start? When does the child vomit — directly after meals, at other times of the day? What does the vomitus look like? What does the vomitus smell like? When the child vomits, does it come out with force or does it just dribble out? How is the baby's energy? Are they restless and agitated or sleepy and somnolent? Do they tend to feel hot or cold? Is their face typically red or pale? What are their bowel movements like? How does the baby's breath smell? All these questions are meant to determine vacuity from repletion and heat from cold.

Establishing a TCM pattern

In TCM as a specific style of Chinese medicine, the hallmark of our methodology is treating on the basis of a pattern discrimination and not just on a disease diagnosis alone. There are ten different methods of pattern discrimination used in TCM:

1. Eight principle pattern discrimination
2. Five phase pattern discrimination
3. Qi & blood pattern discrimination
4. Fluid & humor pattern discrimination
5. Viscera & bowel pattern discrimination
6. Channel & network vessel pattern discrimination
7. Disease caused pattern discrimination
8. Six division pattern discrimination
9. Four division pattern discrimination
10. Three burner pattern discrimination

Frequently more than one of these pattern discrimination methods will be used to describe the total pattern in a given patient. For instance, if we say that our young patient exhibits a spleen qi vacuity, we are using a combination of three different TCM methods of pattern discrimination. Because we have said that the pattern involves the spleen and not any other of the viscera and bowels, we have used viscera and bowel discrimination. Because we have said that the pattern involves the qi and not the blood, we have used qi and blood pattern discrimination. And because we have said that the pattern is one of vacuity and not repletion, we have used eight principle pattern discrimination, vacuity and repletion being one pair of these eight principles.

In TCM as a system, we do not give treatment on the basis of a disease or a main symptom alone. Rather, we give treatment based on the individual patient's individual pattern. That is what makes TCM the safe, holistic, and effective medicine it is. Therefore, whatever methods an individual practitioner chooses to use among the four examinations, these should always be employed with a goal to establishing the patient's TCM pattern of disharmony.

The final TCM pattern discrimination or diagnosis will depend on the synthesis of information gathered by these four examinations. The TCM practitioner may or may not be interested in laboratory tests and cultures. But even if such tests have been done, the TCM pattern discrimination is not made on their basis. Rather, the TCM treatment should be based primarily on the TCM pattern of disharmony. As TCM practitioners, we may choose to take the fact that a baby has tested positive for Streptococcus or has red eardrums into account, but we do not prescribe treatment based solely on such Western medical criteria.

This book describes the main, professionally recognized TCM patterns under each of the diseases discussed and gives representative guiding formulas for the treatment of each of these patterns. However, the practitioner will often need to modify these patterns in order to exactly describe their individual patient. This means that the pattern must be modified to fit the patient and not the patient made to fit a particular textbook pattern. If we modify a pattern, this then means that the formula must be modified as well.

5
Key Points in Treating Children

Just as there are unique characteristics in understanding why young children get sick the way they do and unique methods in pediatric diagnosis, there are also some unique characteristics to the TCM treatment of babies and infants. These can be summarized in four key statements.

1. It is essential to treat in time while the righteous is still firm and being cautious.

This means that treatment should be begun at the first sign of disease. This is based on the assumption that it is better and easier to prevent a disease which has yet to manifest than to treat a disease after its symptoms have already appeared. In actual clinical practice, preventive treatment is often easier to talk about than to do. However, when it comes to children, it is actually possible to provide preventive treatment in a realistic manner.

Since so many infant's and young children's diseases are due to or at least involve poor digestion, practitioners should teach the parents of their young patients how to look for the signs of incipient disease. First of all, if the parent knows that their child has been eating more dairy products, sugars and sweets, chilled fruit juices, or ice cream and frozen yogurt, then immediately they should be warned to be more careful about the child's diet for a few days. This means insuring that the child sticks to a clear, bland diet of cooked, easily digested foods designed to fortify the spleen. In my parent's companion book to this treatment manual, *Keeping Your Child Healthy with Chinese Medicine*, I go to great lengths explaining to parents how to adjust their children's diet and what constitutes the clear, bland diet of Chinese medicine. In addition, my *The Tao of Healthy Eating: A Simple Guide to Healthy Eating According to Traditional Chinese Medicine* also explains the principles of a clear, bland diet for lay readers.

Secondly, if the child's stools become loose, if they lose their appetites, if they develop bad breath or complain of canker sores, or if their nose starts to run with mucus, these are all signs that their spleen has been damaged and has lost control over the transportation and transformation of fluids. In that case, once again the parent should take special care with their child's diet, insuring that it is a clear, bland diet which fortifies and does not damage the spleen and stomach. If parents are able to correct the diet and remedy the very simple or minor symptoms above, then it is less likely spleen dampness will congeal into phlegm and cause inflammation, thus giving rise to earaches, bronchitis, asthma, or tonsillitis. Practitioners may also teach parents how to do some simple Chinese pediatric massage in order to drain the stomach and fortify the spleen or they may choose to give parents some *Bao He Wan* (Protect Harmony Pills) or *Bao Ying Wan* (Protect Babies Pills) which treat food stagnation and the accumulation of phlegm. Armed with knowledge of the signs and symptoms of incipient pediatric disease, knowledge about the role of diet in pediatric disease, and some pediatric massage maneuvers or ready-made formulas for food stagnation, parents can do wonders in preventing the occurrence of disease in their young charges.

2. It is essential to stop treatment in the middle of disease.

As stated above, because children's viscera and bowels are clear and effective, they recuperate from disease very quickly. It is, therefore, one of the unique features of TCM pediatrics that internal medical treatment should be suspended in many cases before a complete cure has been effected. Once the symptoms are clearly moving in the proper direction, treatment should be suspended and the practitioner should rely on the parents instituting a proper diet and lifestyle. If the disease does not continue to abate or reverses itself and gets worse, the practitioner can then always resume administration of internal medicine.

It is my own personal clinical experience in treating babies and toddlers that treatment may improve one symptom and cause some other symptom to crop up. In that case, if one suspends all treatment other than proper diet and lifestyle, commonly all the symptoms then disappear. If one does not suspend all treatment, one may go around and round in a circle. One treats for the original complaint and that complaint goes away but another appears. Then one switches to treat that other complaint and the original complaint comes back. In that case, stop all treatment and see what happens. In my experience, often both complaints go away entirely.

3. One should use suitable methods of administration and even new forms of Chinese medicinals in pediatrics.

4. One should know well the methods of administering Chinese medicine in decoction to children.

In terms of the above two statements, many Chinese as well as Western practitioners think that it is difficult or impossible to give infants and young children Chinese herbal decoctions. However, this is really not so. Yes, if one tries to give a baby or young child a decoction in a teacup and ask them or even try to force them to drink it, they typically will not. First of all, children do not need and, in fact, should not be given the same doses as adults. It is my experience that babies and young children can get very good results with a very small dose of Chinese medicinals in decoction. Chinese books on pediatrics give the following dosage guidelines:

Under 1 year	60-100ml
1-6 years	150-200ml
7-12 years	200-250ml
Over 12 years	adult dose

Prescribing & administering Chinese medicinal decoctions to infants

In our clinic, we have found that the best way to dose and administer internal decoctions for babies and children under six years of age is by a so-called eyedropper. The formula for the decoction is written just as it would be if it were for an adult. Its ingredients are then boiled in 2 cups of water down to 1 cup of medicinal liquid. Then the child is given 1-2 droppers anywhere from 3-8 times per day. Each time the child is to receive a dose, the parent simply squirts it into the child's mouth. Thus there is no pill or capsule to swallow nor is there a large amount of fluid to swallow down. Neither is there any cup or spoon for the child to push away and spill all over the floor.

If the child is very small or the disease is a very light or chronic one, then only one eyedropper is given each time and only a few times each day. If the child is larger or if the disease is either serious or acute, then two eyedroppers of medicinal fluid are given more times each day.

One may question why I have said that the formula should or can be written just as if the formula was being written for an adult. This is because, no matter what the dosages of each individual medicinal ingredient, the child is only going to be given a very small dose each time. Often, one cup of such a decoction will last for several days. In many cases, the formula needs to be changed or suspended before the parent runs out of the full cup of the decoction. This means that, if the decoction is going to be used for more than 48 hours, it should be stored in a refrigerator and either warmed up or allowed to come to room temperature before giving each dose to the child. Except during very hot weather, most decoctions can be stored at room temperature for 48 hours without going bad. If the parent thinks the decoction smells bad or has markedly changed in taste, it should be discarded and a new decoction should be brewed.

Other suitable methods of administration or new forms of Chinese medicine include ear, nose, and eyedrops, compresses, poultices, plasters, washes, soaks, fumigations, and inhalations.

6
Chinese Dietary Therapy & Pediatrics

I believe so strongly in the truth of the above described Chinese theory regarding the spleen and stomach and children's diseases that I have gone to day-care centers to present free in-services trying to change the way we feed infants and toddlers. If our children suffer from a plethora of unnecessary runny noses, coughs, allergies, and earaches, which I believe they most certainly do, it is mainly because we, as a society in the West, have forgotten how to feed babies and young children. What the average Western parent has been led to believe is a healthy diet for infants and children is a dietary disaster according to TCM, and most pediatric diseases can be either completely eliminated or markedly relieved if one simply changes the child's diet. Therefore, although most Chinese pediatric texts do not include a chapter on dietary therapy, I feel I must. Only if the child's diet has been corrected can Chinese herbal medicine, pediatric *tui na*, or acupuncture and moxibustion get complete and lasting effects.

Breast-feeding

Human breast milk is the single best food for babies. It is the right temperature and the right consistency. All other substitutes for human breast milk are second best. That being said, then why do even breast-fed babies develop colic, earaches, coughs, etc.? Typically, the first complaint of very young infants who are brought to my office is colic. Colic refers to stomach cramps with accumulation of gas which worsens in the afternoon and may continue on into the night. The baby cries until or unless they can pass gas and they typically demand to be carried, jiggled, or moved about. Colic is seen as a digestive complaint in TCM pediatrics. Essentially, it is due to food stagnation. This means that food is not transformed and transported properly by the spleen qi but rather gathers and obstructs the stomach and intestines.

Although human breast milk is the perfect food for human babies, even breast-fed children can develop colic. How can this happen? The answer is that too much of a good thing is still too much. In the last few decades, feeding on demand has become the norm.

We have come to believe that feeding whenever the baby demands to be fed is somehow emotionally the right thing to do. However, when we feed on demand, we typically overfeed. When the stomach and spleen are inundated with more food than they can deal with efficiently and effectively, even human breast milk may become stagnant food and thus lead to digestive discomfort.

In Chinese, feeding on demand is called "unregulated feeding" and unregulated feeding is described as the disease cause of colic in the Chinese medical literature. The professional practitioner of TCM trained in pediatrics can tell if colic is due to overfeeding by the smell of the baby's breath, vomit, and stools and by the appearance of the vein at the base of the baby's index finger. When a child's colic or other disease is due to food stagnation, it is extremely important to stop feeding on demand and start feeding less and on a schedule. If the child has just been born, in order to protect the health of the child, it is important to initiate feeding on schedule, not on demand, right from the very beginning.

Feeding on schedule, not on demand

Scheduled feeding is what Western mothers used to do up until only two to three decades ago. Scheduled feeding or what the Chinese call regulated feeding does *not* mean starving the child nor does it mean being unkind. The baby is not any wiser than we adults. In fact, although the baby may be closer to its instinctual needs, it lacks the discipline and judgement of adults based on experience. The parent is in charge of the baby. The parent is supposed to know what is best for the baby better than the baby itself. Babies will feed out of boredom and out of gluttony just as adults do. If there is any single thing I would recommend to parents of newborn infants it would be to breast-feed if at all possible but also to be sure to feed on schedule, not on demand.

If one goes to their local library, one will probably find a whole shelf of books on breast-feeding. Some of these books recommend giving the breast to every baby *every time the baby cries*. One of the rationales of breast-feeding on demand is that babies gain weight faster when fed on demand, but there is no discussion of the assumption that quicker weight gain is actually a good thing for the child long-term. Is it possible that the great rise in obesity among younger Americans is, at least partially, due to having been fed on demand so that they have become habituated to allaying every discomfort by eating something? Certainly proponents of the Japanese diet called Macrobiotics have long held that the increase in size and weight associated with post-World War II overeating and overnutrition is bad for one's health. As a simple guideline for scheduling feedings in newborns, one should consider a regimen of 2-3 ounces of milk every four hours. Although each individual baby has their own nutritional needs based on their own metabolism, this was the schedule that was recommended before breast-feeding on demand became the current dogma.

Feeding on schedule, not on demand, is considered anathema by many breast-feeding advocates. But I have been treating babies for almost two decades, both in the United States and in China, and I feel very positive that feeding on demand is one of the root causes of pediatric diseases in the West. I believe that a return to scheduled feeding as opposed to feeding on demand could significantly decrease colic, earaches, and coughs and colds in infants. These conditions are, to a certain degree, causally related, and avoiding food stagnation and its subsequent colic can change a person's whole childhood health history.

Commercial formulas & other substitutes for human breast milk

If one cannot breast-feed for some reason, what can one do? Obviously, one will have to use a "formula" or some other milk substitute. In Asia, the milk substitute that has traditionally been used is dilute rice soup. This is also the traditional first food other than the mother's breast milk introduced into the baby's diet. This food is nutritious and easy to digest. It is not so sweet as to create an addiction to the sweet flavor. It is also not so supernutritious that it creates excessive stagnant food, dampness, and phlegm. In addition, rice is warm in temperature and thus benefits the baby's digestion, or in Chinese parlance their spleen and stomach yang.

Rice soup is made by putting rice and water in either a crockpot or slow cooker at a ratio of 1 part rice to 6 parts water. This should then be cooked at a low heat for several hours or overnight. At the end of this time, what should be left is a very dilute rice soup, most of the rice starch having dissolved in the process of cooking. If this soup comes out too thick, one can simply add some more hot water to dilute it. Before pouring this soup into a baby bottle, one should strain out the remaining rice kernels through cheesecloth. To make rice soup for babies, one should use white rice which is more easily digestible than brown rice.

One can use cow or goat's milk as a human breast milk supplement for babies. However, since these milks are really not designed for the nutritional needs of human children, they can cause problems. In particular, if cow's milk is used, it should be watered down and not given whole. If using either commercial formulas, cow or goat's milk, or even the dilute rice soup described above, one should be careful not to give the child a bottle every time they cry. In other words, when feeding by a bottle, one should take even more care not to overfeed, thus causing food stagnation.

In particular, one should, in my experience, avoid either soy milk or soy-based formulas as substitutes for human breast milk. According to Chinese medical theory, soybeans are cold. Since the baby's spleen yang qi is itself weak, cold-natured soy milk can easily damage spleen yang and lead more quickly than other milk substitutes to food stagnation.

Further, one should not feed young babies fruit juices, such as apple juice or orange juice. These are too sweet and thus addicting. Anything that is sweet in flavor tends to engender dampness in the body and anything very sweet weakens the Chinese concept of the spleen. Western babies are typically given fruit juices because we think they are nutritious. In a sense they are. But they are supernutritious. They are more nutritious than what the baby actually needs. The intense sweet flavor creates a hankering or addiction on the one hand, while it engenders dampness and weakens the spleen on the other. Other than rice soup or dilute cow's milk, the only thing I recommend parents give their young babies is warm water if they think the baby is genuinely thirsty.

Introducing solid foods

Very young babies do not need anything other than breast milk and possibly a little additional warm water. However, somewhere around five to six months, the baby will start grabbing at food on the parents plates or on the dinner table. When the baby starts itself picking up food and putting it in their mouth, that is the time to begin introducing solid foods into their diet. This juncture is a very important cusp in the baby's development. How it is handled will determine much about the child's health for the next couple of years. The mistake that most Western parents make is introducing solid foods too early in the child's development, introducing too many different foods too rapidly, and introducing the wrong foods at the wrong times. If one introduces solid foods before the baby's digestion is ready to handle them, this will result in their nontransformation and thus the production of food stagnation, dampness, and phlegm. Therefore, it is extremely important to take one's cues from the baby itself.

100 degree soup

In order to understand even more clearly what Chinese medicine has to say about digestion and especially the child's digestion, one should keep in mind that everything the baby eats must be turned into 100° F soup before digestion can take place in the stomach. That means that food should be at the baby's body temperature or just a little above or below this. Most definitely the baby should not be fed chilled, iced, frozen, or cold foods. The process of digestion is a process of warm transformation based on the spleen's yang qi. Cold, chilled, frozen foods weaken and even injure the digestion or spleen because they require so much yang qi to warm them up.

Secondly, food should be pureed so that it is like a thick soup. Babies do not have the back teeth which can mash food into a puree inside the mouth. Unless food is reduced to a mash, it cannot be digested in the stomach. Therefore, everything the baby is given should be cooked into a soup or blended in a blender or food mill.

Third, food should always be cooked. The process of digestion in Chinese medicine is a process of cooking food into soup. The more food is like a 100°F soup when it is eaten, the easier it is to digest. Many people think that raw foods are more nutritious than cooked foods. However, this is only true in a sense. Uncooked foods do have more vitamins and enzymes than cooked foods. However, these nutrients are held within their foods within the walls of the cells. It is the cell walls that keep foods from being a formless puddle. These cell walls are like bags or boxes. In order to get at the nutrients, these bags and boxes must be broken down to get at the nutrients within. This is accomplished by chewing and by the digestive process. Because very young children do not have the teeth to chew efficiently and because their digestive processes are inherently weak and immature, babies are not as efficient at breaking down these cellular bags and boxes as adults.

Cooking is another way humans break down the cellular bags and boxes that surround vital nutrients. Although cooking itself may destroy some of these nutrients, cooking makes the nutrients which are left much more easily assimilable. As an example, an uncooked carrot may have a hypothetical 100 units of some nutrient and a cooked carrot may only have 80 of those same units. If, however, one absorbs only 60 units from the uncooked carrot but 70 from the cooked carrot, the cooked carrot is still more nutritious than the raw carrot. This is the difference between gross nutrients and net absorption.

Cooking is nothing other than predigestion on the outside of the body. Cooking does some of the work of digestion before the food actually enters the stomach. Since babies' stomachs and spleens are weak and immature to begin with, they even more than adults benefit from the predigestion of cooking.

All this means is that whatever the baby is given as their first food should be served warm, mashed or pureed, and cooked, not raw.

What to introduce when

The first food other than mother's milk should be the dilute rice soup described above. This engenders the qi, blood, and body fluids at the same time as it fortifies the spleen, harmonizes the stomach, and seeps out excessive dampness.

Because the baby is new to the world and everything in it, at least this time around, their tastes are not yet jaded. One does not have to vary babies' diets the same way an adult requires. This is good because it is very important that one introduce only a single new food at a time and that one continues feeding this food for some time before introducing another. By introducing one food at a time, one can see whether or not the child can actually digest that food. If the child's digestion is not yet mature and strong enough to digest that food without side effects, there will be some sign of indigestion, such as vomiting, colic, gas, constipation, or loose stools.

If one feeds a baby a new food and consequently there is some sign of indigestion, one should immediately suspend that food *for the time being*. One should wait a couple of weeks or even a month and then try the food again. If there are no signs of indigestion after one week, then it is safe to assume that the child's digestion is capable of handling that food and another food can be tested. If one misses such signs of indigestion as loose stools, constipation, and increased gas, then the undigested food will accumulate in the gut and transform into food stagnation, dampness, and phlegm. At that point, the manifestations will be increased mucus, either mucus in the stools or mucus in the nose and lungs. If one sees such increased mucus after having introduced a new food to the child's diet, once again they should suspend that food for a couple of weeks or even longer before trying it again.

If one introduces several foods at one time or does not allow a week between each new food introduced, one will not know what foods are causing what reactions. Therefore, it is important to go slowly and not rush this process. This is something like an elimination diet for those with allergies. In fact, by introducing foods in this way, one will avoid creating food allergies in their children. According to Chinese medicine, food allergies occur in children because they have been fed too much of difficult to digest foods. These then cause indigestion and the various disease mechanisms which spring from food stagnation, dampness, and phlegm as their root.

In general, after white rice, one should introduce various cooked vegetables. One can next try cooked, mashed carrots. After that, one can try mashed potatoes. Then one can try mashed green beans or peas. One should feed nutritious but not overnutritious, easily digestible foods first, in general, cooked vegetables fill this requirement. Most cooked vegetables are somewhat sweet. They are not greasy, fatty, or too high in hard to digest proteins. Animal proteins, including cheeses, wheat products, and corn should be kept for later when the child's digestion has matured and become stronger. After all, cooked corn will go through the digestive tract in pieces even among many adults.

In particular, wheat is considered cooling and dampening by nature in Chinese medicine. That means that it is more difficult to digest than rice and more likely to cause food stagnation. The Chinese medical classics are full of admonitions not to overeat sodden wheat products which may easily cause food stagnation and injury to the spleen or the process of digestion.

What children should not eat

What babies and young children should not be fed are fruit juices, especially chilled juices out of the refrigerator. These are too sweet and they are too cold. They harm the digestion and cause accumulation of dampness and phlegm. Babies and young children should not eat too much bread. This also harms the spleen and gives rise to dampness and phlegm. Babies and young children should not eat raw vegetables and very much cheese. Nor should they eat all but the smallest amounts of peanut butter. Peanuts generate yin in the body. Dampness and phlegm are both yin. Peanuts are very hard to digest and phlegm-producing according to the logic of Chinese medicine. And children should not be given sweets and ice cream. Sweets damage the spleen and engender dampness, while ice cream is not only too sweet (the sugar), it is also too dampening (the eggs and cream) and too injurious to the spleen yang qi (the freezing cold).

In listing the common foods babies and children *should not be given*, many parents will immediately recognize the typical Western toddler's daily fare. Raw carrots and celery, pieces of cheese, crackers and bread, peanut butter and jelly, chilled milk and fruit juices. These are the foods modern, rushed parents so often feed our children. They are also the staple diet at many day- care centers, where preparing and feeding cooked foods is too difficult. And this is also why our Western children get sick the way they do with earaches, allergies, and chronic coughs.

When parents bring a sick toddler to my clinic, whether with a common cold, tonsillitis, cough, or earache, my first question is whether or not they went to a birthday party right before they got ill. Four times out of five the answer will be yes. How did I know? Well, what do children eat at birthday parties? Sugar and ice cream. That is also why the weeks from Halloween through Christmas are the busiest time of the year for seeing pediatric patients.

How to keep children from getting sick

As both a parent and a practitioner of Chinese medicine, my key advice for keeping children healthy and well is to watch their diet and their stools. By watching their diet, I mean not feeding infants on demand, not introducing solid foods too early or too quickly, and not feeding raw, chilled foods. This also means not feeding too much dairy, meat, eggs, or greasy, fatty foods, and especially not feeding much in the way of sugars and sweets. What it does mean is a diet high in complex carbohydrates and high in vegetables with small amounts of meat, eggs, and dairy just like the U.S. Department of Agriculture's Food Pyramid.

By watching a child's stools, I mean that one can keep tabs on a child's diet by keeping an eye on their feces. If a young child's stools have become loose, it is often a sign that they have been eating too much sugar and sweets. It may also mean they have been eating too much ice cream, the single most delicious and dangerous food I know. When a child overeats sugars and sweets, including ice cream, this injures the spleen and causes the spleen to lose its control over the separation of clear and turbid. The clear and turbid are not separated completely, dampness is engendered, and this dampness and undigested food flow downwards in the form of loose stools or diarrhea. Typically, if one sees that a young child's stools have become loose due to faulty diet, a day or two later one will then see an increase in phlegm and mucus.

Once this increase in damp phlegm becomes apparent, then we say the child has caught a cold, has a runny nose or a wet cough, has swollen glands, or has an earache. In other words, based on my experience, first there is a lapse in dietary wisdom and control, then there are loose stools, and then the child gets sick. If one catches this progression when the stools have become loose but before increased phlegm and dampness have been generated, *and if one can get the diet back on track*, then one can reverse this disease process saving the child from becoming ill. Thus, by keeping an eye on babies' and toddlers' stools, one can adjust their diet before indigestion sets other disease processes in motion.

What to do about sugar & sweets

We all love sugar and sweets, and of course we all love to see the smile on children's faces when we give them something sweet to eat. It is such an easy way to make our little friends happy. And please be sure, I am not saying that we should never allow our little charges to eat a piece of candy, cake, or ice cream. This is not a perfect world and I am not counseling perfection in this regard. Of course we should allow our children to eat sweets from time to time. However, as their guardians, it is up to us to monitor the amount and to control this if it becomes excessive to the point of setting disease mechanisms in process.

As stated above, one can tell if the child's diet is within reasonable limits or not by their stools. If the stools are healthy and formed and the child is not producing a superabundance of mucus, then their diet is probably not too far out of line. If their stools get loose after eating sugar or ice cream, then it's time to tell the child that he or she cannot have that piece of candy or ice cream they are asking for. In other words, I am not talking about abstinence, but rather pacing. To never allow one's child to eat a piece of sweet would have its own harmful repercussions.

What if one's been feeding a child all wrong and they have developed some unfortunate addictions?

Many parents bring their children to acupuncturists and practitioners of Chinese medicine only after they have become ill. These children have become ill mostly because of faulty diet. By the time they make it into the office of a Chinese medical practitioner, they may already have become addicted to sweet foods and drinks. When the Chinese medical practitioner tries to explain what a healthy diet is for the child, frequently the parent says that their child will not eat this or that. At that point, what's to be done?

There's the saying that, "Two wrongs don't make a right." If the child has become ill because of faulty diet, there is no way they are going to get well by continuing to eat the wrong foods. Just like with any addiction, there is going to be a period of "biting the bullet" and "going cold turkey." The child may refuse to eat the healthy food they are offered. They may cry and whine for what they are addicted to. But as long as the parents do not give in, eventually the child is going to eat. They may complain about it, they may make a fuss, but they will not starve themselves to death.

Unfortunately, such situations, are not fun. But a mistake has been made and a correction is necessary. The child is by nature childish and cannot be expected to see the bigger picture and defer immediate gratification of their senses. But the parent is an adult and is the child's guardian. No matter how painful it is, it is the parent's duty to change the child's diet and see that they stick to this new, healthier way of eating. Everything passes and nothing lasts forever. Eventually the crying and stubbornness will give way to at least grudging compliance. On the other hand, the parent always has the option of letting the child eat what they want and continue to be sick. Each family has to make their own decisions. However, everyone needs to be clear that in such situations, one cannot have it both ways — a healthy child willfully eating sugars and sweets.

Conclusion

In the following chapters, we will discuss other ways to treat disease and promote health according to the 2000 plus years of accumulated wisdom of Chinese medicine. However, I cannot overemphasize the importance of diet in young children's health. As my first mentor in Chinese medicine, Dr. (Eric) Tao Xi-yu, used to say, "Children only have one disease — indigestion." Of course, here we are not talking about congenital abnormalities, traumatic injuries, or unusual epidemic diseases. What Dr. Tao was talking about was the common pediatric diseases of colic, cough, swollen glands, earaches, allergies, vomiting, diarrhea, and indigestion. Nine times out of ten, these are the things parents bring their children in to be treated for. Once these diseases have occurred, professional medical treatment may be needed remedially. But in the overwhelming majority of these cases, changes in diet can allow for natural and effective treatment and prevent their relapse.

The key points in Chinese dietary therapy for babies and young children are contained in the following verses. These are from *Pediatric Bronchitis: Its TCM Cause, Diagnosis, Treatment & Prevention* by Xiao Shu-qin et al. translated by Gao Yu-li and myself (Blue Poppy Press, 1991):

> Food and drink should be clear, light, and tasty;
> It should not be uncooked, chilled, or greasy.
> It should be easy to absorb and assimilate, disperse and transform.
> Eat few tough, solid, difficult-to-digest foods.
> Be careful of sour, astringent, fishy smelling, and dry things.
> Do not eat more than the proper amount, stuffing oneself too full.

7
Chinese Herbal Medicine

I have already mentioned that, in TCM pediatrics, the main treatment modality is internally administered herbal medicine, and I have also given guidelines on dosing and administering decoctions to babies and young children. In Book Two, which is the section on the treatment of specific diseases based on TCM pattern discrimination, the reader will typically find more than one formula given under each pattern, and I would, therefore, like to give some hints on how to use this information.

First of all, the formulas listed are prefaced by the words, "guiding formulas." In one of his essays, Qin Bo-wei, one of the great mid-century architects of contemporary TCM, says something to the effect that, "When I say to use *Liu Wei Di Huang Wan* (Six Flavors Rehmannia Pills), I don't mean that you should administer exactly *Liu Wei Di Huang Wan* but rather that you should write your prescription based on the *idea* of *Liu Wei Di Huang Wan*." Likewise, the formulas in this book are not meant to be prescribed by rote copying. Instead, these formulas are only meant as armatures for one's final composition. They are the skeleton of one's actual prescription. The exact prescription for the individual patient should be a modification of the prescriptions listed in this book designed to fit the particular patient's exact signs and symptoms.

Since two different patients suffering from the same disease and even exhibiting basically the same TCM pattern will still differ in regard to their exact specifics, no single formula given for a pattern under a disease is going to be just right and effective for all patients with that pattern and that disease. All individual TCM patterns are made up of multiple signs and symptoms, and no one patient has all the symptoms listed in a textbook under a given pattern. Usually patients only have 60-70% of the listed symptoms. This means that even with the same basic pattern, patients' signs and symptoms differ. As an extension of this, one formula may be better for a pattern with a preponderance of certain symptoms than another listed under that same pattern.

In addition, most real-life patients exhibit patterns which are themselves complex and made up of more than a single element. For instance, a child may have a weak, vacuous spleen with internal dampness, a hot and/or dry, replete stomach, an element of food stagnation, some phlegm, the presence of internal heat, and some liver depression. This is not at all an uncommon complex TCM pattern discrimination in a real-life child (or a real-life adult for that matter). Although this overall complex pattern is relatively common, individuals will vary in many ways. In some cases, spleen vacuity will be more pronounced. In others, there will be more heat or dryness in the stomach. In yet other cases, food stagnation is the main thing. And yet in other cases, phlegm, heat, or dampness may each be more marked. In each instance, one may have to pick a different guiding formula, and in almost every case, one will have to either add ingredients to the base formula or both add and subtract ingredients in order to craft a prescription that matches the child's exact pattern of signs and symptoms. A number of years ago, I attended a workshop where Ted Kaptchuk said that the final prescription is the most complete and accurate statement of a patient's diagnosis, and my experience is that this is very true.

Many Chinese TCM treatment manuals only give a single formula under each pattern of each disease, and experienced practitioners will know that no single formula is effective for all patients even with the same pattern. Therefore, I have listed a number of different formula options under each pattern. Some of these options are only minor variations, while others contain completely different ingredients. When a number of formulas under a given pattern of a particular disease all contain the same basic ingredients, then the reader should know that the majority of Chinese TCM practitioners have found these ingredients to be the most empirically effective and trustworthy for that pattern of that disease. For instance, under the replete heat pattern of pneumonia, the overwhelming majority of Chinese authorities choose *Ma Xing Shi Gan Tang* (Ephedra, Armeniaca, Gypsum & Licorice Decoction). Therefore, one can feel quite certain that this is an empirically effective formula for this pattern of pneumonia *as long as one's pattern discrimination is correct.*

The necessary prerequisites to using this book successfully

Thus, in order to use this book successfully, one must have certain information already in place. In order to choose the most appropriate formula under a given pattern of a disease, one must be able to "read the formula." This means that one must be able to recognize why each ingredient is in the formula and what its role and functions are. Until or unless one knows this information, one has no basis on which to judge whether a formula or any of the formula's specific ingredients are right or wrong for a particular patient. This means that before attempting to use a TCM treatment manual such as this, one must have already completed courses in *ben cao xue* or the study of the materia medica and *fang ji xue*, the study of formulas and prescriptions. One should not use *any formula* which contains *any ingredient* whose nature, flavor, functions, indications, contraindications, and dosage parameters one does not know. Therefore, readers who have not yet studied and gained this basic, fundamental knowledge should first go back and complete this part of their TCM education before attempting to use this book.

Why there are almost no dosages given for individual ingredients

As the reader will see, there are no dosages given for the vast majority of ingredients listed under formulas in the treatment sections below. This is for two reasons. First and foremost, the absence of dosages is meant to dissuade the rote application of the formulas in this book by untrained practitioners. There is nothing safe about the medicinals of Chinese medicine because they are Chinese or because they mostly come from plant sources. If a medicine can cure disease when used correctly, it must be able to cause disease when used erroneously. The medicinals in this book are only safe when prescribed by trained professionals, and trained professionals should already know the appropriate dosage parameters of these medicinals.

Secondly, the exact dose of any given ingredient depends not only on its known safe and effective dosage ranges but also on its role and importance in a particular formula. For instance, in order for *Pu Gong Ying* (Radix Taraxaci) to be effective for clearing heat and resolving toxins, its dosage levels need to be fairly high: 15, 30, or even 45g per formula, while *Xi Xin* (Herba Asari) is usually dosed less than 6g. These differences have to do with these ingredients' inherent strengths and liabilities at their various dosage levels. On the other hand, if *Jin Yin Hua* (Flos Lonicerae) and *Lian Qiao* (Fructus Forysthiae) are the ruling ingredients in a formula, their doses may be larger than most of the other ingredients, while *Gan Cao* (Radix Glycyrrhizae), meant primarily to harmonize the other ingredients, may be dosed less. Therefore, the actual dosage of any given ingredient entirely depends on the known empirically effective dosage ranges of a given ingredient *and* its role or function in a particular formula.

However, the reader will see that, in a few instances, I have given specific dosage instructions. This is when formulas are meant for external application. Without such exact instructions on such a formula's method of preparation, it would be difficult for anyone, even a well-trained practitioner, to know how to make these. However, even these formulas for external medications are not sacrosanct and may be modified as the case at hand warrants. In addition, I have given the doses for the formulas for first aid or emergency use in order that they may be used as quickly and efficiently as possible.

A word about processing medicinals

For the most part, I have refrained from giving too many instructions on the processing of medicinals in the formulas contained in this book. In a few instances, I have given such instructions where to use the wrong form of a processed ingredient would mean using the wrong ingredient. For instance, uncooked *Sheng Gan Cao* (Radix Glycyrrhizae) is a different ingredient than mix-fried *Gan Cao* (Radix Glycyrrhizae) and *Sheng Jiang* (uncooked Rhizoma Zingiberis) is a different ingredient than dry *Gan Jiang* (Rhizoma Zingiberis) which is yet again different from blast-fried *Pao Jiang* (Rhizoma Zingiberis).

The processing of medicinals prior to decocting them is called *pao zhi* in Chinese, and this is normally a part of every Chinese-trained TCM practitioner's basic education. Processing includes many different methods and materials. For instance, one can dry stir-fry, earth stir-fry, bran stir-fry, or rice stir-fry *Bai Zhu* (Rhizoma Atractylodis Macrocephalae) in order to enhance one or more of its specific functions. In the same way, one can vinegar stir-fry, wine stir-fry, ginger juice stir-fry, or carbonize *Dang Gui* (Radix Angelicae Sinensis) in order to enhance one of its specific functions or to modify one of its liabilities or side effects. Although such processing can make one's prescriptions even more clinically effective, I have left it to individual readers to decide if, when, and how they might process particular ingredients in specific formulas. For more information on the use of processed Chinese medicinals, the reader should see Philippe Sionneau's *An Introduction to the Use of Processed Chinese Medicinals* (Blue Poppy Press).

A word about toxicity

The reader will note that there are a number of potentially toxic ingredients in the formulas given in this book. As stated above, there is nothing inherently safe about Chinese medicinals. It is the methodology by which they are prescribed that make them safe. *Fu Zi* (Radix Lateralis Praeparatus Aconti Carmichaeli), *Zhu Sha* (Cinnabar), *Quan Xie* (Scorpio), *Wu Gong* (Scolopendra), and even *Shi Chang Pu* (Rhizoma Acori Tatarinowii) are all potentially toxic when 1) inappropriately prescribed, 2) at the wrong dose, 3) with the wrong complementary ingredients, 4) without the proper processing, or 5) if administered for too long. Each individual practitioner must take responsibility for deciding the benefit/risk ratio when using such ingredients.

There is also nothing inherently safe about hundreds of Western pharmaceutical compounds which Western physicians prescribe every day. Those physicians must analyze and weigh the benefits of such potentially dangerous drugs against their possible risks. In some cases, less dangerous medicinals can be substituted for potentially toxic ones. In other cases, ingredients like Cinnabar may be deleted altogether. And yet in other cases, one may choose to use potentially toxic ingredients at nontoxic doses or for a short period of time before toxicity accumulates to dangerous levels.

Since children are far more susceptible to heavy metal and pesticide poisoning than adults, practitioners may want to ask companies for product testing information, especially when prescribing prepared medicines or extract powders to children. Many Western companies test every batch of every powdered single ingredient or formula for heavy metals and pesticide residues, and guidelines for safe limits on these substances are set by both the publishers of the US Pharmacopoeia and the Australian TGA (their version of the FDA). These limits are listed below in parts per million (PPM).

> **Lead:** less than 10 PPM (USP); less than 5 PPM (Australian TGA)
> **Mercury:** less than 3 PPM
> **Arsenic:** less than 3 PPM
> **Cadmium:** less than 3 PPM

Good product lines should have no detectable pesticide residues, especially if being used with children.

Endangered species

It is one of the great embarrassments of Chinese medicine that it is directly responsible for the threatened extinction of several important species, such as the tiger, rhinoceros, and scaly anteater. As publisher of Blue Poppy Press and a professional practitioner of TCM, I do not believe TCM practitioners should prescribe medicinals from endangered species. Therefore, the reader will note that in formulas titled "Rhinoceros Horn & (something else)" or "Antelope Horn & (something else), I have changed those two ingredients for their non-endangered, domestic substitutes. This means that instead of listing *Xi Jiao* (Cornu Rhinocerori), I have substituted *Shui Niu Jiao,* water buffalo horn (Cornu Bubali), and instead of listing *Ling Yang Jiao* (Cornu Antelopis Saiga-tatarici), I have substituted *Shan Yang Jiao*, goat horn (Cornu Caprae). Otherwise, how could I tell the little friends I treat that I was, in part, responsible for the extinction of tigers and rhinoceroses?

How to prescribe & administer Chinese herbs to children

Many practitioners of Chinese medicine may think that it is difficult to prescribe and administer Chinese herbal medicinals internally to infants and children. However, that is far from my experience. For older children who can swallow them, I recommend administering Chinese herbal medicinals in the form of powdered extracts in capsules or ready-made medicines in pill form. In this case, all one needs to do is reduce the dosage proportionately according to the child's age and/or body weight. The following table shows suggested dosages based on age.

0-1 month	1/18-1/14 of adult dose
1-6 months	1/14-1/7 of adult dose
6-12 months	1/7-1/5 of adult dose
1-2 years	1/5-1/4 of adult dose
2-4 years	1/4-1/3 of adult dose
4-6 years	1/3-2/5 of adult dose
6-9 years	2/5-1/2 of adult dose
9-14 years	1/2-2/3 of adult dose

The next table bases children's dosages on their body weight.

30-40 lbs.	20-27% of adult dose
40-50 lbs.	27-33% of adult dose
50-60 lbs.	33-40% of adult dose

60-70 lbs.	40-47% of adult dose
70-80 lbs.	47-53% of adult dose
80-100 lbs.	53-67% of adult dose
100-120 lbs.	67-80% of adult dose
120-150 lbs.	80-100% of adult dose

Even more ideal than using a powdered extract in capsule form would be to use a powdered extract administered in a glycerin base. They are easy to administer and often have doses already adjusted for children. I recommend a glycerin base for pediatric formulas because it tastes good, children don't mind taking it, and it doesn't contain any alcohol.

If the child is willing to drink a bulk-dispensed, water-based decoction, then I suggest adjusting the normal dosages per ingredient by the above fractions or percentages and prescribing each packet accordingly. However, if the child is an infant, I recommend using a different method of prescribing and administration. In this case, one can write the prescription for bulk-dispensed medicinals just the same as if prescribing for an adult patient. Also, make the water-based decoction the same as usual. However, instead of trying to administer a teacup of the resulting medicine 2-3 times per day, administer 1-2 droppers full numerous times per day. Using this method, one literally squirts the medicine into the baby's mouth. If necessary, one can hold the baby's mouth closed until they swallow. Even if the child spits or dribbles out some of this medicine, the practitioner and parent should not worry. Because babies react so much quicker to treatment and medication than adults, it is my experience that numerous, small doses are more important than the total amount of medicine ingested. Further, it is also my experience that babies are not as reluctant to swallow a bitter decoction as are older children and even adults. Therefore, the parent and practitioner should not have any preconceptions about the child's potential reaction to the medicine. If one uses some common sense and is not shy about prescribing and administering Chinese medicinals to babies and children, they will find this is not as difficult as many (including some doctors of Chinese medicine) might imagine.

8
Acupuncture & Moxibustion

Acupuncture is the best known treatment modality of Chinese medicine *in the West*. In China, Chinese medicine primarily means the prescription of internally administered herbal medicines mostly in the form of decoctions taken orally. For various historical reasons, however, acupuncture and moxibustion have gained a foothold in the West and are what most Westerners immediately think of when they think of Chinese medicine. Although one may treat infants and small children with acupuncture, it is not my treatment of choice. I much prefer and recommend treating children and small infants with Chinese dietary therapy, Chinese herbal medicine, and Chinese pediatric massage.

That being said, sometimes it is necessary or appropriate to treat children, even very small children, with acupuncture. Acupuncture can be used to either provide immediate first aid relief or can be used when Chinese herbal medicines or pediatric *tui na* are otherwise not available. However, when doing acupuncture on babies and young children, one should remember that the qi and blood of children are, by nature, scanty and weak, and their channels and network vessels are not entirely complete and may be easily damaged.

Therefore, I typically use acupuncture in my pediatric practice only in the following instances and ways. First of all, if there is toxic heat causing an acute, emergency condition I do use and do suggest bleeding. For instance, if there is tonsillitis with a very sore, swollen throat potentially causing respiratory distress, then bleeding *Shao Shang* (Lu 11) is a very effective and immediate way of clearing heat and dispersing swelling. It results in an almost immediate reduction in swelling of the tonsils and throat due to replete heat. Likewise, if there is high fever causing convulsions or loss of consciousness, bleeding *Shi Xuan* (M-UE-1) can quickly bring down a high fever due to internal heat.

Secondly, if a child has been overfed, sometimes even to the point of perpetual somnolence and clouding of the spirit, one can needle *Si Feng* (M-UE-9). Most Chinese textbooks say to needle these points with a thick needle and deeply into the joint capsule.

One then squeezes out a yellow serous fluid for best results. However, even without needling with such a fat needle or so deeply, and even without expressing some yellow fluid, needling these points can treat chronic and enduring food stagnation causing diarrhea, vomiting, lack of appetite, somnolence, and clouding of the spirit. Some Chinese acupuncturists also use these points to stimulate growth in children who are growing too slowly. However, although this makes some theoretical sense to me, I have never had occasion to use these points in this way.

And third, if I want to stimulate a viscus or bowel using acupuncture, I recommend the advice of my first acupuncture teacher, Dr. (Eric) Tao Xi-yu. Dr. Tao always suggested needling only the back transport or *shu* points in young children. Remember, children's viscera are clean and efficient. Therefore, even seemingly slight or light stimulation of them can produce quick results. Conversely, children's qi and blood are scanty and weak and their channels are incomplete. Therefore, needling channel points may not be as effective.

Whether one needles back *shu* or channel points, in general, I recommend very short needle retention. One should stimulate the needle to obtain the qi and then withdraw the needle. Again, children respond to light stimulation very quickly, more quickly than adults. Because most children will cry when receiving acupuncture, I try to use the least possible points, points like the back transport points which the child cannot see, and to needle as quickly as possible with the shortest needle retention.

Although I personally do not favor the use of acupuncture when treating infants and small children, because most Western practitioners of Chinese medicine are primarily trained in acupuncture and both they and the public conceive of them as acupuncturists (as opposed to Chinese medicine doctors), I have included acupuncture treatments under most of the disease categories discussed in this book. In general, I have taken these from Chinese pediatric texts.

Other acupuncture techniques & related modalities

Some Japanese acupuncture practitioners use a whole array of point stimulating "needles" called *shonishin*. This is only the Japanese pronunciation of the Chinese, *xiao er zhen*, pediatric needles. In any case, *shonishin* practitioners use a variety of scrapers, brushes, combs, and blunt probes to provide noninvasive stimulation to acupuncture points and channels. This stimulation can be used remedially for the treatment of disease or preventively in regularly scheduled visits for otherwise healthy children. Although this method can be highly effective in trained hands, it is not a part of Chinese TCM and is, therefore, beyond the scope of this book.

Likewise, some practitioners use laser acupuncture, electroacupuncture, and magnetotherapy to provide noninvasive stimulation of acupuncture points. These methods each have their merit and do seem to be effective. However, these, too, are beyond the scope of this book.

9
Antibiotics & Immunizations

Just as Chinese pediatric texts do not have a chapter on dietary therapy, they also do not have chapters on antibiotics and immunizations. In my experience, next to faulty diet, the overuse or wrongful use of antibiotics is the second most important factor in most of the commonly seen pediatric complaints in the West. Therefore, no pediatric text intended for Western practitioners is, in my opinion, complete without addressing this extremely important issue.

Although the evidence is not conclusive, there is a growing concern among many Western parents about the possible long- and short-term deleterious effects of pediatric immunization. This concern is especially greatest in the Western patient population most likely to seek treatment from a TCM practitioner, *i.e.*, those interested in or committed to so-called alternative medicine. At this point in time, I do not believe that a coherent theory concerning the effects of pediatric immunization has yet been written within the confines of TCM logic in either the Western nor the Chinese TCM literature, and it is important to remember that Chinese doctors have used immunization for more than a thousand years. So immunization is a historical part of Chinese medicine. Nevertheless, I do believe that every Western TCM practitioner should be informed about the possible negative side effects of pediatric immunization and their shortcomings and limitations.

Antibiotics

Antibiotics are wonderful, life-saving medicines when used correctly and in moderation. Unfortunately, antibiotics have been irresponsibly overprescribed and erroneously prescribed for conditions which they cannot treat, such as viral infections. This has led to the development of many new strains of infectious bacteria which are resistant to antibiotic treatment. However, even if that were not the case, antibiotics should be reserved for the few cases in which they are truly necessary. This is because antibiotics are so powerful. Not only do they kill disease-producing bacteria, but they commonly kill off the good bacteria upon which our health is founded.

Our bodies are home to many bacteria which actually work for us in healthy ways. In particular, our digestive tracts are homes to all sorts of bacteria and fungi which are commensal, meaning they live within our house, and which are symbiotic, meaning that both sides benefit from their presence. These bacteria help break down foods and the waste products of digestion. Others of these bacteria help keep populations of various yeast and fungi in proper proportions. These yeast and fungi also live within us symbiotically and provide us with certain necessary services.

If, however, antibiotics wipe out these healthy bacteria along with disease-producing ones, it upsets the balance of power within our system and especially within our guts. This then sets in motion a series of events which have profound negative repercussions on our long-term health and well-being. If the bacteria which keep the yeasts and fungi in our intestinal tracts under control are harmed, these populations explode. When they do, they do three important things. First, they invade the interior of the body by moving out of the intestinal tract (which is technically outside the body). Once inside the body, they must protect themselves from attack by the body's immune system. After all, these now are foreign cells which should not be inside the body. In order to defend against the host body's immune response, these fungi very cleverly manufacture and release certain hormone-like substances that 1) weaken the immune system, making it less efficient, and 2) upset the delicate balance between the various hormones of the body. These hormones are the messengers of the body which help keep the body's homeostasis healthy and normal.

Secondly, eventually these yeast and fungi die. When they die, they break down into foreign molecules. The body's immune system recognizes these foreign molecules as foreign and mounts an immune response or attack. Thus, although these yeast and fungi weaken the immune system by confusing it, they also cause it to be perpetually fighting their breakdown products.

Third, when these yeast and fungi move through the intestinal wall, they allow the intestinal wall to become permeable to other things which should not be allowed into the interior of the body. This is called "leaky gut syndrome." These other things are large, undigested molecules of food. If these get into the interior of the body, the body's defense or immune system recognizes these large, undigested food molecules as foreign and so also mounts an immune response or attack. Thus the body becomes allergic to these large food molecules passing undigested through the guts, since an allergy is nothing other than an immune response to a substance which, in healthy people, does not normally cause an immune reaction.

Therefore, the net result of killing off the healthy bacteria in our guts by wrong or repeated use of antibiotics is to lead to 1) leaky guts, 2) hormonal dysregulation of the immune system, and c) perpetual allergic responses. These perpetual allergic responses eventually exhaust the immune system, making the host more and more susceptible to germs it would ordinarily take care of without symptoms of disease. Finally, the body's immune system gets so overworked and so out of balance that it loses all sense of what is foreign and what is self. At that point it may even start attacking itself and cause autoimmune diseases, such as rheumatoid arthritis, multiple sclerosis, and lupus erythematosus.

This scenario is involved in the disease mechanisms of most of the diseases with which people in developed countries are more and more concerned: allergies, immune deficiencies, and autoimmune diseases, but also many viral conditions, including diabetes. As a TCM gynecologist, I also see this scenario playing a part in endometriosis, immunological infertility, and even PMS and menopausal syndrome through autoimmune thyroiditis and ovaritis. This scenario even plays its part in the development and progression of many cancers. Therefore, this scenario is a key one in understanding and successfully treating a whole host of diseases, including chronic, recurrent earaches, chronic, recurrent tonsillitis, and chronic allergies, including eczema and allergic asthma, in children.

Chinese medicine & antibiotics

For the last several paragraphs, I have been talking about antibiotics and their side effects in terms of Western biology. However, Chinese medicine has its own description of these same events. In Chinese medicine, herbs which have pronounced antibacterial, antimicrobial, and anti-inflammatory abilities are usually described as being very "cold." This is because most microbial infections result in some sort of inflammation. Such symptoms of inflammation are seen as the pathogenic or evil presence of heat in the body. Since cold is what clears heat, therefore, medicinals which have pronounced antimicrobial, anti-inflammatory effect on the body are described as being cold in nature.

The logic of this description is supported by another factor. Since digestion in Chinese medicine is believed to be a process of warm transformation, excessively cold medicinals may damage this process. In Chinese medicine this is described as damaging the spleen. If the spleen becomes damaged by wrong or overuse of cold, anti-inflammatory medicinals, then the symptoms that appear are various digestive complaints such as diarrhea and loose stools and gas and abdominal distention after eating. These are exactly the kinds of side effects many antibiotics have. Because the spleen in Chinese medicine is associated with the production of healthy or righteous qi in the body, damage to the spleen also results in fatigue, cold hands and feet, reduced appetite, and a pale or sallow complexion. Further, because the righteous qi is what fights evil or pathogenic qi in the body, if the spleen becomes weak, the body cannot fight off invasion or infection as efficiently as it should. Thus it is said in Chinese that assailing evils take advantage of this deficiency and repeatedly enter the body. In addition, because the spleen is responsible for the transportation and transformation of body fluids and liquids in the body, if cold medicinals damage spleen yang qi, water and dampness accumulate and transform and congeal into phlegm.

Therefore, one can see that even from the TCM point of view, wrong or overuse of antibiotics can lead to damage of the spleen with repeated susceptibility to disease, such as earaches, tonsillitis, and various allergies, and the abnormal production and accumulation of phlegm and mucus, *i.e.*, colds, coughs, and asthma. If the spleen is strong, a person may be treated with antibiotics and bounce back quickly without much in the way of side effects or lingering repercussions. But if the spleen is weak or if antibiotics are used repeatedly, the spleen is weakened even and ever further. Thus infections recur, more antibiotics are given, and the circle goes round and round and round.

The implications of this are that antibiotics should only be used when they are truly necessary. Just two days ago (January 16, 1996), a spokesperson for the American Medical Association went on TV and asked physicians the same thing — not to prescribe antibiotics unless truly necessary. The AMA may have a different interpretation of what is truly necessary, but at least some Western MDs are waking up to the fact that wrong and overuse of antibiotics is creating a major health care problem in the world.

I believe that antibiotics should be seen as the top rung on a ladder of graduated responses. If there is an infection, one should first try to use weaker, less drastic methods of treatment. If those do not work, one should then work their way up this ladder of graduated responses. If the condition is truly serious and potentially life-threatening or if there is the *likelihood* (not just the outside chance) of serious, long-term damage, then yes, that is the time that antibiotics are truly and correctly warranted. In other words, antibiotics should be held as the trump card in case other treatments with less side effects fail. They are there, held in reserve if necessary, but used *only* when necessary.

Avoidance of immunizations, perhaps

Many parents assume that having their children immunized is unquestionably the correct thing to do. However, there is a growing body of literature that proves there are real risks with routine vaccinations. Some of these risks, such as death due to anaphylactic shock, are immediate and catastrophic. Other of these risks consists of possible lifelong damage and disease. Further, statistics do not confirm that the death rate for some of the diseases for which we regularly immunize went down *because of* immunization. In some cases, these rates seem to have declined even before immunization was adopted or simultaneously declined in societies that did not adopt immunization. Further, there are very real questions about how effective these vaccines are in providing immunity against these diseases. The U.S. Congress has created a Vaccine Injury Compensation Program for the compensation of victims of the side effects of immunization. So it is absolutely clear and uncontestable that there is a risk to be run in getting vaccinated. Otherwise there would be no reason to have a compensation program. In other words, the whole subject of immunizations is a tricky one, and there are many parents who are confused about whether or not to immunize.

Since it is not clear to me that immunizations do not have long-term health consequences and since we know that a certain percentage of children *will* be seriously harmed by prophylactic immunizations, I generally counsel against them. However, this must remain the parents' decision and it is a decision with no perfect answers. In other words, one runs certain risks whether one does or does not immunize. Since this is not a perfect world and "nobody gets out alive", this should not be a surprising situation. But parents want only the best for their children and want to protect them against every possible harm. Unfortunately, we cannot do that, and often, trying to do that creates its own problems.

DPT

DPT stands for diphtheria, pertussis, and tetanus. Hence the DPT shot is a combination immunization against these three diseases. This is one of the very first immunizations a baby usually gets, receiving the first shot as young as two weeks of age. Although these three immunizations are usually given as a single injection, depending on one's locale and the willingness of the physician, one can get one or more of these shots by themselves. For instance, one can get just a tetanus shot or one can get a DT shot.

Diphtheria

Diphtheria is a very virulent and dangerous disease. Diphtheria leads to death in one in 10 cases. However, in developed countries in the West, it is very rare. In 1992, there were four reported cases of diphtheria in the United States. If one lives or travels in countries where diphtheria is a present danger, then immunization makes sense. Otherwise, I do not believe it is necessary. If an outbreak or epidemic was moving towards one's place of residence, then one should get this vaccine. Unfortunately, an FDA-sponsored vaccine review has concluded that "for several reasons, diphtheria toxoid, fluid or absorbed, is not as effective an immunizing agent as might be anticipated." Chinese medicine does treat this disease. However, it should be treated with a combination of Chinese and Western medicine, not just Chinese medicine alone.

Pertussis

Pertussis is also called whooping cough. It does exist within developed Western societies. In 1992, there were 3,359 cases of pertussis in the U.S. Seventy percent of these cases were in children under five years of age. The death rate for whooping cough is one case in 100. In infants under six months, three out of four cases require hospitalization, one out of 20, intensive care, and one in five develops pneumonia. Whooping cough is a serious health risk to children under one year of age. However, the pertussis vaccine can definitely cause lifelong damage. The Institute of Medicine of the National Academy of Science, comprised of 11 leading pediatricians in the United States, spent 20 months reviewing hundreds of scientific studies on the safety and efficacy of immunizations. This panel concluded that the pertussis vaccine can cause a number of health problems. In addition, the Vaccine Advisory Committee of the U.S. Congress produced a wealth of data about recurring problems with this vaccine. This vaccine was created in 1912 and has not been changed since. This vaccine has never been tested for safety in the U.S. and especially has never been tested for safety at the current dosage in children as young as six weeks of age or younger. The statistics also do not prove that this vaccine works particularly well in preventing this disease. In recent outbreaks of whooping cough, half or more of all sufferers had been fully vaccinated. According to Prof. Gordon Stewart writing on the pertussis vaccine in *The Lancet*, "No protection by vaccination is demonstrable in infants", while Dr. Morris, testifying before the Subcommittee on Investigations &

General Oversight in May 1982, stated that the pertussis vaccination has only been shown to be *between* 63-93% effective.

The side effects of the pertussis vaccine are as follows: one in 25 children will develop a fever over 102. One in 333 will develop a fever of over 105. One in 100 develop a persistent, unusual, high-pitched cry. One in 1,667 develops convulsions. One in 10,000 develops severe brain problems, while permanent brain damage occurs in one in 310,000 of children vaccinated. Anaphylactic shock and residual seizure disorders do happen, but are even rarer.

That being said, Chinese medicine does treat pertussis. Therefore, I do not advise taking the risk of the pertussis vaccine when Chinese medicine does treat this disease. My own son has never been vaccinated against this disease. If, however, professional Chinese medical treatment is not locally available, one should also take that into account when making a decision about this vaccine. Among those who are against routine childhood vaccinations, this particular vaccine is considered the most dangerous even though, statistically, permanent brain damage is pretty rare. On the other hand, when one thinks that millions of children are routinely given this vaccine, then there are a definite number of permanently brain-damaged children from this vaccine out there.

Tetanus

Tetanus infection is usually the result of an unclean puncture wound or cut. It is caused by germs which live in dirt. Unless a wound is contaminated by contact with dirt, tetanus is not very likely. According to Dr. Velia Hempel of Germany, the immunity provided by tetanus shots wears off after 10 years. In the U.S., if one gets a serious cut requiring medical attention, the doctor will want to give a "booster" shot in any case. According to Dr. Hempel, such booster shots are not given in Europe and cannot provide any immunity for a cut which has already occurred since it takes a number of days before immunity is established. That means that all adults who think they have a lifetime immunity to tetanus are wrong. Again according to Dr. Hempel, this is the same situation with most other immunizations — they do not confer lifetime immunity; their effect wears off. This raises a very large question, at least in my mind. It means that most of us probably do not have the immunity that we think we do. Although Chinese medicine does have treatments for tetanus, it should be treated by a combination of Chinese and Western medicines.

The Institute of Medicine (IOM) study cited above has concluded that the DPT vaccine *definitely* can cause numerous health problems, including death. There is evidence that "indicates a causal relation" between administration of this vaccine and anaphylactic shock. Anaphylactic shock is an extreme allergic reaction which, if not treated immediately can lead to death. This same study found that this vaccine also caused extended periods of inconsolable crying and screaming lasting up to 24 hours. Harris L. Coulter and Barbara Joe Fisher in *DPT: A Shot in the Dark* say this crying resembles the so-called *cri encephalique* which accompanies some cases of encephalitis. Encephalitis or meningitis, an inflammation of the brain, may result in either permanent brain damage or death, and the IOM study did find a link between DPT vaccination, acute encephalopathy, and shock. A group called Dissatisfied Parents Together (DPT) believes their children have been permanently harmed in this way by this vaccine. Other possible side effects of the DPT vaccine are chronic neurologic disease, Guillain-Barre syndrome (a type of paralysis), juvenile diabetes, learning disabilities, attention deficit disorder (ADD), infantile convulsions, and sudden infant death syndrome (SIDS). From January through August of 1991, the Vaccine Adverse Event Reporting System set up by the Compensation Act received 3,447 reports of DPT reactions. Included were 398 cases of convulsions, 218 cases of shock, 72 cases of febrile seizures, and 75 cases of sudden infant death syndrome. Thus clearly there are risks associated with the DPT shot which every parent must carefully weigh before having their child immunized.

Polio

Mine was the first generation mass immunized against polio. Growing up I had a friend who had one leg smaller than the other because of atrophy due to polio. I have also seen many polio patients in Chinese hospitals. So I know polio is real. If one lives in a developed Western country, the incidence of polio is rare. However, the vaccine itself does cause serious and life-threatening effects in a certain percentage of patients. In the United States, virtually the only cases of polio which occur — 5-10 per year — are caused by either the vaccine itself or infection from someone who recently received the vaccine. The last naturally occurring case of poliomyelitis in the United States occurred in 1972. Based on my experience in China, I do not think TCM alone is sufficient treatment for polio. Nevertheless, I also do not recommend this vaccine unless the child is going to travel to underdeveloped countries where polio is a present danger. (The last case in the Americas was recorded in Peru in 1991.) If one does decide to get this vaccine, one should ask for the killed vaccine rather than live vaccine. The killed vaccine has a better safety record. Polio can cause permanent crippling and occasional death. The death rate is 76% in children under two and 7% in those over two. Crippling and death may occur whether the polio is naturally occurring or is the result of immunization.

Measles, rubella & chicken pox

I do not recommend vaccinating for these diseases. In Asia, a childhood bout of any of these three diseases is not considered a bad thing. In Chinese medicine, these diseases are believed to be associated with so-called fetal toxins. It is said in Chinese pediatric books, "Because of fetal toxins accumulated, they are more susceptible to pox." Fetal toxins are toxins which are passed on to the baby at conception or developed in the womb. They lay dormant until they are provoked by some stimulating external pathogen. Then they are expressed to the surface of the body where they manifest as a rash or blisters. If these rashes or blisters are fully expressed and the body then heals correctly, the child is then better off for no longer harboring these fetal toxins. There are case histories in the Chinese medical literature where chronic health problems which develop later in life are associated with incompletely expressed or expelled fetal toxins.

In addition, Chinese medicine does treat these three diseases very well. The main danger from measles is that it may develop into pneumonia. If treated correctly by Chinese medicine, this is very unlikely. However, if one does not choose to immunize their children against these three diseases, they should purposely expose their children to infection when they are still young. Measles and chicken pox tend to be worse for adults than for children, while German measles during pregnancy is associated with certain birth defects. In earlier times, people had measles and chicken pox parties so that their children would get these diseases, and there was wisdom behind that approach.

Mumps

Mumps is another infectious disease for which we can now immunize and which mostly strikes children. Chinese medicine treats mumps very well and this is not a serious disease unless it too is allowed to develop into pneumonia. It can, however, cause sterility in adults and is typically much more uncomfortable in adults than in children. Nonetheless, I do not recommend immunizing against it.

MMR

The MMR vaccine is the name of the vaccine given for measles, mumps, and rubella. As stated above, I do not believe it is necessary or good to vaccinate against these diseases. The side effects of this vaccine are swollen neck glands in one out of seven patients, joint aching and swelling in one out of 100 patients, and rash and slight fever in one out of seven to twenty patients. Anaphylactic shock, though rare, does sometimes occur and encephalitis occurs in one out of 2,500,000 vaccinated with MMR.

Guidelines for making a choice about pediatric immunizations

Miranda Castro, writing in the Summer, 1996 issue of *Mothering*, gives some excellent advice on how to decide whether or not to vaccinate one's children. First she suggests gathering information on the pros and cons of each immunization. Secondly, parents should "take their own beliefs and feelings into account when weighing the risk of contracting each disease versus the efficacy of each vaccination." Third, parents should seek out medical providers who are sympathetic to their needs and wishes. Fourth and perhaps most importantly, parents must recognize that they must live with the consequences of their decisions no matter what the outcome is. That means asking yourself if you are prepared to nurse your child through a childhood disease such as measles or whooping cough *and* how you would feel if your child was one of the few unlucky ones to contract serious, even fatal side effects from a vaccine. Five, wait as long as possible before beginning vaccinations. Six, ask your doctor to administer one at a time and not multiple vaccinations all at once. As Ms. Castro says, "Since we do not contract more than one disease at a time, it makes sense to have only one vaccine at a time." And seven, make peace with the fact that this is a difficult decision and there are risks no matter what you decide. Ms. Castro points out that the goal is to minimize the risks as much as possible.

BOOK TWO

1
The Diagnosis & Treatment of Commonly Encountered Pediatric Diseases

The diseases discussed below are the most commonly encountered complaints among infants and young children. They have been arranged according to what is called a longitudinal approach. This means that they appear roughly in the order they are most likely to arise in terms of the age and development of the child. Under each disease, one will find a brief introduction and its TCM pattern discrimination. Under each pattern, one will find its main signs and symptoms, the treatment principles necessary to restore balance and harmony to the imbalance implied in the name of the pattern, and one or more Chinese medicinal formulas and adjunctive treatments.

1. Neonatal Jaundice

Many babies suffer from varying degrees of jaundice after birth. Jaundice means yellowing of the skin and possibly the whites of the eyes. Usually a small amount of neonatal jaundice is nothing to worry about. It can be treated by giving the baby water to drink and laying them in the sunlight. If, however, jaundice appears either within 24 hours of birth, is too dark a color, or persists too long after birth, Western doctors may want to treat this. Typically, Western medical treatment consists of keeping the baby in the hospital under so-called bilirubin lights and administering frequent feedings in order to help excrete the bilirubin.

Treatment based on pattern discrimination:

1. Yang jaundice

Main symptoms: Brightly colored yellow skin and eyes, deep yellow urine, generalized fever or hot to the touch, possible constipation, spirit clouding, vexation and confusion, fatigue, lack of strength, no desire to eat or drink, abdominal distention and fullness, dry mouth and lips

Treatment principles: Clear heat and eliminate dampness by promoting urination

Guiding formulas:
Yin Chen Hao Tang (Artemisia Scopariae Decoction)
Yin Chen Hao (Herba Artemisiae Scopariae)
Zhi Zi (Fructus Gardeniae)
Da Huang (Radix Et Rhizoma Rhei)

Yin Chen Hao Tang Jia Jian (Artemisia Scopariae Decoction with Additions & Subtractions)
Yin Chen Hao (Herba Artemisiae Scopariae)
Gou Qi Zi (Fructus Lycii)
Hua Shi (Talcum)
Che Qian Zi (Semen Plantaginis)
Da Huang (Radix Et Rhizoma Rhei)

If dampness is more pronounced than heat as evidenced by a lighter yellow color of the skin, consider adding such aromatically drying medicinals as *Hou Po* (Cortex Magnoliae) and *Huo Xiang* (Herba Pogostemonis). One can also use one of the following formulas.

Yin Chen Hao Tang Jia Wei (Artemisia Scopariae Decoction with Added Flavors)
Yin Chen Hao (Herba Artemisiae Scopariae)
Zhi Zi (Fructus Gardeniae)
Fu Ling (Poria)
Zhu Ling (Polyporus)
Ze Xie (Rhizoma Alismatis)
uncooked *Da Huang* (Radix Et Rhizoma Rhei)

If there is no constipation or if there are loose stools, omit the *Da Huang*.

Yin Chen Si Ling Tang (Artemisia Scopariae Four [Ingredients] Poria Decoction)
Yin Chen Hao (Herba Artemisiae Scopariae)
Fu Ling (Poria)
Zhu Ling (Polyporus)
Ze Xie (Rhizoma Alismatis)
Bai Zhu (Rhizoma Atractylodis Macrocephalae)

Gan Lu Xiao Du Dan (Sweet Dew Disperse Toxins Elixir)
Lian Qiao (Fructus Forsythiae)
Huang Qin (Radix Scutellariae)
Bo He (Herba Menthae Haplocalycis)

    She Gan (Rhizoma Belamcandae)
    Chuan Bei Mu (Bulbus Fritillariae Cirrhosae)
    Hua Shi (Talcum)
    Mu Tong (Caulis Akebiae)
    Yin Chen Hao (Herba Artemisiae Scopariae)
    Huo Xiang (Herba Pogostemonis)
    Shi Chang Pu (Rhizoma Acori Tatarinowii)
    Bai Dou Kou (Fructus Cardamomi)

If heat is more pronounced than dampness, as evidenced by fever, constipation, a red tongue, etc., then use *Xi Jiao San Jia Jian* (Rhinoceros Horn Powder with Additions & Subtractions):
    Shui Niu Jiao (Cornu Bubali)
    Yin Chen Hao (Herba Artemisiae Scopariae)
    Long Dan Cao (Radix Gentianae)
    Gan Cao (Radix Glycyrrhizae)
    Sheng Di (uncooked Radix Rehmanniae)
    Tian Hua Fen (Radix Trichosanthis)
    Sheng Ma (Rhizoma Cimicifugae)
    Han Shui Shi (Calcitum)
    Mu Tong (Caulis Akebiae)
    Zhi Zi (Fructus Gardeniae)

2. Yin jaundice

Main symptoms: Dull yellow skin and eyes which endures and does not recede, fatigue, torpid intake, easy vomiting after eating, loose stools, abdominal distention and fullness, cold limbs, a pale tongue

Treatment principles: Fortify the spleen and warm yang while promoting urination

Guiding formulas:
Yin Chen Li Zhong Tang (Artemisia Scopariae Rectify the Center Decoction)
    Yin Chen Hao (Herba Artemisiae Scopariae)
    Gan Jiang (dry Rhizoma Zingiberis)
    Dang Shen (Radix Codonopsitis)
    Bai Zhu (Rhizoma Atractylodis Macrocephalae)
    Fu Ling (Poria)

Yin Chen Li Zhong Tang Jia Jian (Artemisia Scopariae Rectify the Center Decoction with Additions & Subtractions)
    Yin Chen Hao (Herba Artemisiae Scopariae)

Dang Shen (Radix Codonopsitis)
Bai Zhu (Rhizoma Atractylodis Macrocephalae)
Gan Jiang (dry Rhizoma Zingiberis)
Gan Cao (Radix Glycyrrhizae)

If there is concomitant qi and blood vacuity manifest by a pale complexion and lassitude of the spirit, *i.e.*, listlessness, add *Huang Qi* (Radix Astragali) and *Dang Gui* (Radix Angelicae Sinensis).

Yin Chen Li Zhong Tang Jia Wei (Artemisia Scopariae Rectify the Center Decoction with Added Flavors)
Yin Chen Hao (Herba Artemisiae Scopariae)
Dang Shen (Radix Codonopsitis)
Bai Zhu (Rhizoma Atractylodis Macrocephalae)
Fu Ling (Poria)
Gan Jiang (dry Rhizoma Zingiberis)
Gan Cao (Radix Glycyrrhizae)
uncooked *Da Huang* (Radix Et Rhizoma Rhei)

If there is no constipation or if there are loose stools, omit the *Da Huang*.

If there is predominant dampness due to spleen vacuity with cold and dampness internally brewing, *i.e.*, transforming heat from depression, one may use the following unnamed formula:
Cang Zhu (Rhizoma Atractylodis)
Hou Po (Cortex Magnoliae)
Gan Cao (Radix Glycyrrhizae)
Chen Pi (Pericarpium Citri Reticulatae)
Yi Yi Ren (Semen Coicis)
Bai Bian Dou (Semen Dolichoris)
Yin Chen Hao (Herba Artemisiae Scopariae)
Sha Ren (Fructus Amomi)
Zhi Zi (Fructus Gardeniae)

3. Stasis accumulation jaundice

Main symptoms: Yellowing of the skin and eyes. The color of the cheeks is relatively bright but otherwise is dark and lusterless. It gets worse as the sun increases. There is right-sided glomus and lumpiness which is somewhat hard, abdominal distention and fullness, lassitude of the spirit, torpid intake, easy vomiting after eating, short, yellowish urine, greyish white stools, the possible appearance of static macules, ejection of blood, dark red lips, possible static spots on the tongue, and yellow tongue fur.

Treatment principles: Transform stasis and disperse accumulation

Guiding formula:
Xue Fu Zhu Yu Tang **(Blood Mansion Dispel Stasis Decoction)**

Dang Gui (Radix Angelicae Sinensis)
Sheng Di (uncooked Radix Rehmanniae)
Niu Xi (Radix Achyranthis Bidentatae)
Hong Hua (Flos Carthami)
Tao Ren (Semen Persicae)
Chai Hu (Radix Bupleuri)
Zhi Ke (Fructus Aurantii)
Chi Shao (Radix Paeoniae Rubrae)
Chuan Xiong (Rhizoma Chuanxiong)
Jie Geng (Radix Platycodi)
Gan Cao (Radix Glycyrrhizae)

Adjunctive treatment

Generally, this condition is not treated with acupuncture, but rubbing of the abdomen in the direction of peristalsis to increase bowel movements is suggested if there is constipation.

Comments

Severe neonatal jaundice which does not respond to sunlight, water, rubbing of the abdomen, and/or Chinese herbal medicine does need to be treated by Western medicine, possibly including exchange blood transfusion. If left untreated, severe neonatal hyperbilirubinemia may result in brain damage, seizures, and even death. Therefore, if the jaundice is severe, a Western MD should be consulted.

2. Lack of Breast-feeding in a Neonate

If a child is not able to begin to breast-feed within 12-24 hours after birth, this is called lack of breast-feeding or difficulty breast-feeding in Chinese medicine. It is mostly due to former heaven or prenatal insufficiency of natural endowment with viscera and bowel vacuity cold or swallowing of amniotic fluid which then causes heat depression and binding.

Treatment based on pattern discrimination:

1. Vacuity cold

Main symptoms: This may occur in a premature baby or one who has contracted cold during birthing with a weak body, a somber white facial complexion, lack of warmth in the four limbs, cold breath issuing from the mouth and nose, a low, weak cry, weak respiration, and pale lips and tongue

Treatment principles: Bank the origin and warm the center

Guiding formulas:
First administer **Du Shen Tang (Solitary Ginseng Decoction)** to greatly supplement the original qi:
   Ren Shen (Radix Ginseng)

Then administer **Li Zhong Tang (Rectify the Center Decoction)** to fortify the spleen and warm the center:
   Gan Jiang (dry Rhizoma Zingiberis)
   Ren Shen (Radix Ginseng)
   Bai Zhu (Rhizoma Atractylodis Macrocephalae)
   mix-fried *Gan Cao* (Radix Glycyrrhizae)

Si Jun Zi Tang (Four Gentlemen Decoction)
   Ren Shen (Radix Ginseng)
   Bai Zhu (Rhizoma Atractylodis Macrocephalae)
   Fu Ling (Poria)
   mix-fried *Gan Cao* (Radix Glycyrrhizae)

Yun Qi San (Spare Qi Powder)
   Chen Pi (Pericarpium Citri Reticulatae)
   Jie Geng (Radix Platycodi)
   Pao Jiang (blast-fried Rhizoma Zingiberis)
   Sha Ren (Fructus Amomi)
   Mu Xiang (Radix Auklandiae)
   Gan Cao (Radix Glycyrrhizae)
   Da Zao (Fructus Jujubae)

Yun Qi San Jia Jian (Spare Qi Powder with Additions & Subtractions)
   Pao Jiang (blast-fried Rhizoma Zingiberis)
   Gui Zhi (Ramulus Cinnamomi)
   Gan Cao (Radix Glycyrrhizae)
   Da Zao (Fructus Jujubae)
   Sha Ren (Fructus Amomi)
   Chen Pi (Pericarpium Citri Reticulatae)
   Mu Xiang (Radix Auklandiae)

2. Filth & heat congesting & accumulating

Main symptoms: This mostly occurs in babies whose births have been stagnant, *i.e.*, prolonged and difficult, or who have swallowed amniotic fluid. Their abdomens are distended and full and their urination and defecation are not freely flowing. There may also be vomiting, vexation and agitation, distressed rapid dyspneic breathing, an obstructed sound to their cry, and thick, slimy, yellow tongue fur.

Treatment principles: Dispel filth, clear heat, and open the bowels

Guiding formulas:
First administer **Hang Xie Dan (Evening Mist Elixir)** to open and descend filth and turbidity:
   Chuan Xiong (Rhizoma Chuanxiong)
   Da Huang (Radix Et Rhizoma Rhei)
   Huang Qin (Radix Scutellariae)
   Huang Bai (Cortex Phellodendri)
   Hei Chou (Semen Pharbiditis)
   Bo He (Herba Menthae Haplocalycis)
   Shi Gao (Talcum)
   Bing Lang (Semen Arecae)
   Zhi Ke (Fructus Aurantii)
   Lian Qiao (Fructus Forsythiae)
   Chi Shao (Radix Paeoniae Rubrae)

Then administer **Qing Re Xie Pi San (Clear Heat & Drain the Spleen Powder)** in order to clear *yang ming* interior heat:
   Zhi Zi (Fructus Gardeniae)
   Shi Gao (Gypsum Fibrosum)
   Huang Lian (Rhizoma Coptidis)
   Sheng Di (uncooked Radix Rehmanniae)
   Fu Ling (Poria)
   Huang Qin (Radix Scutellariae)

Unnamed formula
   Da Huang (Radix Et Rhizoma Rhei)
   Huang Lian (Rhizoma Coptidis)

Acupuncture & moxibustion

Moxa *Shen Que* (CV 8) for the vacuity cold pattern.

Adjunctive treatment

For filth and heat congesting accumulating and, one can give the baby an enema to induce defecation.

3. Non Free-flowing Defecation in a Neonate

If two days after birth a baby still has not had a bowel movement, this is considered a disease in Chinese medicine and is treated in order to remedy it. There are two basic causes of this condition. Either there is fetal heat congesting and binding or there is insufficiency of the former heaven natural endowment. In the first case, the bowels are blocked, while in the latter case, there is insufficient qi to discharge the feces.

Treatment based on pattern discrimination:

1. Fetal heat congesting & binding

Main symptoms: Non free-flowing bowels after having been given birth, abdominal distention, if severe, vomiting, vexation and agitation, profuse crying, a red face and lips, a dry tongue and mouth

Treatment principles: Clear heat and scatter binding, move the qi and open downward

Guiding formula:
Unnamed formula
   Jin Yin Hua (Flos Lonicerae)
   Gan Cao (Radix Glycyrrhizae)
   Huang Lian (Rhizoma Coptidis)
   Bai Mi (Honey)

2. Fetal endowment insufficiency (a.k.a. original qi vacuity weakness)

Main symptoms: Non free-flowing defecation after having been given birth, a somber white facial complexion, weak, timid spirit qi, a low, feeble voice, a moist, glossy mouth and tongue

Treatment principles: Bank and supplement the original qi, warm, open, and move the qi

Guiding formula:
Du Shen Tang (Solitary Ginseng Decoction)
   Ren Shen (Radix Ginseng)

Acupuncture & moxibustion

Moxa *Shen Que* (CV 8) for babies manifesting fetal endowment insufficiency.

Adjunctive treatment

Give an enema to babies manifesting the fetal heat congesting and binding pattern.

4. Non Free-flowing Urination in a Neonate

If a child does not urinate within 36 hours of having been given birth, this is referred to as non free-flowing urination in a neonate. Like the previous two conditions, it is due either to fetal heat brewing and smoldering in the urinary bladder or former heaven fetal endowment insufficiency.

Treatment based on pattern discrimination:

1. Heat brewing in the urinary bladder

Main symptoms: Non free-flowing urination in a neonate, lower abdominal distention, red lips and a dry mouth, vexation and agitation, profuse crying

Treatment principles: Clear heat and disinhibit urination

Guiding formula:
Dao Chi San Jia Wei (Abduct the Red Powder with Added Flavors)
   Bai Mao Gen (Rhizoma Imperatae)
   Huang Lian (Rhizoma Coptidis)
   Hua Shi (Talcum)
   Che Qian Zi (Semen Plantaginis)
   Sheng Di (uncooked Radix Rehmanniae)
   Mu Tong (Caulis Akebiae)
   Dan Zhu Ye (Herba Lophateri)
   Gan Cao Shao (rootlets of Radix Glycyrrhizae)

2. Original qi vacuity weakness

Main symptoms: Non free-flowing urination in a neonate, lower abdominal distention, a white face and pale lips, bodily qi timorous and weak, the sound of crying weak and feeble

Treatment principles: Bank and supplement the original qi, warm, transform, and disinhibit water

Guiding formula:
Du Shen Tang (Solitary Ginseng Decoction) followed by Wu Ling San (Five [Ingredients] Poria Powder)
   Ren Shen (Radix Ginseng)
   Fu Ling (Poria)
   Zhu Ling (Polyporus)
   Bai Zhu (Rhizoma Atractylodis Macrocephalae)
   Ze Xie (Rhizoma Alismatis)
   Gui Zhi (Ramulus Cinnamomi)

Acupuncture & moxibustion

For original qi vacuity weakness pattern, moxa *Shen Que* (CV 8).

5. Various Umbilical Region Conditions

Some Chinese pediatric texts include a chapter titled as above which includes the diagnosis and treatment of seepage from the navel, umbilical sores, and bleeding from the umbilicus. Except for bleeding from the umbilicus which is divided into two patterns, treatment is given on the basis of disease diagnosis.

Treatment based on pattern discrimination:

1. Umbilical dampness

Main symptoms: Seepage of a pale yellow, fatty liquid from the umbilicus whose exterior surface is slightly red and swollen. The skin surrounding the navel is otherwise normal.

Treatment principles: Contain, restrain, secure, and astringe

External treatment: First, decoct the following in water and use as an external wash of the affected area:
  Cang Zhu (Rhizoma Atractylodis), 9g
  Fang Feng (Radix Saposhnikoviae), 9g
  Ku Shen (Radix Sophorae Flavescentis), 9g
  Jin Yin Hua (Flos Lonicerae), 9g

Then grind into powder **Er Miao San Jia Wei (Two Wonders Powder with Added Flavors)** and apply to the navel 1-2 times each day:
  Cang Zhu (Rhizoma Atractylodis)
  Huang Bai (Cortex Phellodendri)
  Long Gu (Os Draconis)
  Ku Fan (Alumen)
  Hua Shi (Talcum)

2. Umbilical sore

Main symptoms: Redness and swelling of the umbilical region, possible fever, possible ulceration and flowing pus. If evil toxins have penetrated internally, there may be aversion to cold, strong fever, crying, vexation and agitation, red lips, oral thirst, yellow tongue fur, and a rapid pulse.

Treatment principles: Clear heat and resolve toxins, transform dampness and scatter evils

Guiding formulas:
Yin Qiao San Jia Jian (Lonicera & Forsythia Powder with Additions & Subtractions)
Jin Yin Hua (Flos Lonicerae)
Lian Qiao (Fructus Forsythiae)
Dan Dou Chi (Semen Praeparatus Sojae)
Huang Qin (Radix Scutellariae)
Zi Hua Di Ding (Herba Violae)
Jing Jie (Herba Schizonepetae)
Bo He (Herba Menthae Haplocalycis)
Di Fu Zi (Fructus Kochiae)
Xia Ku Cao (Spica Prunellae)
Yi Yi Ren (Semen Coicis)
Gan Cao Shao (rootlets of Radix Glycyrrhizae)

Xi Jiao Xiao Du Yin Jia Jian (Rhinoceros Horn Disperse Toxins Beverage with Additions & Subtractions)
Shui Niu Jiao (Cornu Bubali)
Jin Yin Hua (Flos Lonicerae)
Gan Cao (Radix Glycyrrhizae)
Fang Feng (Radix Saposhnikoviae)
Jing Jie (Herba Schizonepetae)
Niu Bang Zi (Fructus Arctii)

If the disease is mild, omit the Shui Niu Jiao and add *Huang Lian* (Rhizoma Coptidis), *Lian Qiao* (Fructus Forsythiae), and *Zi Hua Di Ding* (Herba Violae). If the disease is severe with spirit dimming and spasms and tremors, add *An Gong Niu Huang Wan* (Quiet the Palace Bezoar Pills, a Chinese patent medicine). If there is constipation with dry, yellow tongue fur, add *Da Huang* (Radix Et Rhizoma Rhei).

Unnamed formula
Huang Lian (Rhizoma Coptidis)
Huang Qin (Radix Scutellariae)
Lian Qiao (Fructus Forsythiae)
Gan Cao (Radix Glycyrrhizae)
Ban Lan Gen (Radix Isatidis/Baphicacanthi)
Zi Hua Di Ding (Herba Violae Yedenositis Cum Radice)
Bo He (Herba Menthae Haplocalycis)
Jing Jie (Herba Schizonepetae)

External treatment: First wash the navel with a decoction of *Fang Feng* (Radix Saposhnikoviae), *Jin Yin Hua* (Flos Lonicerae), and *Ye Ju Hua* (Flos Chrysanthemi Indici) and then apply *Jin Huang San* (Golden Yellow Powder):
Da Huang (Radix Et Rhizoma Rhei), 25g
Huang Bai (Cortex Phellodendri), 25g

Jiang Huang (Rhizoma Curcumae Longae), 25g
   Bai Zhi (Radix Angelicae Dahuricae), 25g
   Nan Xing (Rhizoma Arisaematis), 10g
   Chen Pi (Pericarpium Citri Reticulatae), 10g
   Cang Zhu (Rhizoma Atractylodis), 10g
   Hou Po (Cortex Magnoliae), 10g
   Gan Cao (Radix Glycyrrhizae), 10g
   Tian Hua Fen (Radix Trichosanthis), 50g

Method of preparation & use: Grind the above medicinals into powder, mix with cold, boiled water, and apply to affected area as a paste. Cover with cotton gauze and apply 1 time each day.

3. Umbilical bleeding

A. Qi not containing the blood

Main symptoms: A great amount of blood was lost during birthing and then, 1-2 weeks after birth, a very small amount of blood seeps out from the umbilicus. However, its amount then increases day by day. The infant's facial complexion is lusterless, their lips are pale white, and their four limbs are not warm. The color of the seeping blood is pale. This may be accompanied by hemafecia or hematemesis.

Treatment principles: Boost the qi and contain the blood

Guiding formulas:
Gui Pi Tang Jia Jian (Return the Spleen Decoction with Additions & Subtractions)
   Dang Shen (Radix Codonopsitis)
   Bai Zhu (Rhizoma Atractylodis Macrocephalae)
   Huang Qi (Radix Astragali)
   Fu Ling (Poria)
   mix-fried *Gan Cao* (Radix Glycyrrhizae)
   Suan Zao Ren (Semen Spinosae)
   Dang Gui (Radix Angelicae Sinensis)
   Mu Xiang (Radix Auklandiae)
   E Jiao (Gelatinum Corii Asini)
   Pu Huang (Pollen Typhae)
   Da Zao (Fructus Jujubae)

Gui Pi Tang Jia Wei (Return the Spleen Decoction with Added Flavors)
   Dang Shen (Radix Codonopsitis)
   Bai Zhu (Rhizoma Atractylodis Macrocephalae)
   Huang Qi (Radix Astragali)

Fu Ling (Poria)
mix-fried *Gan Cao* (Radix Glycyrrhizae)
Suan Zao Ren (Semen Spinosae)
Dang Gui (Radix Angelicae Sinensis)
Mu Xiang (Radix Auklandiae)
E Jiao (Gelatinum Corii Asini)
Yuan Zhi (Radix Polygalae)
Da Zao (Fructus Jujubae)
Xue Yu Tan (Crinis Carbonisatus)
carbonized *Ce Bai Ye* (Cacumen Platycladi)

B. Fetal heat internally exuberant

Main symptoms: A red face and red lips, a dry, red tongue, fresh red umbilical blood

Treatment principles: Clear heat and cool the blood

Guiding formulas:
Qian Gen Tang (Rubia Decoction)
Huang Qin (Radix Scutellariae)
Sheng Di (uncooked Radix Rehmanniae)
Qian Cao Gen (Radix Rubiae)
Ce Bai Ye (Cacumen Platycladi)
E Jiao (Gelatinum Corii Asini)
Dang Gui (Radix Angelicae Sinensis)

Qian Gen Tang Jia Jian (Rubia Decoction with Additions & Subtractions)
Qian Cao Gen (Radix Rubiae)
Di Yu (Radix Sanguisorbae)
Sheng Di (uncooked Radix Rehmanniae)
Dang Gui (Radix Angelicae Sinensis)
Zhi Zi (Fructus Gardeniae)
Huang Qin (Radix Scutellariae)
Huang Lian (Rhizoma Coptidis)
Shui Niu Jiao (Cornu Bubali)

Qian Gen Tang Jia Jian (Rubia Decoction with Additions & Subtractions)
Qian Cao Gen (Radix Rubiae)
Di Yu (Radix Sanguisorbae)
Sheng Di (uncooked Radix Rehmanniae)
Dang Gui (Radix Angelicae Sinensis)
Zhi Zi (Fructus Gardeniae)

Huang Qin (Radix Scutellariae)
Huang Lian (Rhizoma Coptidis)
Bai Mao Gen (Rhizoma Imperatae)

6. Colic

Colic may occur anywhere from a few days to a few weeks after birth, and it may last from a couple of weeks to several months. Colic refers to gas pains in infants. The parent knows the baby is having such gas pains because the child cries and characteristically pumps their legs against their abdomen. The baby will want to be carried, held, and moved about. If and when the child passes gas, their crying diminishes or disappears. Usually the crying begins in the late afternoon or early evening and then may continue on through much of the night. In Chinese medicine, colic is traditionally described under the heading, night-crying. As the *Er Ke Zheng Zhi Xin Fa (Heart Methods of Proven Treatments in Pediatrics)* says:

> This disease mainly appears in newborns. During the day they are normal, but as they enter the night there is crying and restlessness. Each evening at the same time there is crying. If severe, this may continue throughout the night until dawn. Thus it is called night-crying.

This is a pretty good description of the timing and main symptoms of colic in young infants.

Colic can be very upsetting for the parents. Their baby is crying for some vague, undetermined reason. It is clear the baby is in pain, but the parent may not know why. Because the baby is crying and refuses to be put down or left alone, one or both parents may become exasperated and lose precious sleep. After a few nights of this, tempers can get short followed by guilty self-recriminations. In an attempt to pacify the baby, many parents try to assuage their child's crying by giving the baby the breast or a bottle. Unfortunately, this usually only makes the colic worse.

As with so many other pediatric complaints among infants and toddlers, colic is essentially a digestive complaint. In fact, it is *indigestion*. If, due to their inherently weak spleen or digestive power, the baby is not able to digest the milk or food that they are given, this accumulates and causes stagnation of the qi in the abdomen. Thus the abdomen becomes distended and the intestines become full of gas. This depressive qi may then manifest as liver signs and symptoms as well as spleen and stomach symptoms and/or may transform into heat. In that case, heat may then counterflow upward disturbing the heart spirit.

Prevention

There are three main ways to prevent colic according to Chinese medicine. The first and most important is to not overfeed the infant. Above we have discussed feeding on demand and the creation of food stagnation. Overfeeding jams the digestive mechanisms and leads to the accumulation of turbid qi and matter within the stomach and intestines. Therefore, feeding on schedule so as not to overstuff the infant's digestion and thus damage their already weak spleen, is the first and most important thing in preventing and treating colic. The fact that feeding should be on schedule and not on demand, according to Chinese medicine, is clearly and unambiguously stated in the following quote from *The English-Chinese Encyclopedia of Practical Traditional Chinese Medicine: Paediatrics* when speaking about the prevention of infantile dyspepsia or indigestion, *i.e.*, colic, "Regular diet [at fixed time and in fixed amount] and breast-feeding should be encouraged."

Secondly, one should rub the infant's abdomen daily. Rubbing the abdomen from right to left following the direction of the large intestine helps to move the food through the digestive tract. This can be done preventively each day but may also be done remedially when and if colic occurs. When treating colic, that there is food stagnation is a given. However, in deciding what direction to rub the small circles, one needs to determine if the child is hot or cold. (See the symptoms of hot and cold colic below.) If the child suffers from hot colic, then the small circles should be in the same direction as the large circles on the abdomen. If the child suffers from cold colic, meaning that their spleen is relatively weaker and needs strengthening beyond just moving stagnant food, then the small circles should go against the direction of the large circles. (For other infant massage techniques to treat this condition, see Fan Ya-li's *Chinese Pediatric Massage Therapy*.)

Third, the mother should avoid certain foods which tend to be gas-producing and colic-aggravating. Foods which the mother should avoid if her child has colic include the cabbage family (cabbage, broccoli, cauliflower, brussel sprouts, etc.), tomatoes, citrus fruits, garlic and onions, chocolate, and coffee. *The Merck Manual* fleshes out this list a bit by adding legumes, *i.e.*, beans, and rhubarb, peaches, and melons.

Treatment based on pattern discrimination:

1. Hot colic (a.k.a. heart channel accumulation & heat or heart/spleen accumulation & heat)

Main symptoms: A red face when crying, hands and feet warm or hot to the touch, a loud, energetic cry, abdominal distention, vexation and agitation, pumping of the legs to the abdomen

Treatment principles: Disperse accumulation and clear heat

Guiding formulas:
Bao He Wan (Protect Harmony Pills)
    Shan Zha (Fructus Crataegi)
    Shen Qu (Massa Medica Fermentata)

Lai Fu Zi (Semen Raphani)
Chen Pi (Pericarpium Citri Reticulatae)
Ban Xia (Rhizoma Pinelliae)
Fu Ling (Poria)
Lian Qiao (Fructus Forsythiae)

To increase the effectiveness of this formula, *Mai Ya* (Fructus Germinatus Hordei) is often added to this formula.

Dao Chi San Jia Jian (Abduct the Red Powder with Additions & Subtractions)
Sheng Di (uncooked Radix Rehmanniae)
Mu Tong (Caulis Akebiae)
Dan Zhu Ye (Herba Lophateri)
Gan Cao Shao (tips of Radix Glycyrrhizae)
Shen Qu (Massa Medica Fermentata)
Shan Zha (Fructus Crataegi)
Mai Ya (Fructus Germinatus Hordei)

2. Cold colic (a.k.a. spleen viscus vacuity cold)

Main symptoms: A pale facial complexion, a blue vein at the bridge of the nose, cold hands and feet, lassitude of the spirit, a forceless cry, possible vomiting of milk after eating, possible loose stools, torpid intake

Treatment principles: Disperse accumulation and fortify the spleen

Guiding formulas:
Xiao Jian Zhong Tang (Minor Fortify the Center Decoction) plus Li Zhong Tang (Rectify the Center Decoction)
Yi Tang (Maltose)
Ren Shen (Radix Ginseng)
Bai Zhu (Rhizoma Atractylodis Macrocephalae)
Gui Zhi (Ramulus Cinnamomi)
Bai Shao (Radix Paeoniae Albae)
mix-fried *Gan Cao* (Radix Glycyrrhizae)
Gan Jiang (dry Rhizoma Zingiberis)
Da Zao (Fructus Jujubae)

Jian Pi Wan Jia Jian (Fortify the Spleen Pills with Additions & Subtractions)
Shan Zha (Fructus Crataegi)
Lai Fu Zi (Semen Raphani)
Hou Po (Cortex Magnoliae)
Mai Ya (Fructus Germinatus Hordei)

Dang Shen (Radix Codonopsitis)
Bai Zhu (Rhizoma Atractylodis Macrocephalae)
Chen Pi (Pericarpium Citri Reticulatae)

Wu Yao San (Lindera Powder)
Wu Yao (Radix Linderae)
Bai Shao (Radix Paeoniae Albae)
Xiang Fu (Rhizoma Cyperi)
Gao Liang Jiang (Rhizoma Alpiniae Officinari)

If there are loose stools due to spleen vacuity, add *Dang Shen* (Radix Codonopsitis), *Bai Zhu* (Rhizoma Atractylodis Macrocephalae), and *Fu Ling* (Poria).

If the colicky baby shows signs of neither hot nor cold, then the practitioner will simply disperse accumulation and harmonize the stomach. For instance, a formula called **Xiao Ru Wan (Disperse Milk Pills)** is often used for just food stagnation without hot or cold:
Shen Qu (Massa Medica Fermentata)
Mai Ya (Fructus Germinatus Hordei)
Sha Ren (Fructus Amomi)
Xiang Fu (Rhizoma Cyperi)
Chen Pi (Pericarpium Citri Reticulatae)

3. Contraction of fear & fright (a.k.a. liver depression with counterflowing upward and harassing of the heart spirit)

Main symptoms: Essence spirit disquietude, *i.e.*, emotional restlessness, night-crying, frightened looking eyes when crying, loose stools which are greenish in color and may smell like rotten eggs, either a red or a greyish, greenish facial complexion

> **Note:** This pattern is also actually a hot pattern of colic involving stagnant food, liver depression transforming heat, and heat then harassing the heart spirit above. The difference between it and hot colic above are the signs of fear and fright associated with the liver/gallbladder. Therefore, this pattern is also sometimes called heart vacuity, timorous gallbladder.

Treatment principles: Settle fright and quiet the spirit, clear heat and disperse accumulation

Guiding formulas:
Zhu Sha An Shen Wan Jia Wei (Cinnabar Quiet the Heart Pills with Added Flavors)
Zhu Sha (Cinnabar)
Huang Lian (Rhizoma Coptidis)
Dang Gui (Radix Angelicae Sinensis)
Sheng Di (uncooked Radix Rehmanniae)

mix-fried *Gan Cao* (Radix Glycyrrhizae)
Shen Qu (Massa Medica Fermentata)
Mai Ya (Fructus Germinatus Hordei)

If there is pronounced abdominal distention with crying diminishing rapidly after passing gas or having a bowel movement, then one can use **Mu Xiang Bing Lang Wan (Auklandia & Betel Nut Pills)**:

Mu Xiang (Radix Auklandiae)
Bing Lang (Semen Arecae)
Chen Pi (Pericarpium Citri Reticulatae)
Lian Qiao (Fructus Forsythiae)
Shan Zha (Fructus Crataegi)
Da Huang (Radix Et Rhizoma Rhei)

Acupuncture & moxibustion

For spleen vacuity with food stagnation, one can also moxa *Shen Que* (CV 8). Needling the *Si Feng* (M-UE-9) every other day is also effective for transforming food and dispersing accumulation.

Adjunctive treatments

For colic due to food stagnation, wrap 60-90g of *Mang Xiao* (Natri Sulfas) in a cotton bag. Place this over the navel and tie in place. If there is food stagnation and heat, one can make a tea out of parsley, hawthorne berries, *i.e.*, *Shan Zha* (Fructus Crataegi), *daikon* radish, and orange peel, *i.e.*, *Chen Pi* (Pericarpium Citri Reticulatae). If there is colic due to food stagnation and internal cold due to spleen vacuity, then one can take 3 scallion stalks, 5 slices of fresh ginger, and 60-90g of wheat bran. Heat these together in a dry wok or fry pan and then wrap them in cotton cloth. While this bundle of herbs is still warm, "iron" around the abdomen with it.

Comments

In my experience, most Western babies with colic have food stagnation and heat. However, it is also often common to see food stagnation, heat, and spleen weakness. In that case, the practitioner will have to craft a prescription which fits this slightly more complex pattern. *The Merck Manual* says that, "Parents should be assured that the colicky infant is basically healthy, that this behavior will cease in a few weeks, and that too much crying is not harmful." On the one hand that is good advice. On the other, Chinese medicine sees colic as one of the first steps in a potential series of health problems which can affect the constitutional balance and predispositions for one's entire life. If colic is treated at its root by using Chinese medicine both preventively and remedially, this can help prevent other health problems from occurring later on which also develop out of food stagnation and a weak spleen engendering dampness, phlegm, and pathological heat.

7. Vomiting of Milk

Vomiting of milk refers to the baby's spitting up some milk after or during each feeding. According to Chinese medicine, this is also associated with the infant's inherently weak spleen and stomach. Just as colic is divided into several different patterns, vomiting in Chinese pediatrics can be subdivided into food stagnation, spleen vacuity cold, spleen and stomach brewing of heat, liver invading the stomach, stomach yin vacuity, and fright and fear patterns. These patterns do not all appear in children of the same age. In infants, the two most commonly seen patterns are food stagnation and spleen deficiency cold types, and these two types are usually quite easy to distinguish. In toddlers and older children, eating solid foods, and especially too much greasy, fatty, spicy, hot foods, stomach heat vomiting is frequently seen. Stomach yin vacuity vomiting is due to recurrent and enduring vomiting exhausting and consuming stomach yin fluids. Liver attacking the stomach is seen in high-strung, highly emotional children. It can occur in very young children and infants and often accompanies infantile convulsions due to startling and fright.

Treatment based on pattern discrimination:

1. Food stagnation (a.k.a. food damage)

Main symptoms: Sour, smelly vomitus comprised of curdled milk which has lain in the child's stomach undigested, acid eructation, no thought for food or drink, possible colic and intestinal gas, abdominal distention and fullness, constipation or diarrhea which is sour or foul-smelling, possible bad breath, thick, slimy tongue fur

> **Note:** It is interesting to note that even the Western medical treatment handbook, *The Merck Manual*, says, "Excessive regurgitation may be due to overfeeding."

Treatment principles: Disperse food and transform stagnation, rectify the qi and downbear counterflow

Guiding formulas:
Bao He Wan Jia Jian (Protect Harmony Pills with Additions & Subtractions)

Shan Zha (Fructus Crataegi)
Bing Lang (Semen Arecae)
Zhi Shi (Fructus Immaturus Aurantii)
ginger-processed *Ban Xia* (Rhizoma Pinelliae)
Chen Pi (Pericarpium Citri Reticulatae)
Lai Fu Zi (Semen Raphani)
Lian Qiao (Fructus Forsythiae)
Mai Ya (Fructus Germinatus Hordei)
Gu Ya (Fructus Germinatus Oryzae)

If there is vexation and agitation with oral thirst, add *Huang Lian* (Rhizoma Coptidis) or *Hu Huang Lian* (Rhizoma Picrorhizae) and *Ye Jiao Teng* (Caulis Polygoni Multiflori). If there is constipation, add *Da Huang* (Radix Et Rhizoma Rhei) and *Mang Xiao* (Natri Sulfas). If there is abdominal distention and pain, add *Mu Xiang* (Radix Auklandiae) and *Qing Pi* (Pericarpium Citri Reticulatae Viride). If urination is reduced, add *Fu Ling Pi* (Cortex Sclerotii Poriae).

Xiao Ru Tang (Disperse Milk Decoction)
Xiang Fu (Rhizoma Cyperi)
Shen Qu (Massa Medica Fermentata)
Mai Ya (Fructus Germinatus Hordei)
Chen Pi (Pericarpium Citri Reticulatae)
Sha Ren (Fructus Amomi)
mix-fried *Gan Cao* (Radix Glycyrrhizae)
Sheng Jiang (uncooked Rhizoma Zingiberis)

If there is constipation, add *Zhi Shi* (Fructus Immaturus Aurantii) and *Da Huang* (Radix Et Rhizoma Rhei).

2. Spleen vacuity cold (a.k.a. stomach cold)

Main symptoms: Vomiting back up the milk which has just been ingested, this vomitus looking just like the milk and not having any bad smell, slow or insidious arising of this disease, relatively prolonged course. The hands and feet are usually cold, the facial complexion is a somber white, and there is typically a visible blue vein at the bridge of the nose. Other symptoms include lassitude of the essence spirit, lack of warmth in the four limbs, abdominal pain desiring pressure and warmth, loose stools, long, clear urination, a pale tongue with white fur, and a deep, fine, not very forceful pulse. In addition, the vomiting is without force. The food wells back up but is not forcefully spit out.

> **Note:** This last sign shows that the baby's spleen is too weak and cold to accept and digest the milk or other food.

Treatment principles: Warm the center and scatter cold, fortify the spleen and harmonize the stomach

Guiding formulas:
Shen Xiang Tang (Ginseng & Aquilaria Decoction)
Ren Shen (Radix Ginseng)
Chen Xiang (Lignum Aquilariae)
Ding Xiang (Flos Caryophylli)
Mu Xiang (Radix Auklandiae)
Huo Xiang Gen (Caulis Pogostemonis)
Mu Gua (Fructus Chaenomelis)

Ding Chen Si Jun Zi Tang (Cloves & Aquilaria Four Gentlemen Decoction)
    Ren Shen (Radix Ginseng)
    Bai Zhu (Rhizoma Atractylodis Macrocephalae)
    Fu Ling (Poria)
    mix-fried *Gan Cao* (Radix Glycyrrhizae)
    Ding Xiang (Flos Caryophylli)
    Chen Xiang (Lignum Aquilariae)

Ding Yu Li Zhong Tang Jia Wei (Cloves & Evodia Rectify the Center Decoction with Added Flavors)
    Ding Xiang (Flos Caryophylli)
    Wu Zhu Yu (Fructus Evodiae)
    Tai Zi Shen (Radix Pseudostellariae)
    Bai Zhu (Rhizoma Atractylodis Macrocephalae)
    Gan Jiang (dry Rhizoma Zingiberis)
    Mu Xiang (Radix Auklandiae)
    Sha Ren (Fructus Amomi)
    ginger-processed *Ban Xia* (Rhizoma Pinelliae)
    Chen Pi (Pericarpium Citri Reticulatae)

If there is vomiting of clear water, insidious abdominal pain, and lack of warmth in the four limbs, add *Gui Xin* (Cortex Cinnamomi) and *Fu Zi* (Radix Lateralis Praeparatus Aconiti Carmichaeli).

Li Zhong Tang Jia Jian (Rectify the Center Decoction with Additions & Subtractions)
    Dang Shen (Radix Codonopsitis)
    Bai Zhu (Rhizoma Atractylodis Macrocephalae)
    Gan Jiang (dry Rhizoma Zingiberis)
    Sha Ren (Fructus Amomi)
    Shen Qu (Massa Medica Fermentata)
    ginger-processed *Ban Xia* (Rhizoma Pinelliae)

If the vomiting still will not stop, add *Wu Zhu Yu* (Fructus Evodiae) and *Gao Liang Jiang* (Rhizoma Alpiniae Officinari).

3. Spleen & stomach brewing heat (a.k.a. stomach heat)

Main symptoms: Vomiting of food upon eating, sour, foul-smelling vomitus, possible projectile vomiting, possible generalized fever or bodily heat, vexation and agitation, oral thirst, desire to drink, foul-smelling stools or constipation, yellowish red urination, dry, red lips, yellow tongue fur, a slippery, rapid pulse

Treatment principles: Clear heat and harmonize the stomach, downbear counterflow and stop vomiting

Guiding formulas:
Huo Po Huang Lian Tang Jia Jian (Pogosternon & Magnolia Coptis Decoction with Additions & Subtractions)
Huang Lian (Rhizoma Coptidis)
Huo Xiang (Herba Pogostemonis)
Hou Po (Cortex Magnoliae)
Zhu Ru (Caulis Bambusae In Teaniis)
Sheng Jiang (uncooked Rhizoma Zingiberis)
ginger-processed *Ban Xia* (Rhizoma Pinelliae)

If there is concomitant constipation, add *Da Huang* (Radix Et Rhizoma Rhei).

Da Huang Gan Cao Tang (Rhubarb & Licorice Decoction)
Da Huang (Radix Et Rhizoma Rhei)
Gan Cao (Radix Glycyrrhizae)

If there is incessant vomiting, add *Dai Zhe Shi* (Haematitum). If oral thirst is severe, add *Tian Hua Fen* (Radix Trichosanthis).

Jia Wei Wen Dan Tang (Added Flavors Warm the Gallbladder Decoction)
Chen Pi (Pericarpium Citri Reticulatae)
Fu Ling (Poria)
ginger-processed *Ban Xia* (Rhizoma Pinelliae)
Zhi Shi (Fructus Immaturus Aurantii)
Zhu Ru (Caulis Bambusae In Taeniis)
Huang Lian (Rhizoma Coptidis)
Deng Xin Cao (Medulla Junci)

Huo Lian Tang (Pogosternon & Coptis Decoction)
Huang Lian (Rhizoma Coptidis)
Huo Xiang (Herba Pogostemonis)
Hou Po (Cortex Magnoliae)
ginger-processed *Ban Xia* (Rhizoma Pinelliae)
Dai Zhe Shi (Haemititum)
Zhu Ru (Caulis Bambusae In Taeniis)

4. Stomach yin vacuity (a.k.a. vacuity fire)

Main symptoms: If enduring, recurrent vomiting has damaged stomach yin which has become vacuous and insufficient, then there will be no desire for food or drink, nausea upon eating, vomiting of clear drool, a dry, parched mouth and throat, dry, constipated stools, red cheeks, heat in the hands, feet, and heart or tidal fever in the afternoon each day, red lips, a scarlet red tongue, if severe, peeled fur, and a fine, rapid pulse

Treatment principles: Enrich and nourish stomach yin

Guiding formulas:
Sha Shen Mai Dong Tang Jia Jian (Glehnia & Ophiopogon Decoction with Additions & Subtractions)
Bei Sha Shen (Radix Glehniae)
Mai Men Dong (Tuber Ophiopogonis)
Tian Hua Fen (Radix Trichosanthis)
Sang Ye (Folium Mori)
Yu Zhu (Rhizoma Polygonati Odorati)
Shi Hu (Herba Dendrobii)
Zhu Ru (Caulis Bambusae In Taeniis)
Sheng Gan Cao (uncooked Radix Glycyrrhizae)

If the vomiting still does not stop, add *Chen Xiang* (Lignum Aquilariae).

Sha Shen Mai Dong Tang Jia Jian (Glehnia & Ophiopogon Decoction with Additions & Subtractions)
Bei Sha Shen (Radix Glehniae)
Yu Zhu (Rhizoma Polygonati Odorati)
Tian Men Dong (Tuber Asparagi)
Mai Men Dong (Tuber Ophiopogonis)
Shi Hu (Herba Dendrobii)
Zhu Ru (Caulis Bambusae In Taeniis)
Bai Bian Dou (Semen Dolichoris)
Gan Cao (Radix Glycyrrhizae)

If there is fever, add *Qing Hao* (Herba Artemisiae Annuae) and *Bai Wei* (Radix Cynanchi Atrati). If there is constipation, add *Yi Li Ren* (Semen Pruni) and *Huo Ma Ren* (Semen Cannabis).

Ju Pi Zhu Ru Tang Jia Wei (Orange Peel & Caulis Bambusae Decoction with Added Flavors)
Chen Pi (Pericarpium Citri Reticulatae)
Zhu Ru (Caulis Bambusae In Taeniis)
Ren Shen (Radix Ginseng)
Sheng Jiang (uncooked Rhizoma Zingiberis)
Gan Cao (Radix Glycyrrhizae)
Da Zao (Fructus Jujubae)
Shi Hu (Herba Dendrobii)
Tian Hua Fen (Radix Trichosanthis)

Zhi Mu (Rhizoma Anemarrhenae)

5. Liver qi attacking the stomach (a.k.a. fear & fright vomiting)

Main symptoms: Vomiting of sour water, burping and belching, chest and lateral costal distention and pain, essence spirit depression and oppression, easy anger, excessive crying, restless sleep, sudden jerking movements while asleep, a red tongue with thin, slimy fur, and a wiry pulse

Treatment principles: Course the liver and rectify the qi, harmonize the stomach and stop vomiting

Guiding formulas:
Jie Gan Jian (Resolve the Liver Decoction)
Bai Shao (Radix Paeoniae Albae)
Zi Su Ye (Folium Perillae)
Sha Ren (Fructus Amomi)
Hou Po (Cortex Magnoliae)
Chen Pi (Pericarpium Citri Reticulatae)
ginger-processed *Ban Xia* (Rhizoma Pinelliae)

If there is vexation and agitation and a red tongue with yellow fur, add *Huang Lian* (Rhizoma Coptidis) and *Wu Zhu Yu* (Fructus Evodiae).

Si Qi Tang (Four [To] Seven Decoction) plus Zuo Jin Wan (Restore the [Left] Pills)
Ban Xia (Rhizoma Pinelliae)
Fu Ling (Poria)
processed *Hou Po* (Cortex Magnoliae)
Zi Su Ye (Folium Perillae)
Huang Lian (Rhizoma Coptidis)
Wu Zhu Yu (Fructus Evodiae)

Ding Tu Wan (Calm Vomiting Pills)
Quan Xie (Scorpio)
Ding Xiang (Flos Caryophylli)
ginger-processed *Ban Xia* (Rhizoma Pinelliae)

If there is dizziness and vertigo, add *Ju Hua* (Flos Chrysanthemi) and *Tian Ma* (Rhizoma Gastrodiae). If there is fright and restlessness, add *Ci Shi* (Magnetitum) and *Zhu Sha* (Cinnabar).

Acupuncture & moxibustion

The main points are *Nei Guan* (Per 6), *Zhong Wan* (CV 12), and *Zu San Li* (St 36). Add

Tai Chong (Liv 3) for the liver invading the stomach. Add *Nei Ting* (St 44) for food stagnation and/or stomach heat. Add *Yin Tang* (M-HN-3) for fear and fright.

Adjunctive treatments

One simple home remedy for treating food stagnation vomiting is to make a tea out of 25g of grated fresh ginger and 50g of dried orange peel. This can then be given to the child through a bottle instead of or before breast-feeding. In the case of spleen vacuity cold, it is especially important to feed the child small, frequent, easily digestible foods. Here one should remember the concept of 100 degree soup. The spleen deficient child should not be given anything dry and hard to digest, nor should they be given anything chilled or raw. All their food should be cooked and served warm. As for spices, a little dry ginger powder, some cardamon powder, or a little cinnamon powder can help strengthen the spleen and warm deficiency cold. A simple home remedy for this type of vomiting is to make a tea out of 5 black dates and a few whole cloves. Crush the cloves and boil with the dates in water.

Spleen and stomach brewing heat vomiting is more commonly met with in a somewhat older toddler or young child. Usually these children have begun eating solid foods and have developed a taste for greasy foods, such as chips, peanut butter, hot dogs and hamburgers, etc. Such greasy, fried, fatty foods are, according to Chinese dietary therapy, inherently hot but also hard to digest. If the child eats too much of this sort of food, it may sit in the stomach and smolder and brew into a type of damp heat. Spleen and stomach brewing heat should first be treated by identifying the offending foods. These then should be removed from the child's diet. In my experience, children with this pattern also eat a lot of sugar which, according to Chinese medicine, is also very dampening. Once the offending foods have been removed, it is wise to feed the child what the Chinese call a clear, bland diet for several days. This means a vegetarian diet consisting of rice porridge and steamed and mashed vegetables without any fat or grease or hot spices. A simple home remedy is to make a "tea" out of a little umeboshi paste, grated ginger, and some kudzu root powder (also available at health food stores).

Stomach yin deficiency vomiting describes a child who has vomited so much or for so long that they have developed dry heaves. Therefore, this pattern typically describes a chronic condition, not an episodic or acute one. Cooked applesauce or cooked mashed pears can be useful foods to help the child recuperate from this pattern.

Comments

It is especially important in the case of vomiting to administer Chinese medicinal decoctions in very small, repeated doses or the decoctions themselves may provoke vomiting. In this case, administering the decoction by eyedropper is extremely effective and appropriate.

If there is repeated projectile vomiting, meaning that the vomit launches out of the child's mouth with great force and carries for some distance, this may signal a more serious condition, such as pyloric stenosis or gastroesophageal reflux. I have treated several cases of projectile vomiting in toddlers whose pattern was damp heat brewing in the spleen and stomach due to eating too many greasy, fatty foods. However, if dietary changes and some Chinese herbal medicine do not bring projectile vomiting quickly to an end, the child should be taken to see a Western MD.

8. Diarrhea

Diarrhea in infants and children is a commonly seen complaint. Often in the West, however, it is not the major presenting complaint but is rather a concomitant complaint or symptom. Because diarrhea is evidence that food and liquids are not being transformed and transported correctly, it is important to treat diarrhea even if it is only persistent loose stools which neither the parent or child are particularly concerned about. Long-term diarrhea or loose stools, according to Chinese medical theory, must result in eventual diminished qi and blood. Pediatric diarrhea is commonly divided into six main patterns.

Treatment based on pattern discrimination:

1. Food stagnation (a.k.a. food damage)

Main symptoms: Abdominal pain and distention, pain relieved by diarrhea, sour, foul-smelling stools, bad breath, acid eructation, possible desire to vomit, no thought for food or milk, restless sleep, possible night-crying, thick, slimy or slightly yellow tongue fur, a slippery pulse or a purplish, engorged vein at the wind bar

Treatment principles: Disperse food, abduct stagnation, and stop diarrhea

Guiding formulas:
Bao He Wan (Protect Harmony Pills)
Shan Zha (Fructus Crataegi)
Shen Qu (Massa Medica Fermentata)
Mai Ya (Fructus Germinatus Hordei)
Fu Ling (Poria)
Ban Xia (Rhizoma Pinelliae)
Chen Pi (Pericarpium Citri Reticulatae)
Lian Qiao (Fructus Forsythiae)

Bao He Wan Jia Jian (Protect Harmony Pills with Additions & Subtractions)
Shan Zha (Fructus Crataegi)
Shen Qu (Massa Medica Fermentata)
Ban Xia (Rhizoma Pinelliae)
Fu Ling (Poria)
Lai Fu Zi (Semen Raphani)

Zhi Shi (Fructus Immaturus Aurantii)
Chen Pi (Pericarpium Citri Reticulatae)

If there is abdominal pain and distention, add *Mu Xiang* (Radix Auklandiae) and *Hou Po* (Cortex Magnoliae).

Xiao Ru Wan (Disperse Milk Decoction)
Xiang Fu (Rhizoma Cyperi)
Shen Qu (Massa Medica Fermentata)
Mai Ya (Fructus Germinatus Hordei)
Chen Pi (Pericarpium Citri Reticulatae)
Sha Ren (Fructus Amomi)
mix-fried *Gan Cao* (Radix Glycyrrhizae)
Sheng Jiang (uncooked Rhizoma Zingiberis)

Shang Shi Fu Tong Zhi Xie Tang (Food Damage Abdominal Pain, Stop Diarrhea Decoction)
Cang Zhu (Rhizoma Atractylodis)
Huo Xiang (Herba Pogostemonis)
Chen Pi (Pericarpium Citri Reticulatae)
Hou Po (Cortex Magnoliae)
Fu Ling (Poria)
Sha Ren (Fructus Amomi)
Gan Cao (Radix Glycyrrhizae)
wine-processed *Da Huang* (Radix Et Rhizoma Rhei)

Administer 2 packets of this decoction. If the diarrhea is not markedly better, add *Ren Shen* (Radix Ginseng).

Xiao Shi Hua Ji Yin (Disperse Food & Transform Accumulation Beverage)
uncooked *Shan Zha* (Fructus Crataegi)
Shen Qu (Massa Medica Fermentata)
Mai Ya (Fructus Germinatus Hordei)
Ji Nei Jin (Endothelium Corneum Gigeriae Galli)
Mu Xiang (Radix Auklandiae)
Sha Ren (Fructus Amomi)
Long Dan Cao (Radix Gentianae)
Gan Cao (Radix Glycyrrhizae)

If milk or meat has been excessive, double the amount of *Shan Zha*. If cereal foods have been excessive, double the amount of *Mai Ya*. If greasy, fatty foods have been excessive, double the amount of *Shen Qu*. If there is nausea and vomiting, add ginger-processed *Ban Xia* (Rhizoma Pinelliae) and *Chen Pi* (Pericarpium Citri Reticulatae). If abdominal pain is relatively pronounced, add *Yan Hu Suo* (Rhizoma Corydalis) and *Xi Xin* (Herba Asari).

2. Wind cold

Main symptoms: A somber white facial complexion, lassitude of the spirit, chilled limbs, abdominal pain, intestinal noises, clear, watery stools with no foul odor, possible aversion to cold with fever, thin, white or white, slimy tongue fur, a soggy, fine pulse

Treatment principles: Course wind, scatter cold, and stop diarrhea

Guiding formulas:
Huo Xiang Zheng Qi San Jia Jian (Pogosternon Correct the Qi Powder with Additions & Subtractions)
Huo Xiang (Herba Pogostemonis)
Zi Su Ye (Folium Perillae)
Ban Xia (Rhizoma Pinelliae)
Fu Ling (Poria)
Bai Zhu (Rhizoma Atractylodis Macrocephalae)
Chen Pi (Pericarpium Citri Reticulatae)
Pao Jiang (blast-fried Rhizoma Zingiberis)

If abdominal pain is relatively severe, add *Mu Xiang* (Radix Auklandiae) and *Sha Ren* (Fructus Amomi).

He Qi Yin (Harmonize the Qi Beverage)
Cang Zhu (Rhizoma Atractylodis)
Fu Ling (Poria)
Hou Po (Cortex Magnoliae)
Chen Pi (Pericarpium Citri Reticulatae)
Pao Jiang (blast-fried Rhizoma Zingiberis)
Zi Su Ye (Folium Perillae)
Fang Feng (Radix Saposhnikoviae)
Gan Cao (Radix Glycyrrhizae)

If there is serious watery diarrhea with reduced urination, add *Ze Xie* (Rhizoma Alismatis) and *Zhu Ling* (Polyporus). If there is a concomitant common cold or rhinitis with clear nasal discharge, add *Qiang Huo* (Radix Et Rhizoma Notopterygii) and *Xi Xin* (Herba Asari).

Wei Ling Tang (Stomach Poria Decoction)
Cang Zhu (Rhizoma Atractylodis)
Hou Po (Cortex Magnoliae)
Chen Pi (Pericarpium Citri Reticulatae)
Gan Cao (Radix Glycyrrhizae)
Bai Zhu (Rhizoma Atractylodis Macrocephalae)
Gui Zhi (Ramulus Cinnamomi)
Zhu Ling (Polyporus)
Ze Xie (Rhizoma Alismatis)

Sheng Jiang (uncooked Rhizoma Zingiberis)
Da Zao (Fructus Jujubae)

If there is marked nasal obstruction, add *Fang Feng* (Radix Saposhnikoviae), *Jing Jie* (Herba Schizonepetae), and *Zi Su Ye* (Folium Perillae).

Cang Ling Tang (Atractylodis & Poria Decoction)
Cang Zhu (Rhizoma Atractylodis)
Gan Jiang (dry Rhizoma Zingiberis)
Hou Po (Cortex Magnoliae)
Chen Pi (Pericarpium Citri Reticulatae)
Gan Cao (Radix Glycyrrhizae)
Fu Ling (Poria)
Huo Xiang (Herba Pogostemonis)
Mu Xiang (Radix Auklandiae)
Sha Ren (Fructus Amomi)
Che Qian Zi (Semen Plantaginis)

3. Damp heat (a.k.a. summerheat abdominal diarrhea)

Main symptoms: Watery, thin stools colored deep yellow with a foul odor, possible explosive discharge, redness and burning around the anus, occasional abdominal pain, devitalized desire for food, possible nausea, fever or no fever, oral thirst, short, yellow urine, bodily fatigue, slimy, yellow tongue fur, a slippery, rapid pulse

Treatment principles: Clear heat, disinhibit dampness, and stop diarrhea

Guiding formulas:
Ge Gen Qin Lian Tang Jia Wei (Pueraria, Scutellaria & Coptis Decoction with Added Flavors)
Ge Gen (Radix Puerariae)
Huang Qin (Radix Scutellariae)
Huang Lian (Rhizoma Coptidis)
Jin Yin Hua (Flos Lonicerae)
Hua Shi (Talcum)
Gan Cao (Radix Glycyrrhizae)
Che Qian Zi (Semen Plantaginis)
fresh *He Ye* (Folium Nelumbinis)

If dampness is more pronounced than heat, add *Fu Ling* (Poria), *Ze Xie* (Rhizoma Alismatis), and *Yi Yi Ren* (Semen Coicis).

Ge Gen Qin Lian Tang Jia Wei (Pueraria, Scutellaria & Coptis Decoction with Added Flavors)
Ge Gen (Radix Puerariae)

Huang Qin (Radix Scutellariae)
Huang Lian (Rhizoma Coptidis)
Gan Cao (Radix Glycyrrhizae)
Chen Pi (Pericarpium Citri Reticulatae)
Hou Po (Cortex Magnoliae)
Fu Ling (Poria)
Mu Xiang (Radix Auklandiae)
Sha Ren (Fructus Amomi)
Huo Xiang (Herba Pogostemonis)
Che Qian Zi (Semen Plantaginis)

Ge Gen Qin Lian Tang Jia Jian (Pueraria, Scutellaria & Coptis Decoction with Additions & Subtractions)
Ge Gen (Radix Puerariae)
Huang Qin (Radix Scutellariae)
Jin Yin Hua (Flos Lonicerae)
Huang Lian (Rhizoma Coptidis)
Che Qian Zi (Semen Plantaginis)

Qing Re Li Shi Tang (Clear Heat & Disinhibit Dampness Decoction)
Jin Yin Hua (Flos Lonicerae)
Qin Pi (Cortex Fraxini)
Bai Bu (Radix Stemonae)
Shan Zha (Fructus Crataegi)
Bai Zhu (Rhizoma Atractylodis Macrocephalae)
Fu Ling (Poria)
Che Qian Zi (Semen Plantaginis)
Ai Ye (Folium Artemisiae Argyii)
Gan Cao (Radix Glycyrrhizae)

4. Spleen vacuity

Main symptoms: Enduring diarrhea which does not heal, loose stools, undigested water and grains, diarrhea after eating, light colored stools with no foul odor, a sallow yellow facial complexion, emaciated, thin muscles and flesh, lassitude of the spirit, listlessness, a pale tongue with white fur, a soft, forceless pulse or a prominent blue vein at the root of the nose

Treatment principles: Fortify the spleen, warm the center, and stop diarrhea

Guiding formulas:
Qi Wei Bai Zhu San Jia Wei (Seven Flavors Atractylodes Powder with Added Flavors)
Dang Shen (Radix Codonopsitis)
Bai Zhu (Rhizoma Atractylodis Macrocephalae)

Fu Ling (Poria)
Ge Gen (Radix Puerariae)
Huo Xiang (Herba Pogostemonis)
Bai Bian Dou (Semen Dolichoris)
Mu Xiang (Radix Auklandiae)
Gan Cao (Radix Glycyrrhizae)
Pao Jiang (blast-fried Rhizoma Zingiberis)

Shen Ling Bai Zhu San (Ginseng, Poria & Atractylodes Powder)
Ren Shen (Radix Ginseng)
Bai Zhu (Rhizoma Atractylodis Macrocephalae)
Fu Ling (Poria)
Gan Cao (Radix Glycyrrhizae)
Yi Yi Ren (Semen Coicis)
Jie Geng (Radix Platycodi)
Shan Yao (Radix Dioscoreae)
Bai Bian Dou (Semen Dolichoris)
Sha Ren (Fructus Amomi)
Lian Zi Rou (Semen Nelumbinis)
Da Zao (Fructus Jujubae)

If there is abdominal pain, one can add *Gui Zhi* (Ramulus Cinnamomi) and *Sheng Jiang* (uncooked Rhizoma Zingiberis). If there is enduring, incessant diarrhea with no evidence of accumulation and fullness, one may add *He Zi* (Fructus Terminaliae) and *Chi Shi Zhi* (Hallyositum Rubrum).

If there is primarily spleen vacuity but slight heat, one can use **Shen Zhu Tang (Ginseng & Atractylodes Decoction)**:
Hong Shen (red Radix Ginseng)
earth stir-fried *Bai Zhu* (Rhizoma Atractylodis Macrocephalae)
Fu Ling (Poria)
Lian Zi Rou (Semen Nelumbinis)
Bai Bian Dou (Semen Dolichoris)
Sha Ren (Fructus Amomi)
Shan Yao (Radix Dioscoreae)
Da Zao (Fructus Jujubae)
Huang Lian (Rhizoma Coptidis)
Chen Pi (Pericarpium Citri Reticulatae)
Gan Cao (Radix Glycyrrhizae)

If there is primarily spleen vacuity but concomitant food stagnation, one can use **Yi Qi Bu Pi Tang (Boost the Qi & Supplement the Spleen Decoction)**:
Huang Qi (Radix Astragali)
Dang Shen (Radix Codonopsitis)
Bai Zhu (Rhizoma Atractylodis Macrocephalae)

Fu Ling (Poria)
Shan Yao (Radix Dioscoreae)
Shan Zha (Fructus Crataegi)
Shen Qu (Massa Medica Fermentata)
Mai Ya (Fructus Germinatus Hordei)
Ji Nei Jin (Endothelium Corneum Gigeriae Galli)
Che Qian Zi (Semen Plantaginis)
Gan Cao (Radix Glycyrrhizae)

If there is spleen vacuity combined with fright tremors and spasms, sudden crying while asleep, and greenish stools, one can use **Yi Pi Zhen Jing San (Boost the Spleen & Settle Fright Powder)**:

Dang Shen (Radix Codonopsitis)
Shan Yao (Radix Dioscoreae)
Fu Ling (Poria)
Gou Teng (Ramulus Uncariae Cum Uncis)
Zhu Sha (Cinnabar)
Gan Cao (Radix Glycyrrhizae)

5. Spleen-kidney yang vacuity

Main symptoms: Enduring diarrhea which will not stop, if severe, possible anal prolapse, diarrhea after eating, clear, watery stools, undigested food in the stools, a cold body and chilled limbs, a somber white facial complexion, lassitude of the essence spirit, a fat, pale tongue with thin, white fur, a fine, weak, or deep, weak pulse or a blue vein at the root of the nose

Treatment principles: Warm and supplement the spleen and kidneys, secure and astringe and stop diarrhea

Guiding formula:
Fu Zi Li Zhong Tang (Aconite Rectify the Center Decoction) plus *Si Shen Wan* (Four Spirits Pills) with additions and subtractions

Fu Zi (Radix Lateralis Praeparatus Aconiti Carmichaeli)
Pao Jiang (blast-fried Rhizoma Zingiberis)
Wu Wei Zi (Fructus Schisandrae)
Wu Mei (Fructus Mume)
Wu Zhu Yu (Fructus Evodiae)
Dang Shen (Radix Codonopsitis)
Bai Zhu (Rhizoma Atractylodis Macrocephalae)
Bu Gu Zhi (Fructus Psoraleae)
Rou Dou Kou (Semen Myristicae)
He Zi (Fructus Terminaliae)

If the defensive is insecure with unchecked perspiration, add *Long Gu* (Os Draconis), *Mu Li* (Concha Ostreae), and *Huang Qi* (Radix Astragali).

6. Damaged yin

Main symptoms: Enduring diarrhea which has damaged yin fluids, lassitude of the essence spirit, vexation and agitation, dry, parched skin, sunken eyes and fontanel, diarrhea of yellow water, short, scanty urination, dry mouth, red lips, a scarlet red tongue with no fluids, a minute, rapid pulse

Treatment principles: Clear heat, nourish yin, and stop diarrhea

Guiding formula:
Lian Mei Tang Jia Jian (Coptis & Mume Decoction with Additions & Subtractions)
Huang Lian (Rhizoma Coptidis)
Wu Mei (Fructus Mume)
Bai Ren Shen (white Radix Ginseng)
Shi Hu (Herba Dendrobii)
Bai Shao (Radix Paeoniae Albae)
Gan Cao (Radix Glycyrrhizae)

Acupuncture & moxibustion

The main points are *Zu San Li* (St 36) and *Tian Shu* (St 25). If there is food stagnation, add *Nei Ting* (St 44). If there is wind cold, add *He Gu* (LI 4). If there is damp heat, add *Yin Ling Quan* (Sp 9). If there is spleen and/or kidney vacuity, add moxibustion at *Shen Que* (CV 8). If there is vomiting, add *Nei Guan* (Per 6). If there are fright tremors or convulsions, add *Tai Chong* (Liv 3). If there is fever, add *Qu Chi* (LI 11). And if there is loss of securing and astringing, add *Chang Qiang* (GV 1).

Adjunctive treatments

In all patterns of pediatric diarrhea, diet is very important. If there is food stagnation, less food or milk should be given. If there is damp heat diarrhea, it is important to feed only a clear, bland diet. The clear, bland diet is also extremely important in the case of spleen qi and/or kidney yang vacuity. This means a diet of cooked, warm foods, no frozen, chilled, or iced foods or liquids, no or very few raw foods, a clear, bland diet, and little or no sugar. In addition, some warming, spleen-strengthening spices may be added to the food, such as cardamom, fennel, dry ginger powder, a little cinnamon, some cloves, and/or a little nutmeg. Practitioners of Chinese medicine may also recommend making a porridge out of any of several, very bland-tasting, spleen-strengthening Chinese herbs which can be ground into powder and cooked into a gruel. These include *Shan Yao* (Radix Dioscoreae), *Fu Ling* (Poria), *Yi Yi Ren* (Semen Coicis), and *Bai Bian Dou* (Semen Dolichoris). Spinal pinch-pull up the spine several times a day can strengthen the spleen and generally strengthen the qi. Another remedy for this type of diarrhea is to pound several cloves of garlic and wrap them in clean cotton gauze. Then tie this herbal compress directly over the navel. And yet another home herbal remedy for this type of deficiency diarrhea is to powder some cloves and cinnamon bark, place this powder in the child's navel, and then hold in place with an adhesive plaster. Children with diarrhea in general and with this pattern of diarrhea in particular should not be allowed to eat honey.

Comments

According to Western medicine, persistent diarrhea in infants may be due to an adverse reaction to wheat gluten, insufficiency in pancreatic enzymes, sugar malabsorption, and food allergies. Pancreatic enzymes are very much related to the Chinese idea of spleen function, some Western authors saying that the Chinese medical concept of the spleen should be called the spleen-pancreas. The clear, bland diet of Chinese medicine for babies is mostly a wheat-free diet, and sugar malabsorption and food allergies are also addressed by the clear, bland diet and Chinese herbal medicine. If there is sudden onset of vomiting, bloody stools, fever, loss of appetite, and listlessness, this suggests dysentery or infectious diarrhea. Even this can be treated with Chinese herbal medicine. This type of diarrhea usually exhibits a damp heat pattern, and Chinese medicinal formulas for damp heat are usually very effective. However, if Chinese medicine does not bring this quickly to a halt, the baby should see a Western MD.

9. Diaper Rash

Diaper rash refers to chapping and chafing of the skin due to wet diapers. In Chinese, this is referred to as *yan kao chuang*, "neglected tailbone sores." It was described in the Chinese medical literature as early as 610 CE. In general, this condition is described as a damp heat pattern. It is a heat pattern because the skin is red in color and hot to the touch. It is damp because there may be small water blisters, wet-looking sores, or the condition is aggravated on exposure to dampness, *i.e.*, the soaking dampness of an unchanged diaper. Chinese medicine primarily treats diaper rash with various external applications. However, if the rash is severe or persistent external treatment should be combined with internal treatment.

Internal treatment:
Ge Gen Qin Lian Tang (Pueraria, Scutellaria & Coptis Decoction)
Ge Gen (Radix Pueraria)
Huang Qin (Radix Scutellariae)
Huang Lian (Rhizoma Coptidis)
Gan Cao (Radix Glycyrrhizae)

External treatments:
Xiao Mi Qing Tang (Millet Clearing Decoction)
Qing Liang Mi (Semen Setariae Italicae), 50g

Method of preparation & use: Cook the millet in 1 liter of water and make into a thin porridge. Strain and reserve the liquid. Allow to cool to body temperature. Then wash the affected area with this liquid. Allow to dry and then powder the affected area using *Fu Long Gan* (Terra Flava Usta) or a combination of *Hua Shi* (Talcum) and *Qing Dai* (Pulvis Indigonis). These last two ingredients are powdered finely and mixed together at a ratio of 5 parts Talcum to 1 part Indigo.

If there is severe diaper rash with red skin, ulceration, and weeping of turbid fluids, one can use **Cang Bai Niu Xi Fang (Atractylodes, Phellodendron & Achyranthes Formula)**:

Cang Zhu (Rhizoma Atractylodis), 10g
Huang Bai (Cortex Phellodendri), 10g
Niu Xi (Radix Achyranthis Bidentatae), 10g
Yin Chen Hao (Herba Artemisiae Scopariae), 10g
Zhi Mu (Rhizoma Anemarrhenae), 10g
Bai Xian Pi (Cortex Dictamni), 10g
Ming Fan (Alumen), 10g
Ku Shen (Radix Sophorae Flavescentis), 30g
Tu Fu Ling (Rhizoma Smilacis), 20g
Di Fu Zi (Fructus Kochiae), 20g
Jin Yin Hua (Flos Lonicerae), 20g

Method of preparation & use: Decoct in water down to 200ml of liquid. Wash the affected area with this liquid up to 10 times per day for 5 minutes each time. Then apply one of the above powders.

If the skin is red, dry, and chapped but there is no fluid exudation, then one can apply *Zi Cao Gao* (Lithospermum Medicinal Ointment) which is a prepared or patent medicine. Another alternative is to apply roasted sesame seed oil. This is even more effective if one cooks till charred *Gan Cao* (Radix Glycyrrhizae) in the roasted sesame oil, then removes the dregs, and applies the resulting medicinal oil.

Comments

In Western medicine, diaper rash is usually seen as a yeast infection or candidiasis. Whenever there is candidiasis, a clear, bland diet should be instituted. In a breast-fed baby, this means that the mother should go on a clear, bland diet. For more information on a clear, bland diet and candidiasis, the reader may see my *The Tao of Healthy Eating: A Simple Guide to Healthy Eating According to Traditional Chinese Medicine*.

10. Prickly Heat

Prickly heat is also called miliaria. It is a commonly seen skin ailment seen in the summertime caused by inadequate perspiration in unduly hot weather. It begins with small little papules or bumps or even tiny little blisters with a red base, each of which has distinct borders but which may blur together gradually into a patch. The skin feels hot to the touch and there is an itchy sensation. Usually prickly heat goes away quickly if one removes tight or hot garments and cools down. A simple home remedy is to wash the affected area with sliced cucumber. However, if severe, prickly heat may be treated as summerheat which is essentially damp heat occurring in the hot, damp weather of summertime.

Internal treatments:
Qing Shu Tang (Clear Summerheat Decoction)
Lian Qiao (Fructus Forsythiae)
Tian Hua Fen (Radix Trichosanthis)
Chi Shao (Radix Paeoniae Rubrae)
Gan Cao (Radix Glycyrrhizae)
Hua Shi (Talcum)
Che Qian Zi (Semen Plantaginis)
Jin Yin Hua (Flos Lonicerae)
Ze Xie (Rhizoma Alismatis)
Dan Zhu Ye (Herba Lophateri)

Pu Di Ren Tang (Dandelion, Viola & Lonicera Decoction)
Pu Gong Ying (Herba Taraxaci)
Zi Hua Di Ding (Herba Violae)
Ren Dong Teng (Caulis Lonicerae)

Lu Dou Tang (Mung Bean Decoction)
Lu Dou (Semen Phaseoli Munginis)
Bo He (Herba Menthae Haplocalycis)
Bai Tang (White sugar)

This "tea" may be given as a beverage in hot summer weather.

External treatments:
San Huang Xi Ji (Three Yellows Wash)
Da Huang (Radix Et Rhizoma Rhei)
Huang Bai (Cortex Phellodendri)
Huang Qin (Radix Scutellariae)
Ku Shen (Radix Sophorae Flavescentis)

Method of preparation & use: Grind equal amounts of the above four medicinals into a fine powder. Mix 10-15g of the resulting powder with 100ml of distilled water and 1ml of carbolic acid. Swab the affected area 4-5 times daily.

Fei Zi Fen (Boiling Seed Powder)
Lu Dou (Semen Phaseoli Munginis), 10g
Bing Pian (Borneol), 2.5g
Hua Shi (Talcum), 87.5g

Method of preparation & use: Grind into powder and mix. Apply this powder to the affected area 2-3 times per day.

Medicinal bath
Hua Shi (Talcum), 180g
Gan Cao (Radix Glycyrrhizae), 30g

Method of preparation & use: Make a decoction of the above two ingredients and bathe the child with the resulting medicinal liquid.

11. Cradle Cap

Cradle cap refers to seborrheic dermatitis in infants. It may develop within the first month of life and is characterized by a thick, yellow, crust on the scalp. If more severe, there can also be cracking and yellow scaling behind the ears and red papules on the face. Many children with cradle cap are also prone to diaper rash, and this fact gives a hint as to its cause and treatment. As we have seen above, diaper rash is due to a damp, hot condition. According to Chinese medicine, children as well as adults typically exhibit a single, overall pattern. That pattern may be complex and multifaceted, but that is the difference between a TCM pattern and a disease. The pattern takes into account all the person's signs and symptoms and tries to recognize the total pattern as a single *gestalt.*

If one analyses the lesions on the top of the head themselves, what one sees in cradle cap is a thick, dry, yellow crust. According to the logic of TCM, such dry, crusty skin lesions suggest a dry disease mechanism. However, if there is damp heat smoldering and brewing within the child, the heat component typically wafts upward because heat inherently rises. This heat then dries out the upper regions of the body even though its origin is a damp heat below. Thus it is not at all uncommon in either children or adults to see damp heat symptoms below and dry heat symptoms above, and, if one understands this aspect of damp heat, one can recognize these two seemingly contradictory manifestations as parts of the same pattern.

Internal treatment:
Ye Ju Niu Zi Tang Jia Wei (Chrysanthemum & Arctium Decoction with Added Flavors)
Ye Ju Hua (Flos Chrysanthemi Indici)
Sheng Di (uncooked Radix Rehmanniae)
Chi Shi Zhi (Hallyositum Rubrum)
Niu Bang Zi (Fructus Arctii)
Dan Pi (Cortex Moutan)
Jing Jie (Herba Schizonepetae)
Fang Feng (Radix Saposhnikoviae)
Yi Yi Ren (Semen Coicis)
Ming Fan (Alumen)

    Gan Cao (Radix Glycyrrhizae)
    Qiang Huo (Radix Et Rhizoma Notopterygii)
    Man Jing Zi (Fructus Viticis)
    Bo He (Herba Menthae Haplocalycis)

If there are red lesions on the face, add *Jin Yin Hua* (Flos Lonicerae), *Lian Qiao* (Fructus Forsythiae), and *Huai Hua Mi* (Fructus Immaturus Sophorae). If there is pronounced dampness, add *Ku Shen* (Radix Sophorae Flavescentis), *Fu Ling* (Poria), and *Hua Shi* (Talcum). If there is concomitant food stagnation which there basically always is in infants with this condition, add *Shan Zha* (Fructus Crataegi).

External treatments: Locally, the parent can massage a small amount of roasted sesame seed oil into the lesion each night. This is left on during sleep and then shampooed out in the morning.

If the cradle cap is more severe, one can use **Zhi Yi Xi Fang (Seborrhea Washing Formula):**
    Cang Er Zi (Fructus Xanthii), 30g
    Wang Bu Liu Xing (Semen Vaccariae), 30g
    Ku Shen (Radix Sophorae Flavescentis), 15g
    Ming Fan (Alumen), 9g

Method of preparation & use: Decoct in water and remove the dregs. While still warm but not too hot, wash the affected area with this liquid, massaging the scalp for 15 minutes each time. Repeat 2-3 times each day.

Adjunctive treatment

If the child is eating solid foods, they should not be fed any sugar or sweets, nor should they be allowed to drink sweet fruit juices. It is important to note that a bottle of fruit juice can have as much or more sugar as a candy bar.

Comments

According to Western medicine, cradle cap is associated with genetic and climactic factors. According to TCM theory, the propensity towards cradle cap is usually developed while the child is in the womb. Commonly, mothers during pregnancy have eaten too many sugars and sweets and/or greasy, spicy, fatty, "hot foods." These types of foods lead to a damp heat condition in the mother which is then passed on to the child. Therefore, eating a nutritious, clear, bland diet during pregnancy is one way to prevent this condition. Although a clear, bland diet is *mainly* a vegetarian diet, it may contain a small, regular amount of animal protein as long as that animal protein is not overeaten or too greasy and fatty. In addition, it is also important for breast-feeding mothers of babies with cradle cap to eat a clear, bland diet.

12. Oral Thrush

Oral thrush refers to an overgrowth of fungus in the mouth. It typically causes creamy or milky patches on the tongue or insides of the mouth with inflammation and even possibly erosion of the underlying tissue. It is also referred to as oral candidiasis. In somewhat older children, candidiasis results in sores or ulcers on the tongue. Most Chinese pediatric texts simply refer to both types of lesions as oral sores and discuss them as a single entity.

Treatment based on pattern discrimination:

1. Spleen-stomach accumulation & heat

Main symptoms: If heat is more pronounced, there are numerous sores and lesions in the oral cavity with red borders, local pain, refusal to eat, vexation and agitation, excessive crying, foul mouth odor, short, yellow urination, dry, bound stools, possible fever and a red face, a red tongue with yellow fur, and a slippery, rapid pulse. If dampness is more pronounced, there is bad breath, loose, foul-smelling stools, a white, slimy coating or membrane over the mouth with possible red borders, excessive crying, and excessive drooling.

Treatment principles: Clear heat and resolve toxins, open the bowels and drain fire

Guiding formulas:
Liang Ge San (Cool the Diaphragm Powder)
Huang Qin (Radix Scutellariae)
Lian Qiao (Fructus Forsythiae)
Zhi Zi (Fructus Gardeniae)
Da Huang (Radix Et Rhizoma Rhei)
Mang Xiao (Natri Sulfas)
Dan Zhu Ye (Herba Lophateri)
Bo He (Herba Menthae Haplocalycis)
Gan Cao (Radix Glycyrrhizae)

Liang Ge San Jia Jian (Cool the Diaphragm Powder with Additions & Subtractions)
Huang Qin (Radix Scutellariae)
Lian Qiao (Fructus Forsythiae)
Zhi Zi (Fructus Gardeniae)
Da Huang (Radix Et Rhizoma Rhei)
Dan Zhu Ye (Herba Lophateri)
Shan Zha (Fructus Crataegi)
Mai Ya (Fructus Germinatus Hordei)
Bing Lang (Semen Arecae)

If there are loose stools, omit the *Da Huang*.

Gan Lu Xiao Du Dan Jia Jian (Sweet Dew Disperse Toxins Elixir with Additions & Subtractions)
Huo Xiang (Herba Pogostemonis)
Yin Chen Hao (Herba Artemisiae Scopariae)
Fu Ling (Poria)
Lian Qiao (Fructus Forsythiae)
Hou Po (Cortex Magnoliae)
Yi Yi Ren (Semen Coicis)
Bai Dou Kou (Fructus Cardamomi)
Ban Xia (Rhizoma Pinelliae)
Tong Cao (Medulla Tetrapanacis)
Shi Chang Pu (Rhizoma Acori Tatarinowii)

If there is constipation, add *Zhi Shi* (Fructus Immaturus Aurantii) and *Da Huang* (Radix Et Rhizoma Rhei).

Zhong Bai Zhu Ye Tang (Sedimen Urinae & Lophaterum Decoction)
Ren Zhong Bai (Sedimen Urinae Hominis)
Dan Zhu Ye (Herba Lophateri)
uncooked *Shi Gao* (Gypsum Fibrosum)
Mu Tong (Caulis Akebiae)
Zhi Mu (Rhizoma Anemarrhenae)
uncooked *Da Huang* (Radix Et Rhizoma Rhei)
Lian Qiao (Fructus Forsythiae)
uncooked *Gan Cao* (Radix Glycyrrhizae)

2. Heart fire upward flaring

Main symptoms: Ulcers and lesions on the tip or top of the tongue which are red in color and are painful, desire to eat but difficulty swallowing, heart vexation, restlessness, dry mouth, desire to drink, short, reddish urination, a red tongue with an even redder tip and thin, yellow fur, a fine, rapid pulse

Note: Many pediatric texts do not separate out this pattern, rather referring to heart/spleen accumulation and heat or heart/spleen depressive heat. In this particular pattern, the disease cause is always a combination of faulty diet and emotional stress, whereas, in the previous pattern, emotional stress typically does not play a significant part. Therefore, this pattern tends to manifest in somewhat older children than the previous pattern.

Treatment principles: Clear the heart and drain fire

Guiding formulas:
Xie Xin Dao Chi Tang (Drain the Heart & Abduct the Red Decoction)
Huang Lian (Rhizoma Coptidis)
Sheng Di (uncooked Radix Rehmanniae)
Dan Zhu Ye (Herba Lophateri)

Mu Tong (Caulis Akebiae)
Zhi Zi (Fructus Gardeniae)
Fang Feng (Radix Saposhnikoviae)
Gan Cao (Radix Glycyrrhizae)

Qing Re Xie Pi San (Clear Heat & Drain the Spleen Powder)
Zhi Zi (Fructus Gardeniae)
Huang Lian (Rhizoma Coptidis)
Sheng Di (uncooked Radix Rehmanniae)
Huang Qin (Radix Scutellariae)
Chi Shao (Radix Paeoniae Rubrae)
Deng Xin Cao (Medulla Junci)

Qing Re Xie Pi San Jia Jian (Clear Heat & Drain the Spleen Powder with Additions & Subtractions)
Huang Qin (Radix Scutellariae)
Huang Lian (Rhizoma Coptidis)
Zhi Zi (Fructus Gardeniae)
Shi Gao (Gypsum Fibrosum)
Sheng Di (uncooked Radix Rehmanniae)
Chi Fu Ling (Red Poria)
Gan Cao (Radix Glycyrrhizae)
Hua Shi (Talcum)
Qing Dai (Pulvis Indigonis)

If there is concomitant constipation, add uncooked *Da Huang* (Radix Et Rhizoma Rhei).

Qing Re Xie Huo Tang (Clear Heat & Drain Fire Decoction)
Ban Lan Gen (Radix Isatidis/Baphicacanthi)
Bo He (Herba Menthae Haplocalycis)
Zhi Zi (Fructus Gardeniae)
Huang Bai (Cortex Phellodendri)

3. Qi & yin dual vacuity (a.k.a. vacuity fire harassing above)

Main symptoms: Mouth and tongue sores and ulcers after a warm disease or in a patient with constitutional insufficiency of yin, small, scattered, pale-colored lesions with no severe aching or pain, clear drool running from the mouth, emaciation, a weak body, lassitude of the spirit, red cheeks, a dry mouth but no thirst, loose stools, pale oral mucosa, a pale tongue with white fur, a fine, soft pulse

Note: These signs and symptoms add up to yin vacuity with simultaneous spleen vacuity.

Treatment principles: Nourish yin and boost the qi

Guiding formulas:
Liu Wei Di Huang Wan Jia Wei (Six Flavors Rehmannia Pills with Added Flavors)

Sheng Di (uncooked Radix Rehmanniae)
Shan Zhu Yu (Fructus Corni)
Shan Yao (Radix Dioscoreae)
Fu Ling (Poria)
Dan Pi (Cortex Moutan)
Ze Xie (Rhizoma Alismatis)
Gui Xin (Cortex Cinnamomi)
Dang Shen (Radix Codonopsitis)
Bai Zhu (Rhizoma Atractylodis Macrocephalae)
Gan Cao (Radix Glycyrrhizae)
Huang Jing (Rhizoma Polygonati)

If there is no spleen qi vacuity, one can use Zhi Bai Di Huang Wan Jia Wei (Anemarrhena & Phellodendron Rehmannia Pills with Added Flavors):

Zhi Mu (Rhizoma Anemarrhenae)
Huang Bai (Cortex Phellodendri)
Sheng Di (uncooked Radix Rehmanniae)
Shan Zhu Yu (Fructus Corni)
Shan Yao (Radix Dioscoreae)
Fu Ling (Poria)
Ze Xie (Rhizoma Alismatis)
Dan Pi (Cortex Moutan)
Xuan Shen (Radix Scrophulariae)

Unnamed formula

Nan Sha Shen (Radix Adenophorae)
Xuan Shen (Radix Scrophulariae)
Shi Hu (Herba Dendrobii)
Shi Gao (Gypsum Fibrosum)
Qing Dai (Pulvis Indigonis)
Hua Shi (Talcum)
Gan Cao (Radix Glycyrrhizae)
Ren Zhong Huang (Pulvis Praeparatus Glycyrrhizae)
Lian Qiao (Fructus Forsythiae)
Lu Gen (Rhizoma Phragmitis)
Bai Mao Gen (Rhizoma Imperatae)
Zhu Ru (Caulis Bambusae In Taeniis)
Dan Zhu Ye (Herba Lophateri)
Gua Lou (Fructus Trichosanthis)

If there is simultaneous fever, add *Dan Dou Chi* (Semen Praeparatus Sojae), *Jin Yin*

Hua (Flos Lonicerae), *Zi Hua Di Ding* (Herba Violae), and *Pu Gong Ying* (Herba Taraxaci). If the mouth is full of red, painful, possibly bleeding ulcers, add *Sheng Di* (uncooked Radix Rehmanniae), *Zhi Mu* (Rhizoma Anemarrhenae), and *Ze Xie* (Rhizoma Alismatis).

Acupuncture & moxibustion

For heart-spleen accumulation and heat, the main points are *Shao Fu* (Ht 8), *Qu Chi* (LI 11), *Nei Ting* (St 44), *Lian Quan* (CV 23), and *Zhao Hai* (Ki 6). If there is restlessness and crying, add *Yin Tang* (M-HN-3). If there is constipation, add *Da Heng* (Sp 15). If there is reduced, yellow-colored urine, add *Yin Ling Quan* (Sp 9). For vacuity fire harassing above, needle *Yin Xi* (Ht 6), *Tao Dao* (GV 13), *Fu Liu* (Ki 7), *Lian Quan* (CV 23), and *Zhao Hai* (Ki 6).

Adjunctive treatments

For best results, external treatments should be combined with internal treatments. One simple external treatment is to sprinkle *Bing Peng San* (Borneol & Borax Powder) onto the lesions. This is made by powdering *Peng Sha* (Borax) and adding to it a small amount of *Bing Pian* (Borneol). Another possibility is to powder *Wu Bei Zi* (Galla Rhois) and *Ming Fan* (Alumen). Then add a small amount of *Bing Pian* (Borneol) and sprinkle this on the lesions. Or one can powder *Qing Dai* (Pulvis Indigonis), 15g, *Huang Lian* (Rhizoma Coptidis), 9g, and *Zhu Sha* (Cinnabar), 4.5g, and apply this to the lesions several times per day. *Xi Gua Shuang* (Watermelon Frost) is a prepared or patent medicine which can also be sprayed into the mouth to treat oral candidiasis. Another external treatment is to powder some *Wu Zhu Yu* (Fructus Evodiae) and mix this with vinegar into a paste. This paste is applied at night before bed to the center of the soles of the feet, covered with gauze, and then washed off in the morning.

Comments

In actual clinical practice, most cases do not divide so neatly into repletion and vacuity patterns. In fact, in my experience, most cases of pediatric thrush are a combination of damp heat in the stomach *with* spleen vacuity. In such cases, the spleen vacuity is due to the spleen's inherent weakness in infants aggravated by faulty feeding or poor diet, while the damp heat is due to overfeeding or faulty diet.

When there is a combination of factors causing oral thrush in infants and toddlers, as there most often is, the accompanying symptoms are also a mixture of repletion and vacuity signs and symptoms. For instance, the lesions are recurring and do not heal, the appetite is not good, the facial complexion is a sallow yellow, and the stools are loose. Therefore, the treatment principles are to supplement the center and boost the qi, suppress and downbear yin fire using a combination of sweet, warm and bitter, cold ingredients. Based on these principles, a modified version of *Bu Zhong Yi Qi Tang* (Supplement the Center & Boost the Qi Decoction) may be prescribed.

Bu Zhong Yi Qi Tang (Supplement the Center & Boost the Qi Decoction)

Huang Qi (Radix Astragali)
Ren Shen (Radix Ginseng)
Bai Zhu (Rhizoma Atractylodis Macrocephalae)
Gan Cao (Radix Glycyrrhizae)
Dang Gui (Radix Angelicae Sinensis)
Chen Pi (Pericarpium Citri Reticulatae)
Chai Hu (Radix Bupleuri)
Sheng Ma (Rhizoma Cimicifugae)

In this case, one should add 1) several ingredients which clear heat and eliminate dampness, such as *Huang Bai* (Cortex Phellodendri), *Huang Lian* (Rhizoma Coptidis), 2) one or more ingredients to transform food and disperse accumulation, such as *Shan Zha* (Fructus Crataegi), and 3) one or more ingredients to aromatically dry dampness and transform turbidity, such as *Huo Xiang* (Herba Pogostemonis).

Because the child has candidiasis, it is usually helpful and important for the mother to go on a clear, bland, anti-candidal, or hypoallergenic diet while the baby is being treated. This is described in some detail below under pediatric allergies. If the mother suffers from polysystemic chronic candidiasis (PSCC), then it is not uncommon for the mother to develop cracked nipples at the same time as the child has oral candidiasis. In that case, besides the mother adopting a clear, bland, yeast-free, sugar-free diet, she should also apply Chinese antifungal medicinals to her cracked nipples. If there is a lot of oozing from the cracks, then a powdered medicine is made from *Bai Zhi* (Radix Angelicae Dahuricae), mixed with breast milk, and applied to the nipples. If the nipples are cracked, dry, and chapped but not oozing or suppurating, then a Chinese herbal salve, such as *Qing Dai Gao* (Indigo Ointment) can be used between feedings.

Because polysystemic chronic candidiasis can play a role in so many other chronic conditions, I believe it is important to treat fungal conditions such as thrush quickly and comprehensively whenever they appear. For me, this always means taking into account the diet as well as any other remedial treatment. This means that both the baby and the breast-feeding mother should be eating a clear, bland diet. What a clear, bland diet means for an infant is either breast milk or, if they are on formula, a formula without added sugar. If they are already on solid foods, they should not be given foods with added sugar or fruits and fruit juices. The best food for an infant other than breast milk is a dilute soup made out of white rice, rice being the most hypoallergenic and easy to digest grain.

13. Teething

Teething is not listed as a disease in Chinese pediatric books. Rather, teething is a normal physiological event in the process of the child's maturation. However, teething may be accompanied by pain and even fever. In Chinese medicine, physiological changes or transformations are warm transformations. The term for maturation in Chinese is *cheng shu*. The word *cheng* means to become, while the word *shu* means to ripen but also to cook. Its radical is the fire radical implying cooking. As parents know, children do not develop steadily at a single pace. Development comes in fits and starts. There are periods of recuperation and preparation and then periods of rapid growth and change. In Chinese medicine, such periods of accelerated growth and change are associated with extra heat in the body, and this extra heat may cause transient fever. This is referred to as *bian zheng*, change or transformation and steaming. This heat is due to increased activity by the life gate fire or kidney yang.

As we will see below, there are a number of ways of relieving fever, and one or more of these can be used if fever accompanies teething. If the fever which often is associated with teething is not too high and if the child is not in great pain or discomfort, it does not necessarily require treatment. However, I have found in my practice that often a few doses of a very simple Chinese herbal formula called *Suan Zao Ren Tang* (Zizyphus Spinosae Decoction) can reduce the fever, calm the fretfulness, and reduce the excessive drooling of teething.

Suan Zao Ren Tang (Zizyphus Spinosa Decoction)
Suan Zao Ren (Semen Zizyphi Spinosae)
Fu Ling (Poria)
Chuan Xiong (Rhizoma Chuanxiong)
Zhi Mu (Rhizoma Anemarrhenae)
Gan Cao (Radix Glycyrrhizae)

As we will also see below, sometimes this change and fever may set off or aggravate an ear infection and these most definitely can and should be treated by Chinese herbal medicine.

14. Fever

Fever in infants and toddlers usually occurs in combination with some other problem such as a cold or earache. Therefore, many Chinese pediatric texts do not discuss fever as a separate disease category. However, often, fever is the main way a parent knows their child is ill, and childrens' fevers tend to be higher than adults and, therefore, more frightening. It is also possible for the child to manifest a fever first and only some time afterwards the symptoms of other disease. If the fever is promptly treated, these other symptoms may never arise. In Chinese medicine, fevers are divided into two broad categories of patterns. There are patterns associated with invasion of the exterior by external pathogens and there are patterns referred to as internal damage patterns. The first group of patterns are associated with recent onset, acute conditions, while the second group are associated with chronic conditions.

Treatment based on pattern discrimination:

External invasion patterns

1. Wind cold

Main symptoms: Nasal congestion, runny nose, cough, aversion to cold, fever, headache, no sweating, muscular aches and pain, thin, white tongue fur, a floating pulse

Treatment principles: Course wind and scatter cold using acrid, warm medicinals to resolve the exterior

Guiding formulas:
Jing Fang Bai Du San (Schizonepeta & Saposhnikovia Vanquish Toxins Powder)
Jing Jie (Herba Schizonepetae)
Fang Feng (Radix Saposhnikoviae)
Chai Hu (Radix Bupleuri)
Qian Hu (Radix Peucedani)
Chuan Xiong (Rhizoma Chuanxiong)
Qiang Huo (Radix Et Rhizoma Notopterygii)
Du Huo (Radix Angelicae Pubescentis)
Fu Ling (Poria)
Jie Geng (Radix Platycodi)
Zhi Ke (Fructus Aurantii)
Gan Cao (Radix Glycyrrhizae)
Sheng Jiang (uncooked Rhizoma Zingiberis)

If there is sweating, one can use **Gui Zhi Tang (Cinnamon Twig Decoction):**
Gui Zhi (Ramulus Cinnamomi)
Bai Shao (Radix Paeoniae Albae)
Sheng Jiang (uncooked Rhizoma Zingiberis)
Da Zao (Fructus Jujubae)
mix-fried *Gan Cao* (Radix Glycyrrhizae)

2. Wind heat

Main symptoms: Nasal congestion, cough, slight aversion to cold, fever, headache, slight perspiration, a red, painful throat, thin, white or slightly yellow tongue fur, a floating, rapid pulse

Treatment principles: Course wind and clear heat using acrid, cool medicinals to resolve the exterior

Guiding formulas:
Sang Ju Yin (Morus & Chrysanthemum Beverage)
Sang Ye (Folium Mori)

Ju Hua (Flos Chrysanthemi)
Lian Qiao (Fructus Forsythiae)
Bo He (Herba Menthae Haplocalycis)
Jie Geng (Radix Platycodi)
Xing Ren (Semen Armeniacae)
Lu Gen (Rhizoma Phragmitis)
Gan Cao (Radix Glycyrrhizae)

Yin Qiao San (Lonicera & Forsythia Powder)
Jin Yin Hua (Flos Lonicerae)
Lian Qiao (Fructus Forsythiae)
Jie Geng (Radix Platycodi)
Niu Bang Zi (Fructus Arctii)
Bo He (Herba Menthae Haplocalycis)
Dan Dou Chi (Semen Praeparatus Sojae)
Jing Jie (Herba Schizonepetae)
Dan Zhu Ye (Herba Lophateri)
Lu Gen (Rhizoma Phragmitis)
Gan Cao (Radix Glycyrrhizae)

3. Warm heat

Main symptoms: High fever which does not abate, annoying or upsetting thirst, definite perspiration, a red tongue with dry, yellow fur, and a slippery, rapid pulse

> **Note:** In this case, warm heat evils have entered the body more deeply than in the two previous patterns.

Treatment principles: Clear heat and nourish fluids

Guiding formula:
Yin Qiao San (Lonicera & Forsythia Powder) plus Shi Gao Zhi Mu Tang (Gypsum & Fibrosum Decoction)
Jin Yin Hua (Flos Lonicerae)
Lian Qiao (Fructus Forsythiae)
Jie Geng (Radix Platycodi)
Niu Bang Zi (Fructus Arctii)
Bo He (Herba Menthae Haplocalycis)
Dan Dou Chi (Semen Praeparatus Sojae)
Jing Jie (Herba Schizonepetae)
Dan Zhu Ye (Herba Lophateri)
Lu Gen (Rhizoma Phragmitis)
Gan Cao (Radix Glycyrrhizae)
Shi Gao (Gypsum Fibrosum)
Zhi Mu (Rhizoma Anemarrhenae)

4. Damp heat (a.k.a. summerheat)

Main symptoms: Fever which is not very high, fullness or tightness in the head, lack of strength in the four limbs, a tight or heavy feeling in the chest, nausea, a dry mouth but only scanty drinking, a bland taste in the mouth, poor appetite, reddish, *i.e.*, darkish urination, possible loose stools, thick, slimy, white tongue fur, a soggy, rapid pulse

Treatment principles: Clear heat and disinhibit dampness using medicinals which are penetratingly aromatic and which transform turbidity

Guiding formula:
Huo Po Xia Ling Tang (Pogosternon, Magnolia, Pinellia & Poria Decoction) plus San Ren Tang (Three Seeds Decoction)
Huo Xiang (Herba Pogostemonis)
Ban Xia (Rhizoma Pinelliae)
Fu Ling (Poria)
Xing Ren (Semen Armeniacae)
Yi Yi Ren (Semen Coicis)
Bai Dou Kou (Fructus Cardamomi)
Zhu Ling (Polyporus)
Dan Dou Chi (Semen Praeparatus Sojae)
Ze Xie (Rhizoma Alismatis)
Hou Po (Cortex Magnoliae)
Tong Cao (Medulla Tetrapanacis)
Dan Zhu Ye (Herba Lophateri)
Hua Shi (Talcum)

Internal damage patterns

1. Yin vacuity, internal heat

Main symptoms: Tidal fever, night sweats, flushed cheeks, a vexed spirit (meaning an irritated, easily annoyed, restless spirit), a dry cough with little phlegm, a dry throat, dry lips, thirst, short, reddish urination, dry stools, a red tongue with scanty fur or a possibly geographic, peeling tongue fur, a fine, rapid pulse

Treatment principles: Nourish yin and clear heat, moisten dryness and generate fluids

Guiding formula:
Qin Jiao Bie Jia San (Gentiana Macrophylla & Carapax Trionycis Powder) combined with Sha Shen Mai Dong Tang (Glehnia & Ophiopogon Decoction)
Chai Hu (Radix Bupleuri)
mix-fried *Bie Jia* (Carapax Trionycis)
Di Gu Pi (Cortex Lycii)

Qin Jiao (Radix Gentianae Macrophyllae)
Dang Gui (Radix Angelicae Sinensis)
Zhi Mu (Rhizoma Anemarrhenae)
Bei Sha Shen (Radix Glehniae)
Mai Men Dong (Tuber Ophiopogonis)
Yu Zhu (Rhizoma Polygonati Odorati)
Sang Ye (Folium Mori)
Tian Hua Fen (Radix Trichosanthis)
Bai Bian Dou (Semen Dolichoris)
Gan Cao (Radix Glycyrrhizae)

2. Qi & blood dual vacuity

Main symptoms: Low-grade fever which is aggravated by or comes on when there is fatigue, spontaneous perspiration or sweating on slight exertion, scanty appetite, loose stools, lassitude of the spirit, fatigue, a lusterless facial complexion and pale lips, a weak voice or disinclination to speak, a pale tongue with white fur, a fine, soft pulse

Treatment principles: Fortify the spleen and boost the qi while using warm and sweet medicinals to eliminate heat

Guiding formula:
Yi Gong San (Strange Effect Powder) combined with *Bu Zhong Yi Qi Tang* (Supplement the Center & Boost the Qi Decoction)

Huang Qi (Radix Astragali)
Ren Shen (Radix Ginseng)
Bai Zhu (Rhizoma Atractylodis Macrocephalae)
Fu Ling (Poria)
mix-fried *Gan Cao* (Radix Glycyrrhizae)
Dang Gui (Radix Angelicae Sinensis)
Chai Hu (Radix Bupleuri)
Sheng Ma (Rhizoma Cimicifugae)
Chen Pi (Pericarpium Citri Reticulatae)

Acupuncture & moxibustion

For wind heat and warm heat, bleed *Da Zhui* (GV 14). If there is a very high fever, one can add/or bleed *Shi Xuan* (M-UE-1).

Adjunctive treatments

In all four of the external invasion patterns, one should not try to bring down the fever by immersing the child or bathing the child in cold water. Since these are primarily exterior patterns, bathing the child will only close the pores of the skin, while the Chinese medical practitioner is trying to do just the opposite — to open the pores and allow the pathogens to leave the body. One can use the repeated massage down the spine to try to lower the fever in all these cases. One can also scrape the shoulders and back of the neck with a Chinese soup spoon until the skin of the upper back and neck have turned red. This is called *gua sha* and is one way of opening or resolving the exterior to allow for the outward dissipation of the heat. A simple Chinese herbal home remedy for a wind heat pattern of fever is to boil some marjoram in water to make into a "tea." Then drink this to induce perspiration. Marjoram is acrid and cool and thus resolves the exterior while clearing heat. For the wind heat, warm heat, and damp heat types of fever, drinking the juice of 2-3 freshly mashed star fruits or carambola 2-3 times per day is a specific remedy in Chinese dietary therapy for reducing fever. However, these fruits are cold in nature and should not be used in either the wind cold type of fever or the qi and blood deficiency fever. If there is constipation accompanying the fever, parents may give the child a warm water enema. Other adjunctive treatments are to make a paste of *Zhi Zi* (Fructus Gardeniae) and egg white and apply this overnight to *Yong Quan* (Ki 1) or to grind into fine powder *Wu Zhu Yu* (Fructus Evodiae), 10g, *Niu Xi* (Radix Achyranthis Bidentatae), 10g, *Da Huang* (Radix Et Rhizoma Rhei), 10g, *Zhi Zi* (uncooked Fructus Gardeniae), 10g, and *Huang Lian* (Rhizoma Coptidis), 5g. This is mixed with vinegar into a paste and this paste is then applied bilaterally to *Yong Quan* (Ki 1) overnight. Children with a yin vacuity, internal heat pattern should be given pear and/or applesauce and maybe even a little warm milk and sugar. Children with the qi and blood dual vacuity pattern should be fed a warm, nutritious yet nevertheless clear, bland diet, and they should be treated with the spinal pinch-pull maneuver of Chinese pediatric massage every day to strengthen their constitution.

Comments

In terms of the two so-called internal damage patterns of fever in TCM pediatrics, although the word damage may sound dangerous, the use of this word is just technical jargon and does not imply a necessarily dangerous or serious condition. What it means is that a disease has dragged on for some time and has damaged one of the body's righteous energies or substances, and it is this damage of the righteous energy which is making the case hard to heal. These two internal damage patterns are not commonly seen in outpatient practice in the West. Children who have these patterns are ill with some disease, such as rheumatoid arthritis, pertussis, or some other chronic condition for which they are probably already under medical care. These patterns are not associated with high fevers which come out of nowhere in the middle of the night.

That being said, Chinese medicine really excels at treating the two above kinds of vacuity patterns. These are the kinds of patterns that Western medicine typically does not treat very well. Antibiotics usually do not achieve any effect in these types of patterns because the issue is not the presence of pathogens or germs but the run-down strength of the body's immunity. Chinese herbal medicine is extremely effective for promoting the health of the body and for strengthening the immunity. Therefore, parents of children suffering from chronic conditions accompanied by either recurrent or low-grade fevers should definitely give Chinese herbal medicine a try.

15. Infantile Convulsions

Traditionally, infantile convulsions are considered one of the four great pediatric diseases in Chinese medicine. This is because they are associated with diseases or conditions which can be life-threatening. Infantile convulsions are characterized by sudden or violent, irregular motions and spirit dimming or mental cloudiness. They may be simply an exaggerated startle reflex where the child suddenly jerks their four limbs or they may include actual epilepsy. In clinical practice in the West, infantile convulsions most commonly occur in association with high fever. Infantile convulsions primarily occur in children under five years of age with a higher likelihood of incidence the younger the child. The incidence of pediatric convulsions gradually decreases after seven years of age. In Chinese medicine, the diagnosis and treatment of infantile convulsions is divided into acute and chronic convulsions. Acute convulsions are associated with contraction of externally invading season evils and phlegm heat from food stagnation, while chronic convulsions are due to internal stirring of wind due to vacuity.

Treatment based on pattern discrimination:

Acute convulsions

1. Wind cold

> **Main symptoms:** Initially there is aversion to cold, fever, no sweating, vomiting of milk or food, restless spirit and emotions. A relatively older child may report headache. Secondarily there is clamping shut of the teeth, arched back rigidity, spasms and tremors of the four limbs, lack of clarity of the spirit-will, thin, white or slimy, white tongue fur, and a floating, tight, wiry pulse.
>
> **Note:** In this case, if true yin is insufficient and the external evils block the flow of qi and blood, then the sinews and vessels may lose their moistening and nourishment to contraction and stirring of wind.
>
> **Treatment principles:** Resolve the exterior and dispel evils, upbear the fluids and humors and soothe the sinews and vessels
>
> ***Guiding formulas:***
> ***Ge Gen Tang Jia Jian* (Pueraria Decoction with Additions & Subtractions)**
> *Ge Gen* (Radix Puerariae)
> *Ma Huang* (Herba Ephedrae)
> *Bai Shao* (Radix Paeoniae Albae)
> *Gan Cao* (Radix Glycyrrhizae)
> *Fang Feng* (Radix Saposhnikoviae)
> *Gou Teng* (Ramulus Uncariae Cum Uncis)
> *Tian Ma* (Rhizoma Gastrodiae)

  Jiang Can (Bombyx Batryticatus)
  Shi Chang Pu (Rhizoma Acori Tatarinowii)

If the exterior pattern is not resolved, external evils may become depressed and transform heat. In that case, there may be high fever, heart vexation, red eyes, red tongue, and a wiry, rapid pulse. Therefore, delete *Ge Gen* and add *Long Dan Cao* (Radix Gentianae), *Huang Qin* (Radix Scutellariae), *Lian Qiao* (Fructus Forsythiae), and *Ju Hua* (Flos Chrysanthemi).

If there is aversion to cold, fever, and sweating with arched back rigidity, a deep, wiry, tight pulse, or the finger venule is purple and stagnant, then wind evils are even more severe. In that case, use **Gua Lou Gui Zhi Tang (Trichosanthes and Cinnamon Twig Decoction):**
  Tian Hua Fen (Radix Trichosanthis)
  Gui Zhi (Ramulus Cinnamomi)
  Bai Shao (Radix Paeoniae Albae)
  Gan Cao (Radix Glycyrrhizae)
  Jiang Can (Bombyx Batryticatus)
  Gou Teng (Ramulus Uncariae Cum Uncis)
  Tian Ma (Rhizoma Gastrodiae)

2. Wind heat

Main symptoms: Aversion to wind, fever, headache, cough, runny nose, a red throat, vexation and agitation, delirious speech, arched back rigidity, trembling or quivering of the hands and fingers, occasional spirit-will clouding and confusion, thin, yellow tongue fur, a superficial, purple finger vein, a floating, rapid pulse

> ***Note:*** In this case, the spasms and tremors are the result of heat damaging the sinews and vessels and giving rise to internal stirring of liver wind.

Treatment principles: Resolve the exterior and clear heat, assisted by opening the portals and settling fright

Guiding formula:
Yin Qiao San Jia Jian (Lonicera & Forsythia Powder with Additions & Subtractions)
  Jin Yin Hua (Flos Lonicerae)
  Lian Qiao (Fructus Forsythiae)
  Bo He (Herba Menthae Haplocalycis)
  Niu Bang Zi (Fructus Arctii)
  Chan Yi (Periostracum Cicadae)
  Gou Teng (Ramulus Uncariae Cum Uncis)
  Jiang Can (Bombyx Batryticatus)
  Jie Geng (Radix Platycodi)

Gan Cao (Radix Glycyrrhizae)
Shi Chang Pu (Rhizoma Acori Tatarinowii)

If there is high fever which is not abated by sweating with vexation and agitation and oral thirst, add uncooked *Shi Gao* (Gypsum Fibrosum) and *Zhi Mu* (Rhizoma Anemarrhenae). If headache is severe, add *Long Dan Cao* (Radix Gentianae) and *Ju Hua* (Flos Chrysanthemi). If there is repeated vomiting, add *Huang Lian* (Rhizoma Coptidis) and *Zhu Ru* (Caulis Bambusae In Taeniis). If spasms and convulsions are repeated and frequent, add *Shan Yang Jiao* (Cornu Caprae).

3. Summerheat & dampness

Main symptoms: At first there is aversion to cold, fever, no sweating, headache, and bodily hypertonicity. Secondarily there is nausea and vomiting, heart vexation, restlessness, arched neck, and fright inversion with slimy, yellow tongue fur and a slippery, rapid pulse.

> ***Note:*** In this case, the convulsions are due to heat damaging the sinews and vessels and giving rise to internal stirring of liver wind.

Treatment principles: Emit sweat and resolve the exterior, dispel summerheat and transform dampness mainly, while simultaneously settling fright and extinguishing wind

Guiding formula:
Xiang Ru Yin Jia Wei (Elsholtzia Beverage with Added Flavors)
Xiang Ru (Herba Elsholtziae)
Jin Yin Hua (Flos Lonicerae)
Lian Qiao (Fructus Forsythiae)
Hou Po (Cortex Magnoliae)
Bian Dou Hua (Flos Dolichoris)
Shan Yang Jiao (Cornu Caprae)
Gou Teng (Ramulus Uncariae Cum Uncis)
Shi Chang Pu (Rhizoma Acori Tatarinowii)
Jiang Can (Bombyx Batryticatus)
Zhu Ru (Caulis Bambusae In Taeniis)

If nausea and vomiting are repeated and frequent with slimy, white tongue fur due to damp evils obstructing the center, add *Huo Xiang* (Herba Pogostemonis), *Pei Lan* (Herba Eupatorii), and *Yi Yi Ren* (Semen Coicis). If spasms and contractions of the four limbs will not stop, add *Quan Xie* (Scorpio) and *Di Long* (Pheretima).

4. Epidemic pestilence

Main symptoms: The onset of the disease is sudden with high fever, oral thirst, severe headache, agitation, stirring, and restlessness. Very quickly there is spirit-will clouding and confusion with both eyes staring upward and frequent, repeated spasms and tremors. The tongue is dry and scarlet with yellow, coarse fur. The finger vein is blue-green and purple and is found in the qi bar or above. The pulse is wiry and rapid.

Note: In this case, exuberant heat has severely damaged fluids and humors.

Treatment principles: Clear heat and resolve toxins, cool the blood and extinguish wind

Guiding formulas:
Qing Wen Bai Du Yin Jia Jian (Clear the Scourge & Vanquish Toxins Beverage with Additions & Subtractions)
  uncooked *Shi Gao* (Gypsum Fibrosum)
  Zhi Mu (Rhizoma Anemarrhenae)
  Zhi Zi (Fructus Gardeniae)
  Huang Lian (Rhizoma Coptidis)
  Jin Yin Hua (Flos Lonicerae)
  Lian Qiao (Fructus Forsythiae)
  Shui Niu Jiao (Cornu Bubali)
  Sheng Di (uncooked Radix Rehmanniae)
  Dan Pi (Cortex Moutan)
  Gou Teng (Ramulus Uncariae Cum Uncis)

Plus An Gong Niu Huang Wan (Quiet the Palace Bezoar Pills, a Chinese patent medicine)

If breathing is obstructed and there is the sound of phlegm in the throat due to phlegm heat blockage and exuberance, add *Dan Nan Xing* (bile-processed Rhizoma Arisaematis), *Zhu Li* (Succus Bambusae), and *Ban Xia* (Rhizoma Pinelliae). If there is abdominal distention and fullness with constipation, add *Da Huang* (Radix Et Rhizoma Rhei) and *Mang Xiao* (Natri Sulfas). If there is a red rash on the body, use double *Shui Niu Jiao* (Cornu Bubali), *Sheng Di* (uncooked Radix Rehmannia), and *Dan Pi* (Cortex Moutan) and add *Chi Shao* (Radix Paeoniae Rubrae) and *Dan Shen* (Radix Salviae Miltiorrhizae).

If there is burning heat in the chest and abdomen with inversion chilling of the four limbs and clouding and confusion which cannot be aroused, a somber white facial complexion, and a deep, faint pulse due to internal blockage and external desertion, in emergency, use **Shen Fu Tang (Ginseng & Aconite Decoction):**
  Ren Shen (Radix Ginseng)
  Fu Zi (Radix Lateralis Praeparatus Aconiti Carmichaeli)

5. Phlegm heat food reversal

Main symptoms: First there is no thought for food or milk, vomiting, abdominal distention and fullness, non free-flowing stools. Then there is fever and spirit affect torpor and stagnation which quickly give rise to spasms and tremors, spirit clouding, rapid dyspneic breathing, and the sound of phlegm in the throat. The face is bluish green, while the tongue has thick, slimy, yellow fur. The finger vein is purplish and stagnant, and the pulse is wiry, slippery, and rapid.

> **Note:** Again, the convulsions are due to phlegm and heat giving rise to stirring of liver wind.

Treatment principles: Disperse food and abduct stagnation, transform phlegm and clear heat, settle fright and open the portals

Guiding formulas:
Bao He Wan Jia Jian (Protect Harmony Pills with Additions & Subtractions)
Shen Qu (Massa Medica Fermentata)
Shan Zha (Fructus Crataegi)
Zhi Shi (Fructus Immaturus Aurantii)
Da Huang (Radix Et Rhizoma Rhei)
Chen Pi (Pericarpium Citri Reticulatae)
Ban Xia (Rhizoma Pinelliae)
Lian Qiao (Fructus Forsythiae)
Gou Teng (Ramulus Uncariae Cum Uncis)
Lai Fu Zi (Semen Raphani)

Plus **Yu Shu Dan (Jade Axis Elixir, a Chinese ready-made medicine)**

If there is profuse phlegm, spirit clouding, and repeated, frequent spasms and tremors, also administer **Xiao Er Hui Chun Dan (Pediatric Restore Spring Elixir,** a Chinese ready-made medicine).

If arching of the neck and body is pronounced, use **Ding Ming San (Stabilize Destiny Powder)**.

If there is chest fullness and abdominal distention with constipation due to pronounced interior repletion, use **Da Cheng Qi Tang (Major Order the Qi Decoction):**
Da Huang (Radix Et Rhizoma Rhei)
Mang Xiao (Natri Sulfas)
Zhi Shi (Fructus Immaturus Aurantii)
Hou Po (Cortex Magnoliae)

Chronic convulsions

1. Spleen yang vacuity weakness

Main symptoms: Appearance of convulsions after possible prolonged vomiting or diarrhea, forceless, indistinct spasms and tremors, listlessness of the essence spirit, the whites of the eyes showing while asleep, lack of clarity of the spirit will, lack of warmth of the four limbs, loose stools, a sallow yellow facial complexion, a pale tongue with white fur, a pale, bluish green vein on the finger, a deep, weak pulse

Note: These convulsions are due to lack of warmth and nourishment therefore giving rise to vacuity wind stirring internally.

Treatment principles: Warm the center and fortify the spleen

Guiding formula:
Li Zhong Tang Jia Jian (Rectify the Center Decoction with Additions & Subtractions)
Dang Shen (Radix Codonopsitis)
Bai Zhu (Rhizoma Atractylodis Macrocephalae)
Gan Jiang (dry Rhizoma Zingiberis)
Wu Zhu Yu (Fructus Evodiae)
Fu Ling (Poria)
Chen Pi (Pericarpium Citri Reticulatae)
Bai Shao (Radix Paeoniae Albae)
Sha Ren (Fructus Amomi)

If diarrhea is frequent and repeated, in order to restrain, astringe, and stop diarrhea, add *Rou Dou Kou* (Semen Myristicae) and blast-fried *He Zi* (Fructus Terminaliae). If there is simultaneous vomiting, in order to downbear counterflow and stop vomiting, add *Ban Xia* (Rhizoma Pinelliae). If there is counterflow chilling of the four limbs due to yang vacuity with cold exuberance, add *Fu Zi* (Radix Lateralis Praeparatus Aconiti Carmichaeli). If spasms and tremors are relatively frequent, add *Tian Ma* (Rhizoma Gastrodiae) and *Quan Xie* (Scorpio).

2. Spleen-kidney yang vacuity

Main symptoms: Extreme listlessness of the essence spirit, squirming movements of the hands and feet, deep sleep, clouding and confusion, icy chill of the four limbs, profuse sweating from the forehead, clear, watery stools, a somber white facial complexion, a pale tongue with glossy, white fur, a deep, faint pulse

Note: In this pattern, it is again vacuity wind engendered internally which gives rise to the squirming or wriggling hands and feet.

Treatment principles: Warm and supplement the spleen and kidneys, strengthen yang and dispel cold

Guiding formula:
Gu Zhen Tang Jia Jian (Secure the True Decoction with Additions & Subtractions)
Ren Shen (Radix Ginseng)

Huang Qi (Radix Astragali)
Fu Zi (Radix Lateralis Praeparatus Aconiti Carmichaeli)
Rou Gui (Cortex Cinnamomi)
mix-fried *Gan Cao* (Radix Glycyrrhizae)
Pao Jiang (blast-fried Rhizoma Zingiberis)
Bai Shao (Radix Paeoniae Albae)
Long Gu (Os Draconis)
Mu Li (Concha Ostreae)

If there is incessant diarrhea, add *Chi Shi Zhi* (Hallyositum Rubrum) and blast-fried *He Zi* (Fructus Terminaliae).

3. Liver-kidney yin vacuity

Main symptoms: Spasms and tremors occasionally are acute and occasionally are relaxed. There is emaciation, listlessness of the essence spirit, restlessness, low-grade fever, heat in the centers of the hands and feet, easy sweating, dry stools, tremors of the four limbs or rigidity of the body and limbs, a flushed red facial complexion, a dry, bright red tongue with no fur, and a fine, deep, rapid pulse.

Note: Due to liver blood vacuity, the sinews lack nourishment, while vacuity gives rise to wind stirring internally.

Treatment principles: Enrich yin and foster yang, nourish the liver and extinguish wind

Guiding formula:
Da Ding Feng Zhu Jia Jian (Great Stabilize Wind Pearls with Additions & Subtractions)
Gui Ban (Plastrum Testudinis)
Bie Jia (Carapax Trionycis)
Mu Li (Concha Ostreae)
Bai Shao (Radix Paeoniae Albae)
Sheng Di (uncooked Radix Rehmanniae)
Xuan Shen (Radix Scrophulariae)
Mai Men Dong (Tuber Ophiopogonis)
Gan Cao (Radix Glycyrrhizae)
Wu Wei Zi (Fructus Schisandrae)
Gou Teng (Ramulus Uncariae Cum Uncis)
Ji Zi Huang (Egg yolk)

If there is tidal fever and night sweats, add *Di Gu Pi* (Cortex Lycii). If there is pronounced lassitude of the spirit and lack of strength with relatively profuse sweating, add *Dang Shen* (Radix Codonopsitis) and *Huang Qi* (Radix Astragali). If there is the sound of phlegm in the throat, add *Chuan Bei Mu* (Bulbus Fritillariae Cirrhosae) and *Dan Nan Xing* (bile-processed Rhizoma Arisaematis). If the four limbs appear rigid and stiff or there is arched back rigidity, one can add *Quan Xie* (Scorpio) and *Wu Gong* (Scolopendra).

Acupuncture & moxibustion

In exterior patterns and phlegm heat food stagnation, needle *Qu Chi* (LI 11) and *Da Zhui* (GV 14) and bleed *Shi Xuan* (M-UE-1-5) if there is high fever. If there are convulsions, needle *Tai Chong* (Liv 3) through to *Yong Quan* (Ki 1) and *Ren Zhong* (GV 26). If there is lockjaw, needle *Xia Guan* (St 7) and *Jia Che* (St 6). If there is the sound of phlegm in the throat, needle *Feng Long* (St 40). If there is food stagnation, needle *Tian Shu* (St 25) and *Nei Guan* (Per 6). For qi and yang vacuity patterns, moxa from among *Da Zhui* (GV 14), *Pi Shu* (Bl 20), *Ming Men* (GV 4), *Guan Yuan* (CV 4), and *Qi Hai* (CV 6). For yin vacuity patterns, needle *Nei Guan* (Per 6), *Qu Chi* (LI 11), and *He Gu* (LI 4) if the spasms are in the upper limbs. If the spasms are in the lower limbs, needle *Cheng Shan* (Bl 57) and *Tai Chong* (Liv 3).

Adjunctive treatments

As a first aid measure, one can massage *Yong Quan* (Ki 1) strongly on both feet. If there is fever, rub vigorously and continuously down the spine. If there is food stagnation giving rise to high fever and convulsions, give an enema and rub the abdomen to promote bowel movements. If there is bodily vacuity, one can do the spinal pinch-pull massage several times per day in order to strengthen the bodily constitution. In case of either food stagnation or spleen vacuity, a well regulated, clear, bland diet is very important. Children manifesting liver-kidney yin vacuity should be given more easily digestible animal protein, such as eggs and meat broths.

Comments

In the outpatient clinic, many times infants are manifesting what Chinese medicine considers convulsions without the parent even being aware of this. In Chinese, convulsions are referred to as fright convulsions, and in babies, they may simply take the form of a pronounced startle reaction to minor stimuli in sick children. Although it is probably best not to tell the parents that their child is having convulsions, the practitioner should include medicinals to level the liver and extinguish wind while treating the baby's main complaint and pattern of disharmony. If convulsions are frequent and severe but without fever, the child should be referred to a neurologist to check for epilepsy. If they are severe and accompanied by high fever, if the fever refuses to abate despite treatment, the child should be taken to an Emergency Room or Western MD.

Meningitis and encephalitis manifesting as high fever, severe headache, convulsions, arched back rigidity, and loss of consciousness both fall under the category of infantile convulsions when they occur in children.

16. Ear Infections

Ear infections are one of the most common pediatric complaints in the West. These typically occur for the first time around the time of first teething. This is also right around the time that many parents introduce solid foods for the first time. Usually, the parent first notices that the child is crying as if in pain. Secondarily, they may see that the child is pulling on or batting their ear. If one of these two things don't get the parent's attention, then a fever accompanying these other two surely does. If taken to a Western MD, the standard treatment is antibiotics. This does usually put an end to the current acute condition. But, all too often, the child develops another earache soon after the course of antibiotics is over. Again the child is put on antibiotics and again, when they are over, the earache comes back. If this continues enough times, the parents will be advised to have tubes surgically implanted in the child's eardrum to allow drainage and prevent rupture with subsequent possible hearing loss. As a clinician, I have heard this story many, many times.

Below is the Chinese textbook treatment of pediatric earaches. Personally, I find that the following information is not sufficient to treat Western babies with ear infections. This is one area in TCM pediatrics where I have a lot of clinical experience. Therefore, the reader is strongly urged to consider my own experience as described in the section titled Comments below.

Treatment based on pattern discrimination:

1. Acute otitis media

A. Wind heat

Main symptoms: Fever, aversion to cold, sore throat, nasal congestion and runny nose, ear blockage, ear distention, deafness, sounds inside the ear, thin, yellow tongue fur, a floating, rapid pulse

Treatment principles: Course wind, clear heat, and resolve toxins

Guiding formula:
Shu Feng Qing Re Tang Jia Jian (Course Wind & Clear Heat Decoction with Additions & Subtractions)
Jing Jie (Herba Schizonepetae)
Fang Feng (Radix Saposhnikoviae)
Jin Yin Hua (Flos Lonicerae)
Lian Qiao (Fructus Forsythiae)
Gan Cao (Radix Glycyrrhizae)
Jie Geng (Radix Platycodi)
Sang Ye (Folium Mori)
Bo He (Herba Menthae Haplocalycis)
Huang Qin (Radix Scutellariae)
Cang Er Zi (Fructus Xanthii)

B. Liver fire

Main symptoms: Pain in the ear, crying and restlessness, diminished eating and drinking, possible high fever, crying worse when pressure is applied around the ear, a bitter taste in the mouth, a dry throat, yellowish red urination, constipation, a red tongue with yellow, slimy fur, a wiry, rapid pulse

Treatment principles: Clear and discharge dampness and heat, resolve toxins and disperse swelling

Guiding formulas:
Long Dan Xie Gan Tang Jia Jian (Gentiana Drain the Liver Decoction with Additions & Subtractions)
Long Dan Cao (Radix Gentianae)
Huang Qin (Radix Scutellariae)
Chai Hu (Radix Bupleuri)
Zhi Zi (Fructus Gardeniae)
Sheng Di (uncooked Radix Rehmanniae)
Shi Gao (Gypsum Fibrosum)
Ye Ju Hua (Flos Chyrsanthemi Indici)
Pu Gong Ying (Herba Taraxaci)
Da Huang (Radix Et Rhizoma Rhei)

If, after 2-3 days, a pussy fluid is discharged from the ear due to rupture of the eardrum, add *Chuan Shan Jia* (Squama Manitis), *Zao Jiao Ci* (Spina Gleditschiae), *Ru Xiang* (Olibanum), *Mo Yao* (Myrrha), and *Dang Gui* (Radix Angelicae Sinensis). If there are spasms and tremors, *i.e.*, convulsions due to high fever, add *Zhen Zhu Mu* (Concha Margaritiferae), *Shi Jue Ming* (Concha Haliotidis), and *Gou Teng* (Ramulus Uncariae Cum Uncis).

Huang Lian Jie Du Tang (Coptis Resolve Toxins Decoction) plus Bai Hu Tang (White Tiger Decoction) with additions and subtractions
Huang Lian (Rhizoma Coptidis)
Huang Qin (Radix Scutellariae)
Huang Bai (Cortex Phellodendri)
Zhi Zi (Fructus Gardeniae)
Shi Gao (Gypsum Fibrosum)
Zhi Mu (Rhizoma Anemarrhenae)
Gan Cao (Radix Glycyrrhizae)
Geng Mi (Semen Oryzae)
Long Dan Cao (Radix Gentianae)
Chai Hu (Radix Bupleuri)

Xiao Du Yin Jia Jian (Disperse Toxins Beverage with Additions & Subtractions)
Pu Gong Ying (Herba Taraxaci)

    Jin Yin Hua (Flos Lonicerae)
    Xuan Shen (Radix Scrophulariae)
    Chi Shao (Radix Paeoniae Rubrae)
    Lian Qiao (Fructus Forsythiae)
    blast-fried *Chuan Shan Jia* (Squama Manitis)
    Zao Jiao Ci (Spina Gleditschiae)
    Qian Hu (Radix Peucedani)
    Fang Feng (Radix Saposhnikoviae)
    Gan Cao (Radix Glycyrrhizae)
    Long Dan Cao (Radix Gentianae)

Unnamed formula: to be used after pussy fluids have begun to be discharged from the ear and the fever and pain are gradually diminishing:
    Jin Yin Hua (Flos Lonicerae)
    Fang Feng (Radix Saposhnikoviae)
    Bai Zhi (Radix Angelicae Dahuricae)
    Dang Gui (Radix Angelicae Sinensis)
    Chen Pi (Pericarpium Citri Reticulatae)
    Gan Cao (Radix Glycyrrhizae)
    Chai Hu (Radix Bupleuri)
    Bei Mu (Bulbus Fritillariae)
    Tian Hua Fen (Radix Trichosanthis)
    Ru Xiang (Olibanum)
    Mo Yao (Myrrha)
    Chuan Shan Jia (Squama Manitis)
    Zao Jiao Ci (Spina Gleditschiae)
    Che Qian Zi (Semen Plantaginis)
    Ku Shen (Radix Sophorae Flavescentis)

Unnamed formula
    Bie Xie (Rhizoma Dioscoreae Hypoglaucae)
    Yi Yi Ren (Semen Coicis)
    Huang Bai (Cortex Phellodendri)
    Chi Shao (Radix Paeoniae Rubrae)
    Dan Pi (Cortex Moutan)
    Ze Xie (Rhizoma Alismatis)
    Hua Shi (Talcum)
    Gan Cao (uncooked Radix Glycyrrhizae)

2. Chronic otitis media

A. Yin vacuity

Main symptoms: Clear, watery pus sometimes exiting from the ear and sometimes stopping, a long course without healing, low back and knee soreness and weakness, lassitude of the spirit, fatigue, a pale face with flushed cheeks, possible night sweats, a dry mouth and a red tongue with diminished fur or a pale tongue with a red tip and thin, white fur, a fine, rapid pulse

Treatment principles: Enrich yin and downbear fire, support the interior and expel pus

> **Note:** The above signs and symptoms and the first guiding formula below presuppose a combination of yin and qi vacuity. If there are no marked signs of qi vacuity, one can use the second guiding formula below instead.

Guiding formulas:
Zhi Bai Di Huang Wan Jia Jian (Anemarrhena & Phellodendron Rehmannia Pills with Additions & Subtractions)

Dang Shen (Radix Codonopsitis)
Huang Qi (Radix Astragali)
Dang Gui (Radix Angelicae Sinensis)
Chi Shao (Radix Paeoniae Rubrae)
Bai Shao (Radix Paeoniae Albae)
Zhi Mu (Rhizoma Anemarrhenae)
Huang Bai (Cortex Phellodendri)
Sheng Di (uncooked Radix Rehmanniae)
Dan Pi (Cortex Moutan)
Fu Ling (Poria)
Shan Zhu Yu (Fructus Corni)
Jin Yin Hua (Flos Lonicerae)
Ku Ding Cha (Folium Ilicis)

Zhi Bai Di Huang Wan Jia Wei (Anemarrhena & Phellodendron Rehmannia Pills with Added Flavors)

Zhi Mu (Rhizoma Anemarrhenae)
Huang Bai (Cortex Phellodendri)
Shu Di (cooked Radix Rehmanniae)
Shan Yao (Radix Dioscoreae)
Shan Zhu Yu (Fructus Corni)
Fu Ling (Poria)
Dan Pi (Cortex Moutan)
Ze Xie (Rhizoma Alismatis)
Bai Mao Gen (Rhizoma Imperatae)

B. Spleen vacuity

Main symptoms: Recurrent earaches, possible clear, white, watery, thick, yellow, or green pussy fluids exiting from the ear enduring for many days, stopping and starting or stopping and recurring, possible thickening of the skin of the auditory pathway and auricle, increased earwax, a sallow yellow facial complexion, torpid, diminished intake of food, bodily fatigue and lack of strength, a pale tongue with white fur, and a fine, relaxed pulse

Treatment principles: Supplement the spleen and nourish the blood, support the interior and expel pulse

Guiding formulas:
Unnamed formula
Dang Shen (Radix Codonopsitis)
Huang Qi (Radix Astragali)
Bai Zhu (Rhizoma Atractylodis Macrocephalae)
Fu Ling (Poria)
Dang Gui (Radix Angelicae Sinensis)
Bai Shao (Radix Paeoniae Albae)
Chuan Xiong (Rhizoma Chuanxiong)
Jin Yin Hua (Flos Lonicerae)
Bai Zhi (Radix Angelicae Dahuricae)
Gan Cao (Radix Glycyrrhizae)
Zao Jiao Ci (Spina Gleditschiae)
Jie Geng (Radix Platycodi)

Ba Zhen Tang Jia Wei (Eight Pearls Decoction with Added Flavors)
Dang Shen (Radix Codonopsitis)
Fu Ling (Poria)
Bai Zhu (Rhizoma Atractylodis Macrocephalae)
Yi Yi Ren (Semen Coicis)
Gan Cao (Radix Glycyrrhizae)
Lian Zi (Semen Nelumbinis)
Shan Yao (Radix Dioscoreae)
Jie Geng (Radix Platycodi)
Bai Bian Dou (Semen Dolichoris)
Sha Ren (Fructus Amomi)
Dang Gui (Radix Angelicae Sinensis)
Chuan Xiong (Rhizoma Chuanxiong)
Bai Shao (Radix Paeoniae Albae)
Shu Di (cooked Radix Rehmanniae)
Sheng Jiang (uncooked Rhizoma Zingiberis)
Da Zao (Fructus Jujubae)

Ba Zhen Tang Jia Wei (Eight Pearls Decoction with Added Flavors)
Dang Shen (Radix Codonopsitis)
Bai Zhu (Rhizoma Atractylodis Macrocephalae)
Fu Ling (Poria)
mix-fried *Gan Cao* (Radix Glycyrrhizae)
Dang Gui (Radix Angelicae Sinensis)

Chuan Xiong (Rhizoma Chuanxiong)
Bai Shao (Radix Paeoniae Albae)
Shu Di (cooked Radix Rehmanniae)
Yi Yi Ren (Semen Coicis)
Chen Pi (Pericarpium Citri Reticulatae)
Sha Ren (Fructus Amomi)
Chan Yi (Periostracum Cicadae)

If there is hearing loss subsequent to ear infection, use **Tong Ming San (Open Sound Powder):**
Shi Chang Pu (Rhizoma Acori Tatarinowii)
Yuan Zhi (Radix Polygalae)
Chai Hu (Radix Bupleuri)
Mai Men Dong (Tuber Ophiopogonis)
Xing Ren (Semen Armeniacae)
Fang Feng (Radix Saposhnikoviae)
Xi Xin (Herba Asari)
Ci Shi (Magnetitum)
Ting Li Zi (Semen Lepidii/Descurainiae)

Acupuncture & moxibustion

For acute otitis media, needle *He Gu* (LI 4) and *Nei Ting* (St 44) to disperse accumulation and clear heat from the *yang ming* as well as the region of the head. Locally, needle *Feng Chi* (GB 20). If there is high fever, bleed either or both *Shi Xuan* (M-UE-1-5) and *Da Zhui* (GV 14). For restlessness, needle *Yin Tang* (M-HN-3). For chronic otitis media and especially after repeated antibiotic usage, moxa *Shen Que* (CV 8) and needle *Zu San Li* (St 36).

Adjunctive treatments

Adjunctive treatments primarily means local treatments in or around the ear. For acute earaches, first one can use alternating hot and cold compresses on the side of the head of the affected ear. Begin with a hot compress to improve circulation and then apply a cold compress to clear heat. This can be repeated several times in a row and more than once in a day as needed. One can also use just a hot compress soaked in a decoction of 60g each of *Ju Hua* (Flos Chrysanthemi) and *Pu Gong Ying* (Herba Taraxaci). Secondly, one can use various applications to the inner ears themselves. The simplest is warm roasted sesame oil. One can also mash and heat several garlic cloves in sesame oil and then remove the cloves and use this garlic oil. Another possibility is to use warm peppermint oil. Or one can simply crush and express the juice from either garlic or fresh peppermint and use this as eardrops. A more complex heat-clearing ear oil is made by taking 10 grams each of *Huang Lian* (Rhizoma Coptidis), *Huang Bai* (Cortex Phellodendri), *Da Huang* (Radix Et Rhizoma Rhei), and *Zhi Zi* (Fructus Gardeniae) and cooking them in

100ml of sesame oil. Remove the dregs and then add four grams of *Bing Pian* (Borneol). Apply to the inner ear 2-3 times per day. Water-based eardrops for clearing heat and relieving pain can be made by mixing a small amount of *Peng Sha* (Borax), *Ming Fan* or *Ku Fan* (Alumen), and a pinch of *Bing Pian* (Borneol) in distilled water. Shake until all these have dissolved and use as eardrops several times per day. For chronic leakage from the ear in vacuity patterns, one can take nine grams of *Wu Bei Zi* (Galla Rhois) and three grams of *Bing Pian* (Borneol), grind into powder, and blow a little of this powder into the ear several times per day. One can also use some calcined *Long Gu* (Os Draconis) and *Ming Fan* (Alumen), powdered and blown into the ear.

Comments

There are at least two important problems with the above Chinese textbook discrimination of ear infections. First, it is very difficult to accurately identify an exterior pattern in very young infants and children, the patient population most likely to manifest ear infections. This is because they cannot answer questions about sore throat, aversion to cold, etc. Secondly, the liver fire pattern fails to take into account that this heat manifesting in the *shao yang* channels is transformed from food stagnation in the stomach and intestines. Further, it also does not take into account infant's inherently weak spleens which are easily damaged by excessively bitter, cold medicinals. Therefore, when it comes to otitis media in the West, it is my opinion a modified approach is necessary.

When I was studying pediatrics in China, several of my teachers asked one day what were the most commonly seen pediatric conditions in the United States. I unhesitatingly answered ear infections. The good doctors conferred for a moment amongst themselves and then turned to me to say that ear infections were not a very big problem in China. Some Western doctors tell parents that infants and toddlers are prone to ear infections because of the short distance between the nasal cavity and the eustachian canals which lead to the inner ear. Therefore, the thinking goes, germs can more easily travel from the nose to the ear in the very young. Well, I cannot believe that Chinese babies' eustachian canals are located that much further from the nasal cavity than Western babies'. So clearly something else must be at work in Western babies.

According to Chinese medicine, there is an internal pathway or connection between the stomach and intestines and the inner ear. If stagnant food accumulates in the stomach and intestines, this may give rise to transformative heat as described above. If there is fever associated with teething, this heat and the heat associated with the stagnant food may aggravate each other and counterflow upward over this pathway from the intestines to the inner ear. As we have seen, stagnant food in infants is ultimately due to their inherently immature and, therefore, weak spleens. Thus, it is no wonder that food stagnation may be aggravated when some children are given solid, *i.e.*, even more hard to digest, food for the first time. This also explains why Chinese children have less problems with ear infections than do Western children. Although there are plenty of things about Chinese culture I do not like, I have to say that their understanding of what is a healthy diet, both for infants and for adults, is way ahead of us in the West. Since teething is associated with increased heat in the body and since this is often the same general time when solid foods have been introduced, it is also no wonder that food stagnation tends to transform into depressive heat at this juncture of time.

If this heat condition is treated with antibiotics, the antibiotics do clear the heat, and the condition improves, at least temporarily. The problem is that antibiotics do nothing to help the food stagnation that is typically at the bottom of pediatric earaches and, in fact, contribute to its worsening. This is because antibiotics damage the spleen according to Chinese medical theory. They do this by wiping out all the healthy bacteria that are necessary for the stomach and intestines to function in a healthy, efficient manner. Since the net result of unnecessary or prolonged use of antibiotics is weakening of the spleen, it is easy to see that antibiotics perpetuate a cycle of recurrent inflammation due to food stagnation. Thus each round of antibiotics is followed by another ear infection until finally the parents and their physician don't know what to do besides putting tubes into the eardrums.

Before going any further with this discussion, let me say right here that I am not against all use of antibiotics. Antibiotics have and do save lives. They are a life-saver when they are truly necessary. The problem is that they are given before there is a life-threatening situation. Rather, I believe that antibiotics should be held in reserve as a part of a graduating and escalating series of responses. It is my opinion that one should first use safer, more benign, and admittedly less powerful treatments first. Because they are less powerful, they have less potential for unwanted side effects. So first one should use more benign methods like hot and cold compresses and/or Chinese herbal medicine, both taken orally and applied directly into the ear. If these do not achieve their intended effect and the condition is getting dangerously worse, *then* one can use antibiotics as a last resource.

The good news is that Chinese herbal medicine is very effective for both treating acute earaches as well as preventing recurrent earaches. What's even better, one usually does not need to do an elaborate Chinese medical pattern discrimination, since most infants and toddlers with earaches have the same pattern. The formula that I find most effective for acute episodes of recurrent earaches in children who have been previously treated with antibiotics is *Xiao Chai Hu Tang Jia Wei* (Minor Bupleurum Decoction with Added Flavors). Because it contains ingredients to fortify the spleen and supplement the qi, it is not as likely to damage the delicate spleens and stomachs of infants who already have inherently weak spleens and whose spleen may have been further damaged by antibiotic use.

Xiao Chai Hu Tang Jia Wei (Minor Bupleurum Decoction with Added Flavors)

Chai Hu (Radix Bupleuri)
Ren Shen (Radix Ginseng)
Huang Qin (Radix Scutellariae)
Ban Xia (Rhizoma Pinelliae)
mix-fried *Gan Cao* (Radix Glycyrrhizae)
Bai Zhi (Radix Angelicae Dahuricae)

Chuan Xiong (Rhizoma Chuanxiong)
Shi Chang Pu (Rhizoma Acori Tatarinowii)
Shan Zha (Fructus Crataegi)
Shen Qu (Massa Medica Fermentata)
Lian Qiao (Fructus Forsythiae)
Sheng Jiang (uncooked Rhizoma Zingiberis)
Da Zao (Fructus Jujubae)

This formula contains within it medicinals to strengthen the spleen, medicinals to eliminate dampness and stagnant food from the stomach and intestines, and medicinals to clear heat and inflammation. According to Chinese medical theory, these medicinals enter the channels of the stomach and intestines and the gallbladder. These are the channels that encircle and, therefore, treat the ear. If fever is severe, I add *Jin Yin Hua* (Flos Lonicerae), *Dan Zhu Ye* (Herba Lophateri), and even sometimes *Shi Gao* (Gypsum Fibrosum). If the ear is very red, I add *Chi Shao* (Radix Paeoniae Rubrae) and *Dan Pi* (Cortex Moutan).

After the acute phase is over, I then typically prescribe unmodified *Xiao Chai Hu Tang* for several months in order to continue supplementing the spleen, harmonizing the liver and spleen, clearing heat from the stomach and intestines and, therefore from the gallbladder channel locally in the region of the ear, and to transform food and disperse accumulation. At the same time, the baby or young child's diet needs to be regulated and, if they are eating solid foods, a clear, bland, hypoallergenic, yeast-free diet should be instituted. The following year, beginning in October, but before Halloween, I usually prescribe this same formula and continue it through April in order to prevent earaches, colds and flues, and tonsillitis.

When opting to use Chinese medicine, the parent is going to have to break the chain of antibiotic use. Commonly this means that the child will have another ear infection soon after the last antibiotics are finished. This is a crucial juncture. If the parent immediately seeks remedial treatment with their Chinese medical practitioner, be that a specially modified herbal prescription and eardrops, compresses, infant massage, and/or acupuncture, there is an extremely good chance that antibiotics will not be necessary. In other words, the parent is going to have to bite the bullet and not immediately run for the antibiotics. For some parents who have no previous experience with any other form of health care except modern Western medicine, this may be scary. However, if one immediately goes back to antibiotics, the cycle of repeated ear infections will only continue.

Because this is a potentially frightening position for parents to be in, they should discuss all this thoroughly with their Chinese medical practitioner so that each party knows what treatments will be given in what situations and when it is necessary and appropriate to use antibiotics.

When children are given antibiotics over and over again at a young age, it is my experience as a clinician that this can lead to many years if not a lifetime of chronic health problems. In my experience, such children are more prone than others to all sorts of allergies, including hay fever and allergic asthma. They are also more prone to sore throats and tonsillitis. Therefore, I cannot overstress how important it is, in my opinion and experience, not to use antibiotics when not truly necessary.

It is also probably a good idea *not* to have a nurse or MD look into a child's ears too often. Very often, Western medical personnel will decide that a child's ears look infected or on the verge of infection and will prescribe antibiotics when the child displays not a single sign or symptom of an earache other than through an otoscope. Most infants will cry when an otoscope is put in their ear and this crying will immediately turn the membrane of the ear red. Thus, so-called routine inspection of the ears can actually cause problems when there was no real problem to begin with. If a child has constantly bulging eardrums and the doctor says that there is fluid behind the ears and the child shows no other sign or symptom of an infection or inflammation, this can also be treated with Chinese herbal medicine. In this case, I typically prescribe *Wu Ling San Jia Wei* (Five [Ingredients] Poria Powder with Added Flavors) which seeps away excess fluids and fortifies the spleen, thus undercutting the root mechanisms of ear infections in infants and toddlers.

Wu Ling San Jia Wei (Five [Ingredients] Poria Powder with Added Flavors)

Fu Ling (Poria)
Zhu Ling (Polyporus)
Bai Zhu (Rhizoma Atractylodis Macrocephalae)
Ze Xie (Rhizoma Alismatis)
Gui Zhi (Ramulus Cinnamomi)
Shi Chang Pu (Rhizoma Acori Tatarinowii)
Bai Zhi (Radix Angelicae Dahuricae)
Chen Pi (Pericarpium Citri Reticulatae)

If the baby is prone to having recurrent earaches and there is a lot of earwax in the ears, this earwax is a sign of dampness and turbidity since, in Chinese medicine, the earwax is seen as a greasy, fatty substance. In that case, I usually prescribe *Er Chen Tang Jia Wei* (Two Aged [Ingredients] Decoction with Added Flavors).

Er Chen Tang Jia Wei (Two Aged [Ingredients] Decoction with Added Flavors)

Ban Xia (Rhizoma Pinelliae)
Fu Ling (Poria)
Chen Pi (Pericarpium Citri Reticulatae)
Gan Cao (Radix Glycyrrhizae)
Wu Mei (Fructus Mume)
Sheng Jiang (uncooked Rhizoma Zingiberis)
Shi Chang Pu (Rhizoma Acori Tatarinowii)
Bai Zhi (Radix Angelicae Dahuricae)
Shan Zha (Fructus Crataegi)

Shen Qu (Massa Medica Fermentata)

There are also times when an eardrum does burst. In some cases, the parent may not even have realized that their child was suffering from an earache until after they notice some fluids running from the opening of the ear. Actually, this is the final stage of an ear infection and when this occurs, it marks the resolution of the situation. If these fluids are mostly clear and watery and if they tend to continue without stopping as they should, then I generally prescribe *Huang Qi Jian Zhong Tang* (Astragalus Fortify the Center Decoction). This formula is designed to promote healing after infection and inflammation are no longer present. I believe this formula is much more appropriate and digestible for young infants than either *Zhi Bai Di Huang Wan* or the *Ba Zhen Tang* modifications mentioned above, unless, of course, the signs and symptoms of the case truly do warrant one of these.

Huang Qi Jian Zhong Tang (Astragalus Fortify the Center Decoction)
Yi Tang (Maltose)
Huang Qi (Radix Astragali)
Bai Shao (Radix Paeoniae Albae)
Gan Cao (Radix Glycyrrhizae)
Da Zao (Fructus Jujubae)
Gui Zhi (Ramulus Cinnamomi)
Sheng Jiang (uncooked Rhizoma Zingiberis)

Over the years, I have helped numerous patients and their young charges deal with both acute and chronic ear infections. I know that Chinese herbal medicine combined with a clear, bland diet and avoidance of sugar and antibiotics can prevent and cure ear infections. Feeding a child a clear, bland diet who has been accustomed to sugar and sweets, chilled fruit juices and cold cow's milk, peanut butter and jelly on bread, cheese and ice cream is no easy task. However, I can assure the reader that it will make a difference in the child's short- and long-term health. I really know this works.

If, in rare instances, an ear infection does progress to meningitis or encephalitis, their treatment is discussed under infantile convulsions above.

17. Cough (Common Colds & Bronchitis)

When children "catch" the common cold, they usually develop a cough. Cough is one of the most common of all pediatric complaints. Children's coughs often get worse at night. This means that the problem is brought to a head just when the parents are trying to get some much needed sleep. Thus children's coughs are very stressful for the whole family. I have had a lot of clinical experience in treating children's cough, and I feel quite confident in saying that Chinese medicine does a very good job in treating children's cough quickly and effectively and without side effects.

As with fever above, Chinese medicine divides coughs into two broad types — external and internal types. In my experience, however, most infants' coughs are of the internal type. One does not really see the external type until the child is older. This is because the internal patterns mostly have to do with poor spleen function and faulty diet. Therefore, in my practice, what I most often see in infants and toddlers is one of the internal patterns of cough.

Treatment based on pattern discrimination:

External invasion patterns

1. Wind cold assailing the lungs

Main symptoms: Mild fever, aversion to draft and chill, no perspiration, headache, nasal congestion, clear runny nose, sneezing, cough with thin, white or clear mucus, thin, white tongue fur, a floating, tight pulse

Treatment principles: Dispel wind and scatter cold, drain the lungs and stop coughing

Guiding formulas:
Jing Jie Bai Du San Jia Jian (Schizonepeta Vanquish Toxins Powder with Additions & Subtractions)
Chai Hu (Radix Bupleuri)
Qian Hu (Radix Peucedani)
Qiang Huo (Radix Et Rhizoma Notopterygii)
Du Huo (Radix Angelicae Pubescentis)
Jing Jie (Herba Schizonepetae)
Fang Feng (Radix Saposhnikoviae)
Jie Geng (Radix Platycodi)
Chuan Xiong (Rhizoma Chuanxiong)
Bo He (Herba Menthae Haplocalycis)
Fu Ling (Poria)
Gan Cao (Radix Glycyrrhizae)
Sheng Jiang (uncooked Rhizoma Zingiberis)

If there is no fever, omit *Chai Hu*, *Du Huo*, and *Qiang Huo*. If there is nasal congestion and runny nose, add *Xin Yi* (Flos Magnoliae) and *Cang Er Zi* (Fructus Xanthii).

Jing Jie Bai Du San Jia Jian (Schizonepeta Vanquish Toxins Powder with Additions & Subtractions)
Jing Jie (Herba Schizonepetae)
Fang Feng (Radix Saposhnikoviae)
Dan Dou Chi (Semen Praeparatus Sojae)
Zi Su Ye (Folium Perillae)

    Xing Ren (Semen Armeniacae)
    Qian Hu (Radix Peucedani)
    Niu Bang Zi (Fructus Arctii)
    Bo He (Herba Menthae Haplocalycis)
    Xin Yi (Flos Magnoliae)
    Gan Cao (Radix Glycyrrhizae)

If there is headache, add *Bai Zhi* (Radix Angelicae Dahuricae).

Xiao Qing Long Tang Jia Jian (Minor Blue-green Dragon Decoction with additions & subtractions)
    Gui Zhi (Ramulus Cinnamomi)
    Bai Shao (Radix Paeoniae Albae)
    Xi Xin (Herba Asari)
    Gan Jiang (dry Rhizoma Zingiberis)
    Ban Xia (Rhizoma Pinelliae)
    Xing Ren (Semen Armeniacae)
    Gan Cao (Radix Glycyrrhizae)

For a phlegmy sound when breathing, add *Zi Su Zi* (Fructus Perillae), *Bai Jie Zi* (Semen Sinapis), and *Lai Fu Zi* (Semen Raphani).

Xing Su San (Armeniaca & Perilla Powder)
    Zi Su Ye (Folium Perillae)
    Xing Ren (Semen Armeniacae)
    Qian Hu (Radix Peucedani)
    Jie Geng (Radix Platycodi)
    Gan Cao (Radix Glycyrrhizae)
    Chen Pi (Pericarpium Citri Reticulatae)
    Zhi Ke (Fructus Aurantii)
    Ban Xia (Rhizoma Pinelliae)
    Fu Ling (Poria)

Xing Su San Jia Jian (Armeniaca & Perilla Powder with Additions & Subtractions)
    Zi Su Ye (Folium Perillae)
    Xing Ren (Semen Armeniacae)
    Qian Hu (Radix Peucedani)
    Zhi Ke (Fructus Aurantii)
    Ban Xia (Rhizoma Pinelliae)
    Jie Geng (Radix Platycodi)
    Cong Bai (Herba Allii Fistulosi)
    Sheng Jiang (uncooked Rhizoma Zingiberis)

Xing Su San Jia Jian (Armeniaca & Perilla Powder with Additions & Subtractions)

Zi Su Ye (Folium Perillae)
Xing Ren (Semen Armeniacae)
Qian Hu (Radix Peucedani)
Jie Geng (Radix Platycodi)
Jing Jie (Herba Schizonepetae)
Ban Xia (Rhizoma Pinelliae)
Zhi Ke (Fructus Aurantii)
Gan Cao (Radix Glycyrrhizae)

For more serious cough, add *Ma Huang* (Herba Ephedrae). If the exterior symptoms have been relieved but cough persists, add *Zi Wan* (Radix Asteris), *Kuan Dong Hua* (Flos Farfarae), and *Bai Bu* (Radix Stemonae).

2. Wind heat assailing the lungs

Main symptoms: High fever, sweating but no reduction in the fever, yellow, sticky nasal mucus, sore throat, red throat, cough, thin, white or thin, yellow tongue fur with a red tongue tip, a floating, rapid pulse

Treatment principles: Dispel wind and clear heat, transform phlegm and stop coughing

Guiding formulas:
Sang Ju Yin Jia Jian (Morus & Chrysanthemum Beverage with Additions & Subtractions)

Sang Ye (Folium Mori)
Ju Hua (Flos Chrysanthemi)
Lian Qiao (Fructus Forsythiae)
Dan Dou Chi (Semen Praeparatus Sojae)
Bo He (Herba Menthae Haplocalycis)
Gan Cao (Radix Glycyrrhizae)
Lu Gen (Rhizoma Phragmitis)
Jie Geng (Radix Platycodi)
Ban Lan Gen (Radix Isatidis/Baphicacanthi)
Pu Gong Ying (Herba Taraxaci)

If there is profuse phlegm, add *Dong Gua Zi* (Semen Benincasae). If there is sore throat with a red tongue and yellow fur, add *Niu Bang Zi* (Fructus Arctii) and *Huang Qin* (Radix Scutellariae).

Sang Ju Yin Jia Jian (Morus & Chrysanthemum Beverage with Additions & Subtractions)

Sang Ye (Folium Mori)

Ju Hua (Flos Chrysanthemi)
Bo He (Herba Menthae Haplocalycis)
Xing Ren (Semen Armeniacae)
Jie Geng (Radix Platycodi)
Lu Gen (Rhizoma Phragmitis)
Lian Qiao (Fructus Forsythiae)
Bei Mu (Bulbus Fritillariae)
Huang Qin (Radix Scutellariae)

If there is high fever and a sore, swollen throat, add *Zhi Zi* (Fructus Gardeniae) and *Ban Lan Gen* (Radix Isatidis/Baphicacanthi). If there is productive cough with oral thirst, heart vexation, and slimy, yellow tongue fur, add *Sang Bai Pi* (Cortex Mori), *Ban Xia* (Rhizoma Pinelliae), and *Fu Ling* (Poria).

Unnamed formula
Lu Gen (Rhizoma Phragmitis)
Sang Ye (Folium Mori)
Ju Hua (Flos Chrysanthemi)
Lian Qiao (Fructus Forsythiae)
Da Qing Ye (Folium Daqingye)
Xing Ren (Semen Armeniacae)
Jie Geng (Radix Platycodi)
Huang Qin (Radix Scutellariae)
Bo He (Herba Menthae Haplocalycis)

Ma Xing Shi Gan Tang Jia Jian (Ephedra, Armeniaca, Gypsum, & Licorice Decoction with Additions & Subtractions)
Ma Huang (Herba Ephedrae)
Shi Gao (Gypsum Fibrosum)
Xing Ren (Semen Armeniacae)
Gan Cao (Radix Glycyrrhizae)
Huang Qin (Radix Scutellariae)
Lian Qiao (Fructus Forsythiae)
Lu Gen (Rhizoma Phragmitis)
Jie Geng (Radix Platycodi)

If phlegm is profuse, add *Hai Ge Ke* (Concha Cyclinae/Meretricis), *Dan Nan Xing* (bile-processed Rhizoma Arisaematis), *Dong Gua Zi* (Semen Benincasae), and *Hai Fu Shi* (Pumice). If phlegm is profuse and there are dry stools, add *Sang Bai Pi* (Cortex Mori), *Ting Li Zi* (Semen Lepidii/Descurainiae), and whole *Quan Gua Lou* (Fructus Trichosanthis).

Qing Fei Yin (Clear the Lungs Beverage)
Jing Jie (Herba Schizonepetae)
Qian Hu (Radix Peucedani)

Huang Qin (Radix Scutellariae)
Bai Bu (Radix Stemonae)
Ban Lan Gen (Radix Isatidis/Baphicacanthi)
Lian Qiao (Fructus Forsythiae)
Sang Bai Pi (Cortex Mori)
Bei Mu (Bulbus Fritillariae)
Chen Pi (Pericarpium Citri Reticulatae)
Ban Xia (Rhizoma Pinelliae)
Gan Cao (Radix Glycyrrhizae)
Zhi Mu (Rhizoma Anemarrhenae)

For constipation, add uncooked *Da Huang* (Radix Et Rhizoma Rhei).

3. Wind dryness assailing the lungs

Main symptoms: Cough with little or no phlegm, a dry, sore throat, dry nose and mouth, chapped lips, a red tongue with scanty, dryish fur, a floating, fine, rapid pulse

Treatment principles: Clear heat and moisten dryness, dispel wind and stop coughing

Guiding formulas:
Unnamed formula
Bei Sha Shen (Radix Glehniae)
Sang Ye (Folium Mori)
Sang Bai Pi (Cortex Mori)
Xing Ren (Semen Armeniacae)
Di Gu Pi (Cortex Lycii)
Pi Pa Ye (Folium Eriobotryae)
Chuan Bei Mu (Bulbus Fritillariae Cirrhosae)
Mai Men Dong (Tuber Ophiopogonis)
Sheng Di (uncooked Radix Rehmanniae)
Dan Dou Chi (Semen Praeparatus Sojae)

Sang Xing Tang Jia Wei (Morus & Armeniaca Decoction with Added Flavors)
Sang Ye (Folium Mori)
Xing Ren (Semen Armeniacae)
Zhi Zi (Fructus Gardeniae)
Dan Dou Chi (Semen Praeparatus Sojae)
Zhe Bei Mu (Bulbus Fritillariae Thunbergii)
Li Pi (Exocarpium Pyri)
Bei Sha Shen (Radix Glehniae)
Mai Men Dong (Tuber Ophiopogonis)

Internal damage patterns

1. Food damage

Main symptoms: Cough with profuse phlegm, no thought for eating or drinking, foul-smelling breath, abdominal distention and fullness, untransformed grains in the stools, restlessness when lying down at night, possible red tongue and lips with thick, white fur, a deep, slippery pulse or a deep, stagnant looking vein at the wind bar

Treatment principles: Disperse accumulation, transform food, and stop coughing

Guiding formula:
Bao He Wan Jia Jian (Protect Harmony Pills with Additions & Subtractions)
  Shen Qu (Massa Medica Fermentata)
  Mai Ya (Fructus Germinatus Hordei)
  Chen Pi (Pericarpium Citri Reticulatae)
  Ban Xia (Rhizoma Pinelliae)
  Fu Ling (Poria)
  Gan Cao (Radix Glycyrrhizae)
  Qing Dai (Pulvis Indigonis)
  Hou Po (Cortex Magnoliae)
  Lai Fu Zi (Semen Raphani)

2. Heat accumulating in the lungs & stomach

Main symptoms: Cough with profuse yellow, sticky phlegm, possible vomiting of sticky phlegm, red face, hot hands and feet, irritability, poor sleep, kicking off of the covers at night, dry or greenish, loose stools, reduced, yellow urine, red tongue edges with thick, yellow fur, a floating, rapid pulse

Note: This pattern is a food damage pattern but with more depressive heat than the first internal damage pattern above.

Treatment principles: Clear heat from the lungs and stomach, transform food and stop coughing

Guiding formula:
Unnamed formula
  Shan Zha (Fructus Crataegi)
  Zhi Zi (Fructus Gardeniae)
  Huang Lian (Rhizoma Coptidis)
  Lai Fu Zi (Semen Raphani)
  Sang Bai Pi (Cortex Mori)
  Huang Qin (Radix Scutellariae)
  Zi Su Zi (Fructus Perillae)

Xing Ren (Semen Armeniacae)
Zhi Ke (Fructus Aurantii)

3. Phlegm heat accumulating in the lungs

Main symptoms: Cough, white or yellow, sticky phlegm, possible severe, paroxysmal cough, possible high fever, thick, white tongue fur, a red tongue tip and edge, a slippery rapid pulse

Treatment principles: Clear heat, transform phlegm, and stop coughing

Guiding formulas:
Xie Bai San Jia Jian (Drain the White Powder with Additions & Subtractions)
Sang Bai Pi (Cortex Mori)
Di Gu Pi (Cortex Lycii)
Jie Geng (Radix Platycodi)
Zhe Bei Mu (Bulbus Fritillariae Thunbergii)
Huang Qin (Radix Scutellariae)
Ting Li Zi (Semen Lepidii/Descurainiae)
Che Qian Zi (Semen Plantaginis)
Gan Cao (Radix Glycyrrhizae)

If there is cough with hard to expectorate, sticky phlegm, add whole *Quan Gua Lou* (Fructus Trichosanthis) and *Dan Nan Xing* (bile-processed Rhizoma Arisaematis). If there is simultaneous constipation with high fever and rough breathing, add *Bing Lang* (Semen Arecae), *Zhi Shi* (Fructus Immaturus Aurantii), and *Da Huang* (Radix Et Rhizoma Rhei).

Qing Jin Ding Sou Tang (Clear Metal & Calm Coughing Decoction)
Ju Hong (Exocarpium Citri Rubri)
Qian Hu (Radix Peucedani)
Xing Ren (Semen Armeniacae)
Sang Bai Pi (Cortex Mori)
Huang Lian (Rhizoma Coptidis)
Gua Lou (Fructus Trichosanthis)
Jie Geng (Radix Platycodi)
Bei Mu (Bulbus Fritillariae)
Da Zao (Fructus Jujubae)
Sheng Jiang (uncooked Rhizoma Zingiberis)

Unnamed formula
Hai Fu Shi (uncooked Pumice)
Hai Ge Ke (Concha Cyclinae/Meretricis)
Sang Bai Pi (Cortex Mori)
Pi Pa Ye (Folium Eriobotryae)

Bai Bu (Radix Stemonae)
Zi Su Zi (Fructus Perillae)
Xing Ren (Semen Armeniacae)
Huang Qin (Radix Scutellariae)

Wei Jing Tang Jia Wei (Reed Decoction with Added Flavors)
Lu Gen (Rhizoma Phragmitis)
Yi Yi Ren (Semen Coicis)
Dong Gua Ren (Semen Benincasae)
Jie Geng (Radix Platycodi)
Bei Mu (Bulbus Fritillariae)
Yu Xing Cao (Herba Hedyotis Diffusae)
Huang Qin (Radix Scutellariae)
Sang Bai Pi (Cortex Mori)
Xing Ren (Semen Armeniacae)

Unnamed formula
Pi Pa Ye (Folium Eriobotryae)
Dan Dou Chi (Semen Praeparatus Sojae)
Yu Jin (Tuber Curcumae)
Tong Cao (Medulla Tetrapanacis)
She Gan (Rhizoma Belamcandae)
Ban Xia (Rhizoma Pinelliae)

Unnamed formula
Lu Gen (Rhizoma Phragmitis)
Yi Yi Ren (Semen Coicis)
Tao Ren (Semen Persicae)
Dong Gua Ren (Semen Benincasae)
Hua Shi (Talcum)
Xing Ren (Semen Armeniacae)
Pi Pa Ye (Folium Eriobotryae)
Yu Jin (Tuber Curcumae)
Tong Cao (Medulla Tetrapanacis)
Dan Dou Chi (Semen Praeparatus Sojae)

4. Phlegm dampness

Main symptoms: Cough with white, thin, profuse phlegm, the sound of phlegm rattling in the throat when breathing, loss of appetite, lassitude of the spirit, a pale facial complexion, white, slimy tongue fur, a slippery pulse

> **Note:** While this pattern shares some food stagnation symptoms with the first internal damage pattern above, the emphasis in this pattern is on the excessive phlegm and dampness and there are no signs of evil heat.

Treatment principles: Arouse the spleen and dry dampness, transform phlegm and stop coughing

Guiding formulas:
Er Chen Tang Jia Wei (Two Aged [Ingredients] Decoction with Added Flavors)
Fu Ling (Poria)
Ban Xia (Rhizoma Pinelliae)
Chen Pi (Pericarpium Citri Reticulatae)
Xing Ren (Semen Armeniacae)
Jie Geng (Radix Platycodi)
Bei Mu (Bulbus Fritillariae)
Zhi Ke (Fructus Aurantii)
Lai Fu Zi (Semen Raphani)
Zi Su Zi (Fructus Perillae)
Gan Cao (Radix Glycyrrhizae)

Su Zi Jiang Qi Tang (Perilla Downbear the Qi Decoction)
Zi Su Zi (Fructus Perillae)
Ban Xia (Rhizoma Pinelliae)
mix-fried *Gan Cao* (Radix Glycyrrhizae)
Dang Gui (Radix Angelicae Sinensis)
Rou Gui (Cortex Cinnamomi)
Ju Hong (Exocarpium Citri Erythrocarpae)
Qian Hu (Radix Peucedani)
Hou Po (Cortex Magnoliae)

If coughing is severe, add *Gan Jiang* (dry Rhizoma Zingiberis) and *Wu Wei Zi* (Fructus Schisandrae). If spleen vacuity and dampness are severe, add *Fu Ling* (Poria) and *Dong Gua Zi* (Semen Benincasae).

If there is more spleen vacuity with dampness and a minor element of heat, one can use
Jian Pi Hua Tan Tang (Fortify the Spleen & Transform Phlegm Decoction):
Dang Shen (Radix Codonopsitis)
Ban Xia (Rhizoma Pinelliae)
Fu Ling (Poria)
Gan Cao (Radix Glycyrrhizae)
Chen Pi (Pericarpium Citri Reticulatae)
Ban Xia (Rhizoma Pinelliae)
Jie Geng (Radix Platycodi)
Bai Jie Zi (Semen Sinapis)
Zi Su Zi (Fructus Perillae)
Bei Mu (Bulbus Fritillariae)

Gua Lou Pi (Pericarpium Trichosanthis)
Huang Qin (Radix Scutellariae)
Sheng Jiang (uncooked Rhizoma Zingiberis)

5. Spleen dampness, lung heat

Main symptoms: Cough with profuse, white phlegm, heavy breathing, chest oppression, turbid runny nose, excessive sweating, poor appetite, flaccid muscles, a pale facial complexion, possible eczema, loose stools, a desire for cold drinks, a pale tongue with wet, white, slimy fur, a soft, slippery pulse

Treatment principles: Regulate the spleen and eliminate dampness, clear the lungs and stop coughing

Guiding formula:
Er Chen Tang Jia Wei (Two Aged [Ingredients] Decoction with Added Flavors)
Fu Ling (Poria)
ginger-processed *Ban Xia* (Rhizoma Pinelliae)
Chen Pi (Pericarpium Citri Reticulatae)
Zi Su Zi (Fructus Perillae)
Sang Bai Pi (Cortex Mori)
Huang Qin (Radix Scutellariae)
Xing Ren (Semen Armeniacae)
Hai Ge Ke (Concha Cyclinae/ Meretricis)
Hai Fu Shi (Pumice)

6. Phlegm heat damaging yin

Main symptoms: Enduring cough with little or no phlegm which is more severe at night, possible blood-streaked phlegm, a dry throat, red cheeks or flushed face in the late afternoon and evening, heat in the hands, feet, and heart, a red tongue with scanty fluids and fur, a fine, rapid pulse

Treatment principles: Enrich yin and moisten the lungs, cool the blood and stop coughing

Guiding formulas:
Sha Shen Mai Dong Tang Jia Jian (Glehnia & Ophiopogon Decoction with Additions & Subtractions)
Bei Sha Shen (Radix Glehniae)
Mai Men Dong (Tuber Ophiopogonis)
Yu Zhu (Rhizoma Polygonati Odorati)
Tian Hua Fen (Radix Trichosanthis)

Chuan Bei Mu (Bulbus Fritillariae Cirrhosae)
Pi Pa Ye (Folium Eriobotryae)
Bai Bian Dou (Semen Dolichoris)
Gan Cao (Radix Glycyrrhizae)

If there is blood-streaked phlegm, add *Bai Ji* (Rhizoma Bletillae), *Bai Mao Gen* (Rhizoma Imperatae), *E Jiao* (Gelatinum Corii Asini), and *Sheng Di* (uncooked Radix Rehmanniae). If there is tidal fever and night sweats, add *Qing Hao* (Herba Artemisiae Annuae), *Di Gu Pi* (Cortex Lycii), and *Bie Jia* (Carapax Trionycis).

Unnamed formula

Bei Sha Shen (Radix Glehniae)
Bai Mao Gen (Rhizoma Imperatae)
Bai Bu (Radix Stemonae)
Zi Su Zi (Fructus Perillae)
Sang Bai Pi (Cortex Mori)
Huang Qin (Radix Scutellariae)
Xing Ren (Semen Armeniacae)
Mai Men Dong (Tuber Ophiopogonis)
Wu Wei Zi (Fructus Schisandrae)

Unnamed formula

Shi Gao (Gypsum Fibrosum)
Mai Men Dong (Tuber Ophiopogonis)
Huo Ma Ren (Semen Cannabis)
Gan Cao (Radix Glycyrrhizae)
Dang Shen (Radix Codonopsitis)
Xing Ren (Semen Armeniacae)
Pi Pa Ye (Folium Eriobotryae)
E Jiao (Gelatinum Corii Asini)

7. Lung qi vacuity

Main symptoms: Weak but enduring cough with thin, white mucus, shortness of breath and wheezing, lassitude of the spirit, lack of strength, disinclination to speak, spontaneous perspiration, easily catches cold, a pale facial complexion, a pale tongue with thin, white fur, a deep, weak pulse

> **Note:** Although a number of Chinese pediatric texts list this pattern, I have never seen it in clinical practice due to the fact that, in most cases, there is concomitant spleen vacuity and/or kidney vacuity.

Treatment principles: Supplement and boost the lung qi, transform phlegm and stop coughing

***Guiding formulas: Gui Zhi Tang* (Cinnamon Twig Decoction) plus *Ren Shen Wu Wei Zi Tang* (Ginseng & Schisandra Decoction)**

Gui Zhi (Ramulus Cinnamomi)
Bai Shao (Radix Paeoniae Albae)
Gan Cao (Radix Glycyrrhizae)
Sheng Jiang (uncooked Rhizoma Zingiberis)
Da Zao (Fructus Jujubae)
Ren Shen (Radix Ginseng)
Bai Zhu (Rhizoma Atractylodis Macrocephalae)
Fu Ling (Poria)
Wu Wei Zi (Fructus Schisandrae)
Mai Men Dong (Tuber Ophiopogonis)

Unnamed formula

Huang Qi (Radix Astragali)
Dang Shen (Radix Codonopsitis)
Zi Wan (Radix Asteris)
Kuan Dong Hua (Flos Farfarae)
Wu Wei Zi (Fructus Schisandrae)
Xing Ren (Semen Armeniacae)
Zi He Che (Placenta Hominis)

At least one Chinese text lists **Su Zi Jiang Qi Tang (Perilla Downbear the Qi Decoction)** as a prescription appropriate for this pattern, and, in my opinion, it might also be used under lung-kidney vacuity as well. The first formula listed above might also be listed under lung-spleen vacuity, while the second formula could be seen also under lung-kidney vacuity.

8. Lung/spleen dual vacuity

Main symptoms: Cough, dyspnea, and wheezing with thin, white phlegm, easily catches cold, diminished appetite, fatigue, lack of strength, excessive sweating, possible loose stools, a pale, fat tongue with the indentations of the teeth on its edges, slimy, white tongue fur, a deep, relaxed, *i.e.*, slightly slow, pulse

Treatment principles: Supplement the lungs and boost the spleen

Guiding formulas:
***Si Jun Zi Tang Jia Wei* (Four Gentlemen Decoction with Added Flavors)**

Ren Shen (Radix Ginseng)
Bai Zhu (Rhizoma Atractylodis Macrocephalae)
Fu Ling (Poria)
mix-fried *Gan Cao* (Radix Glycyrrhizae)

Mai Men Dong (Tuber Ophiopogonis)
Wu Wei Zi (Fructus Schisandrae)

Liu Jun Zi Tang Jia Jian (Six Gentlemen Decoction with Additions & Subtractions)
Tai Zi Shen (Radix Pseudostellariae)
Fu Ling (Poria)
Bai Zhu (Rhizoma Atractylodis Macrocephalae)
Ban Xia (Rhizoma Pinelliae)
Wu Wei Zi (Fructus Schisandrae)
Huang Qi (Radix Astragali)
Jie Geng (Radix Platycodi)
Gan Cao (Radix Glycyrrhizae)

Liu Jun Zi Tang (Six Gentlemen Decoction) plus *Ping Wei San* (Level the Stomach Powder)
Dang Shen (Radix Codonopsitis)
Bai Zhu (Rhizoma Atractylodis Macrocephalae)
Fu Ling (Poria)
Gan Cao (Radix Glycyrrhizae)
Ban Xia (Rhizoma Pinelliae)
Chen Pi (Pericarpium Citri Reticulatae)
Cang Zhu (Rhizoma Atractylodis)
Hou Po (Cortex Magnoliae)
Da Zao (Fructus Jujubae)

9. Lung-kidney dual vacuity

Main symptoms: Enduring cough and wheezing with profuse, thin, white mucus, profuse sweating, shortness of breath, inability to breathe when lying down, wheezing provoked by movement, fear of cold, fatigue, lassitude of the spirit, cold hands and feet, copious, clear urination, a darkish, dull complexion, a pale tongue, a deep, fine or deep, weak pulse

Treatment principles: Supplement the lungs and boost the kidneys

Guiding formulas:
Unnamed formula
Tai Zi Shen (Radix Pseudostellariae)
Huang Qi (Radix Astragali)
Bai Guo (Semen Gingkonis)
Wu Wei Zi (Fructus Schisandrae)
Bu Gu Zhi (Fructus Psoraleae)
Hu Tao Ren (Semen Juglandis)
uncooked *Mu Li* (Concha Ostreae)

Kuan Dong Hua (Flos Farfarae)
Zi Wan (Radix Asteris)

Mai Wei Di Huang Wan (Ophiopogon & Schisandra Rehmannia Pills)
Mai Men Dong (Tuber Ophiopogonis)
Wu Wei Zi (Fructus Schisandrae)
Shu Di (cooked Radix Rehmanniae)
Shan Yao (Radix Dioscoreae)
Shan Zhu Yu (Fructus Corni)
Fu Ling (Poria)
Dan Pi (Cortex Moutan)
Ze Xie (Rhizoma Alismatis)

Wen Fei Zhi Ke Yin (Warm the Lungs & Stop Cough Beverage)
Fu Zi (Radix Lateralis Praeparatus Aconiti Carmichaeli)
Ma Huang (Herba Ephedrae)
Xi Xin (Herba Asari)
Jiang Can (Bombyx Batryticatus)
Di Long (Pheretima)
Jie Geng (Radix Platycodi)
Bai Bu (Radix Stemonae)
Chuan Bei Mu (Bulbus Fritillariae Cirrhosae)
Gan Cao (Radix Glycyrrhizae)
Xian Ling Pi (Herba Epimedii)

Do not use this formula is there is profuse sweating. It is good for chronic and enduring, spasmodic coughing and wheezing with pronounced cold symptoms.

Acupuncture & moxibustion

For exterior patterns, needle *Feng Men* (Bl 12), *Fei Shu* (Bl 13), *Lie Que* (Lu 7), and *He Gu* (LI 4). If there is wind cold, add moxibustion on the back transport points after needling. For wind heat, add *Chi Ze* (Lu 5). If there is fever add *Qu Chi* (LI 11) and *Da Zhui* (GV 14). As for internal damage patterns, needle *Fei Shu* (Bl 13), *He Gu* (LI 4), and *Nei Ting* (St 44) for food damage cough. If there is profuse phlegm, add *Feng Long* (St 40). If there is heat, add *Chi Ze* (Lu 5). If there is spleen vacuity, needle *Pi Shu* (Bl 20) and *Zu San Li* (St 36). If there is kidney vacuity, add *Shen Shu* (Bl 23). If there is cold phlegm, again moxa the back transport points associated with the lungs. If there is chest oppression, add *Nei Guan* (Per 6) and *Shan Zhong* (CV 17).

Adjunctive treatments

For all patterns of cough, one can seven star hammer the back transport points associated with the lungs. For exterior patterns, one can *gua sha* or cup the same area. For wind cold assailing the lungs, give a tea made out of scallions, fresh ginger, and blanched almonds.

For wind heat assailing the lungs, it is very important not to use a cold bath or cold sponge bath to try to bring down what can be a high fever. What is wanted in this case is for the pores of the skin to be open in order to allow the pathogens to be pushed back out of the body. The application of cold water in this pattern will only shut the pores and drive the evils even deeper into the body. A good home remedy is a tea made from peppermint and blanched almonds. For wind, heat, and dryness, use of a humidifier or an old-fashioned steam tent helps to moisten the dryness in the lungs.

In the case of the internal patterns of pediatric cough, emphasis should be placed on the child's diet. This is because "the spleen is the root of phlegm production, while the lungs are the place where phlegm is stored." One of the reasons children are so prone to coughs is because of their inherently weak spleen function. If there is food damage, simply reduce the amount of food or milk given and rub the abdomen. If there is spleen vacuity, be sure the child avoids any sugar or sweets, any dairy products, and anything cold, chilled, or raw. If there is stomach heat, the child should also avoid anything fried, fatty, greasy, or hot and spicy. A simple Chinese herbal home remedy for lung yin vacuity cough is to make a tea from watercress and blanched almonds. Watercress is cool, clears heat, and moistens the lungs, while almonds transform phlegm, moisten the intestines, and stop coughing. Another simple home remedy is to make a tea from figs, particularly fresh figs if available. Figs clear heat and moisten the lungs and intestines. The child may also eat fresh peaches or pears. If there is lung, spleen, and/or kidney vacuity, children should be fed a diet of cooked, warm, nutritious though nevertheless easily digested foods, such as soups, broths, and stews. In particular, *Yi Yi Ren* (Semen Coicis) is believed to be very beneficial to both the lungs and spleen. Spinal pinch-pull up the back can also increase basic health and resistance. A simple Chinese herbal home remedy for lung-kidney dual vacuity cough is to cook mulberries over a low flame down into a syrup with honey added. Then take 2 teaspoons of this syrup 2 times each day.

Comments

As the reader can see, in most of these internal cough patterns, the spleen and, therefore, diet play an important role. "The spleen is the root of phlegm production, while the lungs are where phlegm is stored." This two line verse is the key to diagnosing and treating pediatric cough in my experience. Children's cough can be prevented by feeding them a diet of primarily warm, cooked food which is not too greasy or fatty, not too hot and spicy, and not too much sugar and sweets. In particular, diary products tend to produce phlegm easily because of their very damp, wet nature. While chilled, frozen, cold foods and drinks easily damage children's fragile spleens and stomachs. So often do children "catch cold" or develop a cough after eating sugars and sweets and soda and ice cream that I routinely ask parents of children with coughs if their child has recently eaten those things. In the United States, I see a huge increase in children's coughs and colds directly after Halloween when children go "trick or treating" for shopping bags of candy and sweets. It is my experience that if parents can control and limit the amounts of sugar and sweets, most pediatric coughs can be prevented.

18. Whooping Cough

Whooping cough or pertussis is an acute, infectious, upper respiratory infection due, according to Western medicine, to the *Bordetella pertussis* bacteria. There is also a milder form of this disease caused by *Bordetella parapertussis*. This milder form is called parapertussis. Children under seven are most susceptible to pertussis, and it occurs more often in the late winter and early spring. Although most Western children are immunized against pertussis, because there is ongoing controversy over the safety and effectiveness of the pertussis vaccine, a substantial number of children are not vaccinated and there are cases of whooping cough in most Western communities. Whooping cough gets its name from the distinctive whooping sound at the end of a series of coughs. There are 5-15 coughs in a row followed by a hurried, deep inhalation or the whoop. These coughs are paroxysmal or spasmodic in nature. Chinese medicine calls whooping cough, *bai ri ke* or hundred day cough. This is because, if left untreated, it tends to persist for three months or 100 days. Whooping cough is a serious disease but it is not necessarily life-threatening. When babies under six months get pertussis, special care must be taken to prevent their inhaling their mucus and vomit and thus asphyxiating themselves. Otherwise, the danger of pertussis is that, *if not properly treated*, it can lead to pneumonia. However, if treated with professionally administered Chinese medicine, that should not happen.

According to Chinese medical theory, whooping cough occurs in children who already have an accumulation of phlegm in their body, and, as we have already seen, such an accumulation of phlegm is due to poor spleen function in turn due to or worsened by faulty diet. If such a child is invaded by an external pathogen, then this external invasion and the accumulation of phlegm already present mutually aggravate each other. Therefore, right away, parents should know that keeping their child's spleen function in healthy shape and keeping phlegm production to a minimum is one way to help prevent children from developing whooping cough.

Treatment based on pattern discrimination:

Chinese medicine approaches the treatment of pertussis by dividing the course of disease into three stages — the initial stage which typically lasts 7-10 days, the second or paroxysmal stage which lasts between 40-60 days, and the recovery or debility and decline stage which lasts between 20-30 days.

1. Initial stage

A. Cold & phlegm fettering the lungs

Main symptoms: Spasmodic cough with thin, watery phlegm, clear runny nose, slight fever and aversion to cold, white, slimy tongue fur, a floating tight pulse

Treatment principles: Warm the lungs and transform phlegm, rectify the qi and downbear counterflow

Guiding formulas:
Xiao Qing Long Tang Jia Wei (Minor Blue-green Dragon Decoction with Added Flavors)

Ma Huang (Herba Ephedrae)
Ban Xia (Rhizoma Pinelliae)
Bai Shao (Radix Paeoniae Albae)
Gui Zhi (Ramulus Cinnamomi)
Wu Wei Zi (Fructus Schisandrae)
Xi Xin (Herba Asari)
Gan Cao (Radix Glycyrrhizae)
Sheng Jiang (uncooked Rhizoma Zingiberis)
Bai Bu (Radix Stemonae)

If there is vomiting of phlegm after coughing, add *Xuan Fu Hua* (Flos Inulae). If there is profuse, sticky phlegm, add *Bai Jie Zi* (Semen Sinapis) and *Zhe Bei Mu* (Bulbus Fritillariae Thunbergii).

San Ao Tang Jia Wei (Three [Ingredients] for Twisting [i.e., Binding] Decoction with Added Flavors)

Ma Huang (Herba Ephedrae)
Xing Ren (Semen Armeniacae)
Gan Cao (Radix Glycyrrhizae)
mix-fried *Bai Bu* (Radix Stemonae)
Bai Qian (Rhizoma Cynanchi Stautoni)
Tian Zhu Zi (Fructus Nandinae Domesticae)

Jin Fu Hua San Jia Jian (Inula Powder with Additions & Subtractions)

Xuan Fu Hua (Flos Inulae)
Qian Hu (Radix Peucedani)
Bai Jie Zi (Semen Sinapis)
Xi Xin (Herba Asari)
mix-fried *Bai Bu* (Radix Stemonae)
Bei Mu (Bulbus Fritillariae)
Ban Xia (Rhizoma Pinelliae)

If there are deep, heavy sounding coughs with aversion to cold and no sweating, add *Ma Huang* (Herba Ephedrae) and *Xing Ren* (Semen Armeniacae). If there are signs and symptoms of wind heat, add *Sang Ye* (Folium Mori), *Ju Hua* (Flos Chrysanthemi), and *Lian Qiao* (Fructus Forsythiae).

Jin Fu Hua San Jia Jian (Inula Powder with Additions & Subtractions)

Xuan Fu Hua (Flos Inulae)
Qian Hu (Radix Peucedani)

Jing Jie (Herba Schizonepetae)
Jie Geng (Radix Platycodi)
Xing Ren (Semen Armeniacae)
Zhe Bei Mu (Bulbus Fritillariae Thunbergii)
Ban Xia (Rhizoma Pinelliae)
Ju Hong (Exocarpium Citri Erythrocarpae)
Fu Ling (Poria)
Bai Bu (Radix Stemonae)

Zhi Ke San Jia Wei (Stop Coughing Powder with Added Flavors)
Jing Jie (Herba Schizonepetae)
mix-fried *Bai Qian* (Radix Peucedani)
Jie Geng (Radix Platycodi)
Gan Cao (Radix Glycyrrhizae)
Huang Qin (Radix Scutellariae)
Ban Xia (Rhizoma Pinelliae)
Xing Ren (Semen Armeniacae)
Bai Jie Zi (Semen Sinapis)

Unnamed formula
Zi Su Ye (Folium Perillae)
Zhi Ke (Fructus Aurantii)
Yu Xing Cao (Herba Hedyotis Diffusae)
Jie Geng (Radix Platycodi)
Bai Qian (Radix Cynanchi Stautoni)
Jing Jie (Herba Schizonepetae)
Zi Wan (Radix Asteris)
Chen Pi (Pericarpium Citri Reticulatae)
Gan Cao (Radix Glycyrrhizae)
Bai Bu (Radix Stemonae)

B. Wind heat

Main symptoms: A heavy sounding cough which is worse at night and which gets worse with every passing day, fever, slight perspiration, oral thirst, possible yellow nasal mucus, possible sore throat, slight or no aversion to cold, thin, white or thin, yellow tongue fur, a floating, rapid pulse

Treatment principles: Clear heat and resolve the exterior, diffuse the lungs and stop coughing

Guiding formulas:
San Ju Yin Jia Jian (Morus & Chrysanthemum Beverage with Additions & Subtractions)
Sang Ye (Folium Mori)

Ju Hua (Flos Chrysanthemi)
　　Niu Bang Zi (Fructus Arctii)
　　Xing Ren (Semen Armeniacae)
　　Gan Cao (Radix Glycyrrhizae)
　　Jie Geng (Radix Platycodi)
　　Hai Ge Ke (Concha Cyclinae/Meretricis)
　　Qing Dai (Pulvis Indigonis)

Ma Xing Shi Gan Tang Jia Wei (Ephedra, Armeniaca, Gypsum & Licorice Decoction with Added Flavors)
　　Ma Huang (Herba Ephedrae)
　　Xing Ren (Semen Armeniacae)
　　Shi Gao (Gypsum Fibrosum)
　　Gan Cao (Radix Glycyrrhizae)
　　Zi Su Zi (Fructus Perillae)
　　Ting Li Zi (Semen Lepidii/Descurainiae)

2. Paroxysmal stage: phlegm attaching to the lungs

Main symptoms: Spasmodic cough with thicker, pastier phlegm which is not easily spit up, cough worse at night, a distinctive whooping sound at the end of a bout of coughing, possible blood-streaked phlegm, possible nosebleed, a dry mouth and tongue, thirst with a desire to drink water, dry tongue fur, a slippery, rapid pulse

Treatment principles: Clear heat and drain the lungs, transform phlegm and stop coughing

Guiding formulas:
Sang Bai Pi Tang (Morus Bark Decoction)
　　Sang Bai Pi (Cortex Mori)
　　Huang Qin (Radix Scutellariae)
　　Huang Lian (Rhizoma Coptidis)
　　Zhi Zi (Fructus Gardeniae)
　　Zi Su Zi (Fructus Perillae)
　　Xing Ren (Semen Armeniacae)
　　Chuan Bei Mu (Bulbus Fritillariae Cirrhosae)
　　Ting Li Zi (Semen Lepidii/Descurainiae)
　　mix-fried *Bai Bu* (Radix Stemonae)
　　Tian Zhu Zi (Fructus Nandinae Domesticae)

Su Ting Gun Tan Wan Jia Jian (Perilla & Descurainia Shift Phlegm Pills with Additions & Subtractions)
　　Zi Su Zi (Fructus Perillae)
　　Ting Li Zi (Semen Lepidii/Descurainiae)

Wu Wei Zi (Fructus Schisandrae)
Meng Shi (Lapis Chloriti)
Ju Hong (Exocarpium Citri Erythrocarpae)
Zhi Shi (Fructus Immaturus Aurantii)
Quan Gua Lou (Fructus Trichosanthis)
Da Zao (Fructus Jujubae)

If spasmodic cough is frequent and violent, add *Jiang Can* (Bombyx Batryticatus) and *Di Long* (Pheretima). If there is scanty phlegm and a red tongue with little fur, add *Nan Sha Shen* (Radix Adenophorae), *Tian Men Dong* (Tuber Asparagi), and *Mai Men Dong* (Tuber Ophiopogonis). If there is hemoptysis or other hemorrhaging, add *Bai Mao Gen* (Rhizoma Imperatae) and *Ce Bai Ye* (Cacumen Platycladi).

Er Dong Tang (Two Dongs Decoction)
Mai Men Dong (Tuber Ophiopogonis)
Tian Men Dong (Tuber Asparagi)
mix-fried *Bai Bu* (Radix Stemonae)
Gua Lou Ren (Semen Trichosanthis)
Sang Bai Pi (Cortex Mori)
Bei Mu (Bulbus Fritillariae)
Xing Ren (Semen Armeniacae)
Huang Qin (Radix Scutellariae)
Ban Xia (Rhizoma Pinelliae)
Gan Cao (Radix Glycyrrhizae)
Bai Tou Weng (Radix Pulsatillae)
Jie Geng (Radix Platycodi)
Ju Hong (Exocarpium Citri Erythrocarpae)

Unnamed formula
Mai Men Dong (Tuber Ophiopogonis)
Tian Men Dong (Tuber Asparagi)
Bai Bu (Radix Stemonae)
Ju Hong (Exocarpium Citri Erythrocarpae)
Ban Xia (Rhizoma Pinelliae)
Gua Lou (Fructus Trichosanthis)
Zhu Ru (Caulis Bambusae In Taeniis)
Pi Pa Ye (Folium Eriobotryae)
Chuan Bei Mu (Bulbus Fritillariae Cirrhosae)
Zi Wan (Radix Asteris)
Kuan Dong Hua (Flos Farfarae)
Yu Xing Cao (Herba Hedyotis Diffusae)
Qing Dai (Pulvis Indigonis)

If there is ejection of blood or hacking of blood, add *Zhi Zi* (Fructus Gardeniae), *Dan*

Pi (Cortex Moutan), and *Bai Mao Gen* (Rhizoma Imperatae). If there is edema of the eyelids, add *Fu Ling* (Poria) and *Sang Bai Pi* (Cortex Mori). If vomiting is severe, add *Bai Zhu* (Rhizoma Atractylodis Macrocephalae) and *Fu Ling* (Poria).

Jing Ke Ling (Spasmodic Cough Efficacious Remedy)
Huang Jing (Rhizoma Polygonati)
Bai Bu (Radix Stemonae)
Bei Sha Shen (Radix Glehniae)
Mai Men Dong (Tuber Ophiopogonis)
Zhi Shi (Fructus Immaturus Aurantii)
Zi Wan (Radix Asteris)
Gan Cao (Radix Glycyrrhizae)
Wu Gong (Scolopendra)

Kuan Dong Hua Tang (Coltsfoot Decoction)
Kuan Dong Hua (Flos Farfarae)
Sang Bai Pi (Cortex Mori)
Wu Mei (Fructus Mume)
Fu Ling (Poria)
Xing Ren (Semen Armeniacae)
Zi Wan (Radix Asteris)
Chuan Bei Mu (Bulbus Fritillariae Cirrhosae)
Wu Wei Zi (Fructus Schisandrae)
Bai He (Bulbus Lilii)
E Jiao (Gelatinum Corii Asini)
Bai Bu (Radix Stemonae)

Zhi Jing Er Chen Tang (Stop Tetany Two Aged [Ingredients] Decoction)
Quan Xie (Scorpio)
Wu Gong (Scolopendra)
Chen Pi (Pericarpium Citri Reticulatae)
Ban Xia (Rhizoma Pinelliae)
Gan Cao (Radix Glycyrrhizae)
Fu Ling (Poria)

If there is phlegm heat, add *Zhu Ru* (Caulis Bambusae In Taeniis), *Chuan Bei Mu* (Bulbus Fritillariae Cirrhosae), and *Gua Lou* (Fructus Trichosanthis). If there is enduring cough which has damaged yin, add *Bei Sha Shen* (Radix Glehniae), *Lu Gen* (Rhizoma Phragmitis), and *Yu Zhu* (Rhizoma Polygonati Odorati). If there is torpid intake, diminished eating, and thick tongue fur, add stir-fried *Lai Fu Zi* (Semen Raphani) and *Xing Ren* (Semen Armeniacae). If spasmodic cough is severe, add *Chan Yi* (Periostracum Cicadae) and *Jiang Can* (Bombyx Batryticatus). If there is nosebleeding, add *Bai Mao Gen* (Rhizoma Imperatae) and *Zhi Zi* (Fructus Gardeniae).

3. Decline & debility stage
A. Lung-spleen qi vacuity

Main symptoms: Diminished coughing, weak voice, disinclination to speak, scanty, watery phlegm, spontaneous perspiration, lack of strength, lassitude and fatigue of the essence spirit, reduced appetite, abdominal distention after eating, loose stools, a white facial complexion, a pale tongue with white fur, a deep, forceless pulse

Treatment principles: Mainly nourish the lungs and supplement the spleen, assisted by clearing remaining evils

Guiding formulas:
Ren Shen Wu Wei Zi Tang (Ginseng & Schisandra Decoction)
Ren Shen (Radix Ginseng)
Wu Wei Zi (Fructus Schisandrae)
Bai Zhu (Rhizoma Atractylodis Macrocephalae)
Fu Ling (Poria)
Gan Cao (Radix Glycyrrhizae)
Mai Men Dong (Tuber Ophiopogonis)
Chen Pi (Pericarpium Citri Reticulatae)
Ban Xia (Rhizoma Pinelliae)

Ren Shen Wu Wei Zi Tang Jia Jian (Ginseng & Schisandra Decoction with Additions & Subtractions)
Ren Shen (Radix Ginseng)
Wu Wei Zi (Fructus Schisandrae)
Bai Zhu (Rhizoma Atractylodis Macrocephalae)
Fu Ling (Poria)
Gan Cao (Radix Glycyrrhizae)
Chen Pi (Pericarpium Citri Reticulatae)
Chuan Bei Mu (Bulbus Fritillariae Cirrhosae)
Xing Ren (Semen Armeniacae)
Yin Guo (Semen Ginkgonis)

B. Lung-kidney yin vacuity

Main symptoms: Cough with no phlegm, tidal fever, night sweats, possible occasional vexation and agitation, a dry throat, heat in the hands, feet, and heart, restless sleep at night, red cheeks, dry lips, a red tongue with scanty fur, a fine, rapid pulse

Treatment principles: Enrich yin and moisten the lungs

Guiding formulas:
Mai Men Dong Tang Jia Jian (Ophiopogon Decoction with Additions & Subtractions)
Mai Men Dong (Tuber Ophiopogonis)

Bei Sha Shen (Radix Glehniae)
Sheng Di (uncooked Radix Rehmanniae)
Di Gu Pi (Cortex Lycii)
Bai Shao (Radix Paeoniae Albae)
Huang Jing (Rhizoma Polygonati)
Tian Men Dong (Tuber Asparagi)
Gan Cao (Radix Glycyrrhizae)
Geng Mi (Semen Oryzae)

Qing Zao Jiu Fei Tang Jia Jian (Clear Dryness & Rescue the Lungs Decoction with Additions & Subtractions)

Nan Sha Shen (Radix Adenophorae)
Da Jiao Ye (Folium Musae)
Xing Ren (Semen Armeniacae)
Mai Men Dong (Tuber Ophiopogonis)
Tian Men Dong (Tuber Asparagi)
Jie Geng (Radix Platycodi)
Hei Zhi Ma (black Semen Sesami)
E Jiao (Gelatinum Corii Asini)
Da Zao (Fructus Jujubae)

Unnamed formula

Gan Cao (Radix Glycyrrhizae)
Yu Zhu (Rhizoma Polygonati Odorati)
Mai Men Dong (Tuber Ophiopogonis)
Bei Sha Shen (Radix Glehniae)
Bia Bian Dou (Semen Dolichoris)
Sang Ye (Folium Mori)
Tian Hua Fen (Radix Trichosanthis)
Bai He (Bulbus Lilii)
Wu Mei (Fructus Mume)

Acupuncture & moxibustion

During the initial stage, needle *Feng Men* (Bl 12), *Fei Shu* (Bl 13), and *Lie Que* (Lu 7). During the spasmodic cough stage, needle *Chi Ze* (Lu 5), *Fei Shu* (Bl 13), and *He Gu* (LI 4). During the later stage when there is bodily vacuity and debility, add *Qi Hai* (CV 6), *Zu San Li* (St 36), and *San Yin Jiao* (Sp 6).

Adjunctive treatments

A simple Chinese herbal home remedy for whooping cough during the spasmodic stage is to boil 15 fresh marigold flower heads in water, mix with a little brown sugar, and drink. Children with lung-spleen qi vacuity obviously need rest and a cooked, warm, nourishing, clear, bland diet. They should not be allowed to eat sugar and sweets or raw, chilled, cold, frozen foods and drinks. Daily administration of spinal pinch-pull massage up the spine several times a day can also strengthen the body and its recuperative powers. For all stages of whooping cough, one can seven star hammer the back transport points associated with the lungs or cup *Shen Zhu* (GV 12) once a day. Other simple Chinese herbal home remedies for whooping cough are cooking carrots and red dates (available at Oriental specialty food shops and Chinese apothecaries) into a soup, steaming a lemon with sugar and eating it every morning for whooping cough with excessive phlegm and taking 2 teaspoons of a 10-20% garlic solution every two hours. Liquid garlic is available at Western health food stores.

Comments

It is interesting to note that Chinese doctors have recently begun adding ingredients to formulas for whooping cough from the antispasmodic category of Chinese medicinals. These are ingredients which are usually used for convulsions, tremors, and paralysis and are not usually thought of for coughs and lung problems. However, modern Chinese doctors have noticed the spasmodic nature of the cough in whooping cough and have added these antispasmodic ingredients on that basis. These ingredients seem to make formulas for pertussis more effective.

19. Pediatric Pneumonia

Pneumonia in children typically occurs in children under two years of age, and it usually occurs in the winter and spring. The general symptoms of pneumonia are fever, a productive cough, shortness of breath, flaring of the wings of the nose when breathing, and cyanotic, *i.e.*, bluish/purplish, lips. Pneumonia, as opposed to bronchitis or bronchial asthma, is diagnosed by the particular crackling, bubbly sounds in the lungs when listened to with a stethoscope and by x-rays showing a cloudy patch on the lungs. In other words, a diagnosis of pneumonia can only be made by a Western MD. There is no traditional Chinese disease category corresponding to pneumonia. Traditionally, it is treated according to the presenting pattern under the heading of cough.

Pneumonia may be due to direct infection by *Streptococcus pneumoniae* or may be a development from some already existing upper respiratory tract infection which either has not been treated in a timely manner or has not been treated correctly. For instance, pneumonia may result as a complication of measles or whooping cough.

Treatment based on pattern discrimination:

1. Wind cold

Main symptoms: Slight fever with no perspiration, aversion to cold, cough, shortness of breath, no particular thirst, thin, white phlegm, thin, white or white, slimy tongue fur, and a floating, tight pulse

Treatment principles: Resolve the exterior with acrid, warm medicinals, diffuse the lungs and transform phlegm

Guiding formulas:
San Ao Tang Jia Wei (Three [Ingredients] for Twisting Decoction with Added Flavors)
Ma Huang (Herba Ephedrae)
Xing Ren (Semen Armeniacae)
Gan Cao (Radix Glycyrrhizae)
Zi Su Zi (Fructus Perillae)
Lai Fu Zi (Semen Raphani)
Bai Jie Zi (Semen Sinapis)
Chen Pi (Pericarpium Citri Reticulatae)
Ban Xia (Rhizoma Pinelliae)

San Ao Tang Jia Wei (Three [Ingredients] for Twisting Decoction with Added Flavors)
Ma Huang (Herba Ephedrae)
Xing Ren (Semen Armeniacae)
Gan Cao (Radix Glycyrrhizae)
Zi Su Zi (Fructus Perillae)
Qian Hu (Radix Peucedani)
Ban Xia (Rhizoma Pinelliae)

Hua Gai San Jia Jian (Florid Canopy Powder with Additions & Subtractions)
Ma Huang (Herba Ephedrae)
Xing Ren (Semen Armeniacae)
Zi Su Zi (Fructus Perillae)
Chen Pi (Pericarpium Citri Reticulatae)
Ban Xia (Rhizoma Pinelliae)
Fu Ling (Poria)
Kuan Dong Hua (Flos Farfarae)
Sheng Jiang (uncooked Rhizoma Zingiberis)

If there is profuse, white phlegm, add *Lai Fu Zi* (Semen Raphani) and *Bai Jie Zi* (Semen Sinapis). If there is counterflow chilling of the four limbs with white, slimy tongue fur, add *Fu Zi* (Radix Lateralis Praeparatus Aconiti Carmichaeli) and *Xi Xin* (Herba Asari).

If there is aversion to cold, fever, and no sweating at the same time that there is vexation and agitation, oral thirst, and a red tongue with thin, white fur, this is wind cold with depressive heat in the interior. For this, use **Da Qing Long Tang Jia Wei (Major Blue-green Dragon Decoction with Added Flavors):**
Ma Huang (Herba Ephedrae)

Gui Zhi (Ramulus Cinnamomi)
Sheng Jiang (uncooked Rhizoma Zingiberis)
Xing Ren (Semen Armeniacae)
Gan Cao (Radix Glycyrrhizae)
Shi Gao (Gypsum Fibrosum)
Sang Bai Pi (Cortex Mori)
Lu Gen (Rhizoma Phragmitis)
Zhu Ru (Caulis Bambusae In Taeniis)

Yin Guo San (Ginkgo Powder)
Bai Guo (Semen Ginkgonis)
Xing Ren (Semen Armeniacae)
Xiao Hui Xiang (Fructus Foeniculi)
Ma Huang (Herba Ephedrae)

If there is simultaneous lung qi vacuity and wind cold damage with fever, aversion to cold, wheezing, and shortness of breath, use the following unnamed formula:
Zi Su Zi (Fructus Perillae)
Xing Ren (Semen Armeniacae)
Chen Pi (Pericarpium Citri Reticulatae)
Qian Hu (Radix Peucedani)
Ban Xia (Rhizoma Pinelliae)
Gan Cao (Radix Glycyrrhizae)
Sang Bai Pi (Cortex Radici Mori)
Qing Pi (Pericarpium Citri Reticulatae Viride)
Dang Shen (Radix Codonopsitis)
Ma Huang (Herba Ephedrae)
Sheng Jiang (uncooked Rhizoma Zingiberis)

2. Wind heat

Main symptoms: Fever with sweating or at least slight sweating, thirst, cough with sticky, yellow phlegm, a red tongue with thin, yellow fur, a floating, slippery, rapid pulse

Treatment principles: Dispel wind and clear heat, diffuse the lungs and transform phlegm

Guiding formulas:
Ma Xing Shi Gan Tang Jia Wei (Ephedra, Armeniaca, Gypsum & Licorice Decoction with Added Flavors)
Ma Huang (Herba Ephedrae)
Xing Ren (Semen Armeniacae)
Shi Gao (Gypsum Fibrosum)
Gan Cao (Radix Glycyrrhizae)

Huang Qin (Radix Scutellariae)
  Lian Qiao (Fructus Forsythiae)
  Ban Lan Gen (Radix Isatidis/Baphicacanthi)
  Jie Geng (Radix Platycodi)
  Gua Lou (Fructus Trichosanthis)
  Sang Bai Pi (Cortex Mori)

If there is severe cough with profuse, thick phlegm, add *Yu Xing Cao* (Herba Hedyotis Diffusae), *Qing Dai* (Pulvis Indigonis), and *Hai Ge Ke* (Concha Cyclinae/ Meretris). If oral thirst is severe, add *Tian Hua Fen* (Radix Trichosanthis). If there is vexation, agitation, and restlessness, double the amount of *Shi Gao* and add *Zhi Zi* (Fructus Gardeniae). If there is a red, dry tongue with dry lips, add *Xuan Shen* (Radix Scrophulariae) and *Sheng Di* (uncooked Radix Rehmanniae).

Ma Xing Shi Gan Tang Jia Wei (Ephedra, Armeniaca, Gypsum & Licorice Decoction with Added Flavors)
  Ma Huang (Herba Ephedrae)
  Xing Ren (Semen Armeniacae)
  Shi Gao (Gypsum Fibrosum)
  Gan Cao (Radix Glycyrrhizae)
  Huang Qin (Radix Scutellariae)
  Yu Xing Cao (Herba Hedyotis Diffusae)

Yin Qiao San (Lonicera & Forsythia Powder) plus *Ma Xing Shi Gan Tang* (Ephedra, Armeniaca, Gypsum & Licorice Decoction) with additions and subtractions
  Jin Yin Hua (Flos Lonicerae)
  Lian Qiao (Fructus Forsythiae)
  Bo He (Herba Menthae Haplocalycis)
  Ma Huang (Herba Ephedrae)
  Xing Ren (Semen Armeniacae)
  Shi Gao (Gypsum Fibrosum)
  Jie Geng (Radix Platycodi)
  Lu Gen (Rhizoma Phragmitis)
  Gan Cao (Radix Glycyrrhizae)

3. Phlegm heat accumulating in the lungs

Main symptoms: High fever, cough, shortness of breath, nasal flaring, restlessness, oral thirst, red, dry, possibly cyanotic lips, the sound of phlegm in the throat when breathing, a red tongue with slimy, yellow fur, a slippery, rapid pulse

Treatment principles: Clear heat and drain the lungs, stop coughing and level wheezing

Guiding formulas:
Ma Xing Shi Gan Tang (Ephedra, Armeniaca, Gypsum & Licorice Decoction) plus Ting Li Da Zao Xie Fei Tang (Descurainia & Dates Drain the Lungs Decoction) with additions and subtractions

Ma Huang (Herba Ephedrae)
Xing Ren (Semen Armeniacae)
Sang Bai Pi (Cortex Mori)
Ting Li Zi (Semen Lepidii/Descurainiae)
Di Gu Pi (Cortex Lycii)
Shi Gao (Gypsum Fibrosum)
Yu Xing Cao (Herba Hedyotis Diffusae)
Huang Qin (Radix Scutellariae)
Gan Cao (Radix Glycyrrhizae)

If there is constipation and abdominal distention, add *Da Huang* (Radix Et Rhizoma Rhei) and *Zhi Shi* (Fructus Immaturus Aurantii). If the face and lips are cyanotic, add *Dan Shen* (Radix Salviae Miltiorrhizae), *Hong Hua* (Flos Carthami), *Tao Ren* (Semen Persicae), and *Chi Shao* (Radix Paeoniae Rubrae). If there is profuse, thick, yellow mucus, add *Dan Nan Xing* (bile-processed Rhizoma Arisaematis) and *Zhe Bei Mu* (Bulbus Fritillariae Thunbergii).

Yin Dai Tang (Ginkgo & Indigo Decoction)

Qing Dai (Pulvis Indigonis)
Yin Xing (Semen Ginkgonis)
Di Gu Pi (Cortex Lycii)
Zi Su Zi (Fructus Perillae)
Tian Zhu Huang (Concretio Silicea Bambusae)
Han Shui Shi (Calcitum)

Ku Jiang Xin Kai Fang (Bitter Downbearing & Acrid Opening Formula)

Huang Lian (Rhizoma Coptidis)
Huang Qin (Radix Scutellariae)
Gan Jiang (dry Rhizoma Zingiberis)
Ban Xia (Rhizoma Pinelliae)
Zhi Ke (Fructus Aurantii)
Yu Jin (Tuber Curcumae)
Lai Fu Zi (Semen Raphani)

4. Damp heat depressing the lungs

Main symptoms: Cough with excessive phlegm, obstructed breathing, wheezing and dyspnea, chest glomus, abdominal distention, a dirty looking facial complexion, a red tongue with slimy, yellow fur, a soggy, rapid pulse, and a green-blue purplish finger vein

Treatment principles: Clear heat and eliminate dampness, loosen the chest and stop coughing

Guiding formula:
Unnamed formula
> *Lu Gen* (Rhizoma Phragmitis)
> *Yi Yi Ren* (Semen Coicis)
> *Tao Ren* (Semen Persicae)
> *Dong Gua Ren* (Semen Benincasae)
> *Hua Shi* (Talcum)
> *Xing Ren* (Semen Armeniacae)
> *Pi Pa Ye* (Folium Eriobotryae)
> *Tong Cao* (Medulla Tetrapanacis)
> *She Gan* (Rhizoma Belamcandae)
> *Yu Jin* (Tuber Curcumae)
> *Dan Dou Chi* (Semen Praeparatus Sojae)
> *Huang Qin* (Radix Scutellariae)

5. Phlegm dampness depressing the lungs

Main symptoms: Cough with copious, white phlegm, shortness of breath, wheezing and dyspnea, the sound of phlegm rattling in the throat, a yellowish face and pale lips, sometimes hot, sometimes cold, a red tongue with slimy fur, a slippery pulse

Treatment principles: Dry dampness and transform phlegm, stop coughing and level wheezing

Guiding formulas:
Xiao Qing Long Tang (Minor Blue-green Dragon Decoction) plus *Er Chen Tang* (Two Aged [Ingredients] Decoction) with additions and subtractions
> *Ma Huang* (Herba Ephedrae)
> *Gui Zhi* (Ramulus Cinnamomi)
> *Xing Ren* (Semen Armeniacae)
> *Ban Xia* (Rhizoma Pinelliae)
> *Chen Pi* (Pericarpium Citri Reticulatae)
> *Ting Li Zi* (Semen Lepidii/Descurainiae)
> *Xi Xin* (Herba Asari)
> *Wu Wei Zi* (Fructus Schisandrae)
> *Gan Cao* (Radix Glycyrrhizae)

6. Yin vacuity, lung heat

Main symptoms: Low-grade fever, night sweats, flushed face, dry cough with scanty or no phlegm, dry mouth with red lips, dry, red tongue with no or scanty fur, a fine, rapid pulse

THE DIAGNOSIS & TREATMENT OF COMMONLY ENCOUNTERED PEDIATRIC DISEASES

Treatment principles: Nourish yin and clear the lungs

Guiding formulas:
Sha Shen Mai Dong Tang Jia Jian (Glehnia & Ophiopogon Decoction with Additions & Subtractions)
Bei Sha Shen (Radix Glehniae)
Mai Men Dong (Tuber Ophiopogonis)
Yu Zhu (Rhizoma Polygonati Odorati)
Sang Bai Pi (Cortex Mori)
Di Gu Pi (Cortex Lycii)
Tian Hua Fen (Radix Trichosanthis)
Bai Bian Dou (Semen Dolichoris)
Xing Ren (Semen Armeniacae)
Gan Cao (Radix Glycyrrhizae)

For severe cough, add *Pi Pa Ye* (Folium Eriobotryae), *Bai Bu* (Radix Stemonae), and *Chuan Bei Mu* (Bulbus Fritillariae Cirrhosae). If there is lack of appetite due to food stagnation, add *Shan Zha* (Fructus Crataegi) and *Mai Ya* (Fructus Germinatus Hordei).

Unnamed formula
Sheng Di (uncooked Radix Rehmanniae)
Xuan Shen (Radix Scrophulariae)
Shi Gao (Gypsum Fibrosum)
Zhi Mu (Rhizoma Anemarrhenae)
Mai Men Dong (Tuber Ophiopogonis)

7. Lung-spleen qi vacuity

Main symptoms: Low-grade fever which comes and goes especially when fatigued, weak cough, disinclination to speak, feeble voice, thin, watery phlegm, a pale facial complexion, lassitude of the spirit, spontaneous perspiration, diminished appetite, loose stools, a pale tongue with white, slimy fur, and a fine, faint pulse

Treatment principles: Boost the qi and arouse the spleen

Guiding formulas:
Ren Shen Wu Wei Zi Tang Jia Jian (Ginseng & Schisandra Decoction with Additions & Subtractions)
Ren Shen (Radix Ginseng)
Huang Qi (Radix Astragali)
Bai Zhu (Rhizoma Atractylodis Macrocephalae)
Fu Ling (Poria)
Wu Wei Zi (Fructus Schisandrae)
Ban Xia (Rhizoma Pinelliae)
Gan Cao (Radix Glycyrrhizae)

If there is a wet, productive cough, add *Zi Wan* (Radix Asteris), *Chen Pi* (Pericarpium Citri Reticulatae), and *Dan Nan Xing* (bile-processed Rhizoma Arisaematis). If there is profuse sweating and shortness of breath due to vacuity of the constructive and defensive, add *Gui Zhi* (Ramulus Cinnamomi), *Mu Li* (Concha Ostrea), and *Long Gu* (Os Draconis).

Shen Ling Bai Zhu San Jia Wei (Ginseng, Poria & Atractylodes Powder with Added Flavors)

Ren Shen (Radix Ginseng)
Fu Ling (Poria)
Bai Zhu (Rhizoma Atractylodis Macrocephalae)
Yi Yi Ren (Semen Coicis)
Shan Yao (Radix Dioscoreae)
mix-fried *Gan Cao* (Radix Glycyrrhizae)
Chen Pi (Pericarpium Citri Reticulatae)
Jie Geng (Radix Platycodi)
Gui Zhi (Ramulus Cinnamomi)
Dang Gui (Radix Angelicae Sinensis)
Yin Chai Hu (Radix Stellariae)
Bai Bu (Radix Stemonae)
Da Zao (Fructus Jujubae)

Shen Ling Bai Zhu San Jia Jian (Ginseng, Poria & Atractylodes Powder with Additions & Subtractions)

Ren Shen (Radix Ginseng)
Fu Ling (Poria)
Bai Zhu (Rhizoma Atractylodis Macrocephalae)
mix-fried *Gan Cao* (Radix Glycyrrhizae)
Yi Yi Ren (Semen Coicis)
Shan Yao (Radix Dioscoreae)
Chen Pi (Pericarpium Citri Reticulatae)
Ban Xia (Rhizoma Pinelliae)

8. Heart yang vacuity & decline

Note: This pattern is seen in extremely severe pneumonia where yang qi has been damaged.

Main symptoms: Cough, shortness of breath, lack of warmth in the four limbs, vacuity vexation and restlessness, a somber, white facial complexion, cyanotic lips, a purplish, dark tongue, a faint, weak, rapid pulse

Treatment principles: Mainly warm and supplement yang qi, assisted by raising and diffusing the lung qi

Guiding formulas:
Shen Fu Tang Jia Wei (Ginseng & Aconite Decoction with Added Flavors)

Ren Shen (Radix Ginseng)
Fu Zi (Radix Lateralis Praeparatus Aconiti Carmichaeli)
Bai Shao (Radix Paeoniae Albae)
Gan Cao (Radix Glycyrrhizae)

If there is a blue-green, purplish, dark tongue and lips and an enlarged liver, add *Dan Shen* (Radix Salviae Miltiorrhizae), *Hong Hua* (Flos Carthami), and *Dang Gui* (Radix Angelicae Sinensis).

Shen Fu Long Mu Jiu Ni Tang (Ginseng, Aconite, Dragon Bone & Oyster Shell Rescue Counterflow Decoction)

Ren Shen (Radix Ginseng)
Fu Zi (Radix Lateralis Praeparatus Aconiti Carmichaeli)
mix-fried *Gan Cao* (Radix Glycyrrhizae)
Bai Shao (Radix Paeoniae Albae)
calcined *Long Gu* (Os Draconis)
calcined *Mu Li* (Concha Ostreae)

Shen Fu Tang Jia Wei (Ginseng & Aconite Decoction with Added Flavors)

Ren Shen (Radix Ginseng)
Fu Zi (Radix Lateralis Praeparatus Aconiti Carmichaeli)
mix-fried *Gan Cao* (Radix Glycyrrhizae)
Xing Ren (Semen Armeniacae)
Jie Geng (Radix Platycodi)

If symptoms of lung qi blockage and obstruction are pronounced, add *Ma Huang* (Herba Ephedrae), *Gui Zhi* (Ramulus Cinnamomi), *Gan Jiang* (dry Rhizoma Zingiberis), and *Wu Wei Zi* (Fructus Schisandrae).

If the child's face is blue-green and grey with great sweating dribbling and dripping, evidencing yang qi vacuity desertion, use **Si Ni Tang Jia Wei (Four Counterflows Decoction with Added Flavors):**

Ren Shen (Radix Ginseng)
Wu Wei Zi (Fructus Schisandrae)
Long Gu (Os Draconis)
Mu Li (Concha Ostreae)
Shan Zhu Yu (Fructus Corni)
Fu Zi (Radix Lateralis Praeparatus Aconiti Carmichaeli)
Gan Jiang (dry Rhizoma Zingiberis)
mix-fried *Gan Cao* (Radix Glycyrrhizae)

Yi Xin Hua Yu Tang (Boost the Heart & Transform Stasis Decoction)

Huang Qi (Radix Astragali)
Dang Shen (Radix Codonopsitis)

Chuan Xiong (Rhizoma Chuanxiong)
Sheng Di (uncooked Radix Rehmanniae)
Mai Men Dong (Tuber Ophiopogonis)
Dan Shen (Radix Salviae Miltiorrhizae)
Shui Zhi (Hirudo)
Jin Yin Hua (Flos Lonicerae)
Da Qing Ye (Folium Daqingye)
Jie Geng (Radix Platycodi)
Che Qian Zi (Semen Plantaginis)
Gan Cao (Radix Glycyrrhizae)

Ding Chuan Er Hao (Level Asthma No. 2)
Huang Qi (Radix Astragali)
Dan Shen (Radix Salviae Miltiorrhizae)
Tao Ren (Semen Persicae)
Hong Hua (Flos Carthami)
Gua Lou (Fructus Trichosanthis)
Yu Xing Cao (Herba Hedyotis Diffusae)
Xi Xin (Herba Asari)

9. Evils falling into the *jue yin* (a.k.a., stirring internally of liver wind, evils entering the original spirit)

Note: This pattern describes convulsions due to high fever in a deteriorated case.

Main symptoms: High fever, vexation and agitation, spirit dimming, delirious speech, spasms and tremors of the four limbs, teeth clenched tightly shut, both eyes staring upward, arched neck rigidity, a scarlet red tongue with dry, yellow fur, a wiry, rapid pulse

Treatment principles: Clear the heart and open the portals, level the liver and extinguish wind

Guiding formulas:
Ling Jiao Gou Teng Tang Jia Jian (Antelope Horn & Uncaria Decoction with Additions & Subtractions)
Shan Yang Jiao (Cornu Caprae)
Gou Teng (Ramulus Uncariae Cum Uncis)
Sheng Di (uncooked Radix Rehmanniae)
Bai Shao (Radix Paeoniae Albae)
Chuan Bei Mu (Bulbus Fritillariae Cirrhosae)
Sang Bai Pi (Cortex Mori)
Shi Chang Pu (Rhizoma Acori Tatarinowii)

Ling Jiao Gou Teng Tang Jia Jian (Antelope Horn & Uncaria Decoction with Additions & Subtractions)

Shan Yang Jiao (Cornu Caprae)
Gou Teng (Ramulus Uncariae Cum Uncis)
Sheng Di (uncooked Radix Rehmanniae)
Bai Shao (Radix Paeoniae Albae)
Shi Gao (Gypsum Fibrosum)
Zhi Mu (Rhizoma Anemarrhenae)
Lian Qiao (Fructus Forsythiae)
Shi Chang Pu (Rhizoma Acori Tatarinowii)

Ling Jiao Gou Teng Tang (Antelope Horn & Uncaria Decoction) plus *An Gong Niu Huang Wan* (Quiet the Palace Bezoar Pills) with additions and subtractions

Shan Yang Jiao (Cornu Caprae)
Gou Teng (Ramulus Uncariae Cum Uncis)
Fu Shen (Sclerotium Pararadicis Poriae)
Bai Shao (Radix Paeoniae Albae)
Zhu Ru (Caulis Bambusae In Taeniis)
Shi Chang Pu (Rhizoma Acori Tatarinowii)
Yu Jin (Tuber Curcumae)
Zhi Zi (Fructus Gardeniae)
Huang Qin (Radix Scutellariae)

Acupuncture & moxibustion

For wind cold, needle *Feng Men* (Bl 12), *Fei Shu* (Bl 13), and *Lie Que* (Lu 7). For wind heat, add *Chi Ze* (Lu 5). For phlegm heat and damp heat, needle *Fei Shu* (Bl 13), *Chi Ze* (Lu 5), and *Feng Long* (St 40). For phlegm dampness, needle *Fei Shu* (Bl 13), *Pi Shu* (Bl 20), and *Feng Long* (St 40). For yin vacuity, needle *Fei Shu* (Bl 13), *Lie Que* (Lu 7), and *Zhao Hai* (Ki 6). For lung-spleen vacuity, needle *Fei Shu* (Bl 13), *Pi Shu* (Bl 20), and *Zu San Li* (St 36). For internal stirring of liver wind, needle *Ren Zhong* (GV 26), *Bai Hui* (GV 20), and bleed the twelve *jing* well points. And for heart yang vacuity, moxa *Bai Hui* (GV 20), *Shen Que* (CV 8), *Guan Yuan* (CV 4), and *Zu San Li* (St 36).

Adjunctive treatments

For wind cold pneumonia, scrape (*gua sha*) the upper back. The patient should be kept under cover in order both to avoid further chill and to promote sweating. Hot, dilute rice soup can also help promote sweating and improve the effect of internally administered medicinals. A home remedy for all upper respiratory tract infections characterized as wind cold patterns is to boil several pieces of scallions with some fresh ginger and brown sugar. For wind heat, *gua sha* of the upper back and shoulders can be used to help resolve the exterior more effectively and rubbing down the center of the spine can help reduce the fever which is higher in this second pattern than the first. For any kind of wind heat pattern of upper respiratory infection, one can make a tea out of fresh peppermint and drink this frequently. In the case of phlegm dampness depressing the lungs or phlegm heat blocking the lungs, one must remember that, "The spleen is the root of phlegm production, while the lungs are where phlegm is stored." Therefore, in these patterns, a clear, bland diet is especially important as are cooked, warm foods which strengthen the spleen. Dairy products and sugars and sweets as well as raw, cold, chilled, and frozen foods and drinks should be strictly avoided. In the lung-spleen qi vacuity pattern, since the spleen is the root of engenderment of the lung qi, once again care must be taken to enforce a warm, nourishing but nevertheless clear, bland diet. Spinal pinch-pull massage several times daily is also helpful for strengthening the righteous qi. And in the case of yin vacuity due to enduring heat consuming yin fluids, a small amount of dairy products and sugar can actually be useful to nourish and engender yin fluids. In addition, one should eat some nourishing meat broths and eggs. In both these patterns, adequate rest is absolutely necessary.

For wind cold, phlegm dampness, and lung and spleen dual vacuity patterns of pneumonia, one can crush and pound together fresh buttercup (Ranunculus) with sugar at a ratio of 10 to 1 respectively. Buttercup is a common perennial garden flower (which should never be taken internally!). This paste is then spread over the area of the chest corresponding to the shadow on the x-ray. This paste should be aged for 1-2 months before use. Otherwise it will tend to cause blisters on the skin. However, since one does not know 1-2 months in advance that they may need this paste, one can still make and use this paste, however knowing in advance that it may cause blistering. As long as such blisters are kept clean and uninfected, this "counterirritation" is actually healing for the pneumonia. For all types of pneumonia, one can cup directly over the area where rales are heard or a shadow appears on the x-ray.

Comments

In the internal treatment of pneumonia, it is important to use medicinals with a known empirical effect on the treatment of pneumonia, such as *Yu Xing Cao* (Herba Hedyotis Diffusae). It is also important for parents to know that Chinese medicine does treat pneumonia without necessarily resorting to antibiotics. As the reader is by now aware, I really do counsel avoiding antibiotics unless truly necessary. Many parents and their MDs, as soon as a diagnosis of pneumonia is made, assume there is no other alternative to antibiotics. Chinese herbal medicine is such an alternative as long as the case is closely monitored by a Western MD. If and when antibiotics become necessary, then they can be used.

20. Pediatric Asthma

Pediatric asthma is mostly an allergic disease. It occurs most frequently in children four or more years of age and occurs more often in the spring and fall. It is characterized by recurrent bouts of an oppressive feeling of tightness in the chest and throat followed by wheezing, shortness of breath, and difficulty breathing. During an attack, the child will not be able to calmly rest while lying down on their back but must often sit up in order to facilitate breathing. Frequently, the asthma spontaneously improves as the child grows older, but may relapse again as an adult if one becomes stressed, run down, has a poor diet, or as one ages. Thus asthma which begins in childhood may often become a lifelong problem. This condition is also characterized by its acute bouts separated by periods of remission, and its TCM treatment takes this into account in terms of pattern discrimination and treatment.

Treatment based on pattern discrimination:

During acute attacks

1. Hot asthma

Main symptoms: Cough, panting, and wheezing, thick, yellow-colored phlegm, fever, a red face, a stuffy, oppressed feeling in the chest, thirst with a desire to drink, reddish yellow urine, dry stools or constipation, a red tongue with thin, yellow or slimy, yellow fur, a slippery, rapid pulse

Treatment principles: Clear the lungs, transform phlegm, and stabilize the asthma

Guiding formulas:
Ding Chuan Tang (Calm Asthma Decoction)

Sang Bai Pi (Cortex Mori)
Huang Qin (Radix Scutellariae)
Ban Xia (Rhizoma Pinelliae)
Ma Huang (Herba Ephedrae)
Xing Ren (Semen Armeniacae)
Gan Cao (Radix Glycyrrhizae)
Zi Su Zi (Fructus Perillae)
Kuan Dong Hua (Flos Farfarae)
Yin Guo (Semen Ginkgonis)

Ding Chuan Tang Jia Jian (Calm Asthma Decoction with Additions & Subtractions)

Ma Huang (Herba Ephedrae)
Xing Ren (Semen Armeniacae)
Sang Bai Pi (Cortex Mori)
Huang Qin (Radix Scutellariae)
Shi Gao (Gypsum Fibrosum)
Ting Li Zi (Semen Lepidii/Descurainiae)
Ban Xia (Rhizoma Pinelliae)
Kuan Dong Hua (Flos Farfarae)
Yin Guo (Semen Ginkgonis)
Gan Cao (Radix Glycyrrhizae)

If there is phlegm congestion in the lungs, add *Yu Xing Cao* (Herba Hedyotis Diffusae), and *Bai Jiang Cao* (Herba Patriniae Heterophyllae Cum Radice). If panting is heavy, add *Dai Zhe Shi* (Haemititum) and *Bai Shao* (Radix Paeoniae Albae). If there is itchy nose as in allergy, add *Fang Feng* (Radix Saposhnikoviae), *Xin Yi* (Flos Magnoliae), *Xia Ku Cao* (Spica Prunellae), *Cang Er Zi* (Fructus Xanthii), and *Wu Mei* (Fructus Mume). If sleep at night is restless or asthma gets worse in the nighttime, add *Ye Jiao Teng* (Caulis Polygoni Multiflori), *Zhen Zhu Mu* (Concha Margaritiferae), and *Ci Shi* (Magnetitum). If there is constipation, add *Da Huang* (Radix Et Rhizoma Rhei).

Ma Xing Shi Gan Tang Jia Wei (Ephedra, Armeniaca, Gypsum & Licorice Decoction with Added Flavors)

mix-fried *Ma Huang* (Herba Ephedrae)
Shi Gao (Gypsum Fibrosum)
Xing Ren (Semen Armeniacae)
Gan Cao (Radix Glycyrrhizae)
Sang Bai Pi (Cortex Mori)
Bai Bu (Radix Stemonae)
Huang Qin (Radix Scutellariae)
Lian Qiao (Fructus Forsythiae)
Bei Mu (Bulbus Fritillariae)
Ju Hong (Exocarpium Citri Erythrocarpae)
Bai Jie Zi (Semen Sinapis)

Ma Xing Shi Gan Tang Jia Wei (Ephedra, Armeniaca, Gypsum & Licorice Decoction with Added Flavors)

Ma Huang (Herba Ephedrae)
Xing Ren (Semen Armeniacae)
Shi Gao (Gypsum Fibrosum)
Gan Cao (Radix Glycyrrhizae)
Bo He (Herba Menthae Haplocalycis)
Gua Lou (Fructus Trichosanthis)
Qian Hu (Radix Peucedani)
Sang Bai Pi (Cortex Mori)
Kuan Dong Hua (Flos Farfarae)

Er Huang Er Zi Tang (Two Yellows & Two Seeds Decoction)

mix-fried *Ma Huang* (Herba Ephedrae)
uncooked *Da Huang* (Radix Et Rhizoma Rhei)
Zi Su Zi (Fructus Perillae)
Ting Li Zi (Semen Lepidii/Descurainiae)
Zhe Bei Mu (Bulbus Fritillariae Thunbergii)
Xing Ren (Semen Armeniacae)
Ju Hong (Exocarpium Citri Erythrocarpae)

If there is damp heat asthma as evidenced by phlegm congestion causing labored breathing, chest glomus and abdominal distention, fatigue, not eating, loose stools, yellow, diminished urination, a dirty colored face and red lips, a red tongue with white or thick, slimy, yellow fur, a soggy, rapid pulse, or a purplish, stagnant finger vein, use the following unnamed formula:

Wei Jing (Rhizoma Phragmitis)
Yi Yi Ren (Semen Coicis)
Tao Ren (Semen Persicae)
Dong Gua Ren (Semen Benincasae)
Hua Shi (Talcum)
Xing Ren (Semen Armeniacae)

If there is phlegm heat with simultaneous qi and yin vacuity as evidenced by cough, rapid dyspneic breathing, vomiting a small amount of sticky phlegm, a dry mouth and throat, lassitude of the spirit, shortness of breath, a somber white facial complexion with red cheeks, a red tongue with diminished fur, a fine, rapid, forceless pulse, use **Jin Shui Liu Jun Jian (Metal Water Six Gentlemen Decoction)** plus **Sheng Mai San (Engender the Pulse Powder) with additions and subtractions:**

Tian Men Dong (Tuber Asparagi)
Mai Men Dong (Tuber Ophiopogonis)
Sheng Di (uncooked Radix Rehmanniae)
Shu Di (cooked Radix Rehmanniae)
Tai Zi Shen (Radix Pseudostellariae)
Wu Wei Zi (Fructus Schisandrae)
Gua Lou (Fructus Trichosanthis)
Fu Ling (Poria)
Gan Cao (Radix Glycyrrhizae)
Qian Hu (Radix Peucedani)
Chuan Bei Mu (Bulbus Fritillariae Cirrhosae)
Xing Ren (Semen Armeniacae)

2. Cold asthma

Main symptoms: Cough with rapid breathing, the sound of phlegm rattling in the throat, cough with clear, watery, white-colored phlegm, a cold body and no perspiration, a dull, lusterless, stagnant facial complexion which may even be a bit bluish green, lack of warmth in the four limbs, no thirst or thirst with a desire for hot drinks only, thin, white or white, slimy tongue fur, a floating, slippery pulse

Treatment principles: Warm the lungs, transform phlegm, and stabilize asthma

Guiding formulas:
Xiao Qing Long Tang (Minor Blue-green Dragon Decoction)
Ma Huang (Herba Ephedrae)
Gui Zhi (Ramulus Cinnamomi)
Bai Shao (Radix Paeoniae Albae)
Xi Xin (Herba Asari)
Ban Xia (Rhizoma Pinelliae)

Gan Jiang (dry Rhizoma Zingiberis)
Wu Wei Zi (Fructus Schisandrae)
mix-fried *Gan Cao* (Radix Glycyrrhizae)

If panting is severe and phlegm is profuse, add *Bai Jie Zi* (Semen Sinapis), *Yuan Zhi* (Radix Polygalae), and *Zao Jia* (Fructus Gleditschiae).

Xiao Qing Long Tang Jia Jian (Minor Blue-green Dragon Decoction with Additions & Subtractions)

Ma Huang (Herba Ephedrae)
Xing Ren (Semen Armeniacae)
Ban Xia (Rhizoma Pinelliae)
Wu Wei Zi (Fructus Schisandrae)
Kuan Dong Hua (Flos Farfarae)
Zi Su Zi (Fructus Perillae)
Bai Guo (Semen Ginkgonis)
Sang Bai Pi (Cortex Mori)
Di Long (Pheretima)
Yu Xing Cao (Herba Hedyotis Diffusae)
Gan Cao (Radix Glycyrrhizae)

If there is exterior cold and internal heat, add *Huang Qin* (Radix Scutellariae), *Ban Lan Gen* (Radix Isatidis/Baphicacanthi), and *Shi Gao* (Gypsum Fibrosum). If there is cough with profuse phlegm, add *Qian Hu* (Radix Peucedani), *Bei Mu* (Bulbus Fritillariae), and *Jie Geng* (Radix Platycodi). If asthma is severe, add *Lai Fu Zi* (Semen Raphani), *Bai Jie Zi* (Semen Sinapis), and *Zhi Ke* (Fructus Aurantii).

For wind cold asthma with phlegm and dampness, use **Ma Xing Shi Gan Tang Jia Jian (Ephedra, Armeniaca, Gypsum & Licorice Decoction with Additions & Subtractions):**

Ma Huang (Herba Ephedrae)
Xing Ren (Semen Armeniacae)
Zi Su Zi (Fructus Perillae)
mix-fried *Gan Cao* (Radix Glycyrrhizae)
Chen Pi (Pericarpium Citri Reticulatae)
Fu Ling (Poria)
Sang Bai Pi (Cortex Mori)
Bai Jie Zi (Semen Sinapis)
Ban Xia (Rhizoma Pinelliae)

Ding Chuan Tang Jia Jian (Calm Asthma Decoction with Additions & Subtractions)

Bai Guo (Semen Ginkgonis)
mix-fried *Ma Huang* (Herba Ephedrae)
Zi Su Zi (Fructus Perillae)
Gan Cao (Radix Glycyrrhizae)

    Ban Xia (Rhizoma Pinelliae)
    Xing Ren (Semen Armeniacae)
    mix-fried *Sang Bai Pi* (Cortex Mori)
    Huang Qin (Radix Scutellariae)
    Zhe Bei Mu (Bulbus Fritillariae Thunbergii)
    Ju Hong (Exocarpium Citri Erythrocarpae)

Jie Xiao Tang (Cut in Two Wheezing Decoction)
    mix-fried *Ma Huang* (Herba Ephedrae)
    Xing Ren (Semen Armeniacae)
    Sang Bai Pi (Cortex Mori)
    Fang Feng (Radix Saposhnikoviae)
    Bai Guo (Semen Ginkgonis)
    Quan Gua Lou (whole Fructus Trichosanthis)
    Xuan Fu Hua (Flos Inulae)
    Di Long (Pheretima)
    processed *Jiang Can* (Bombyx Batryticatus)
    Quan Xie (Scorpio)

Wen Fei Kang Min Tang (Warm the Lungs & Combat Allergy Decoction)
    Fu Zi (Radix Lateralis Praeparatus Aconiti Carmichaeli)
    Ma Huang (Herba Ephedrae)
    Xi Xin (Herba Asari)
    Huang Qi (Radix Astragali)
    Wu Gong (Scolopendra)
    Di Long (Pheretima)
    Jiang Can (Bombyx Batryticatus)
    Da Huang (Radix Et Rhizoma Rhei)
    Gan Cao (Radix Glycyrrhizae)

During the remission stage

1. Lung qi vacuity

Main symptoms: A dull white or somber white facial complexion, shortness of breath and disinclination to speak, a soft, low voice, fatigue, lack of strength, spontaneous perspiration or sweating on slight movement, fear of chill, lack of warmth in the four limbs, a pale tongue with thin fur, a fine, forceless pulse

Treatment principles: Supplement the lungs and secure the defensive

Guiding formulas:
Yu Ping Feng San (Jade Wind Screen Powder) plus *Gui Zhi Tang* (Cinnamon Twig Decoction)
    Huang Qi (Radix Astragali)

Bai Zhu (Rhizoma Atractylodis Macrocephalae)
Fang Feng (Radix Saposhnikoviae)
Gui Zhi (Ramulus Cinnamomi)
Bai Shao (Radix Paeoniae Albae)
Gan Cao (Radix Glycyrrhizae)
Sheng Jiang (uncooked Rhizoma Zingiberis)
Da Zao (Fructus Jujubae)

Gui Zhi Jia Huang Qi Tang Jia Jian (Cinnamon Twig Plus Astragalus Decoction with Additions & Subtractions)
Huang Qi (Radix Astragali)
Bai Zhu (Rhizoma Atractylodis Macrocephalae)
Wu Wei Zi (Fructus Schisandrae)
Gui Zhi (Ramulus Cinnamomi)
Bai Shao (Radix Paeoniae Albae)
Fang Feng (Radix Saposhnikoviae)
Sheng Jiang (uncooked Rhizoma Zingiberis)
Da Zao (Fructus Jujubae)

2. Spleen vacuity weakness

Main symptoms: Cough with profuse phlegm, diminished appetite, a full feeling in the upper abdomen, a yellow, lusterless facial complexion, incomplete stools or loose stools, emaciation, fatigue, lack of strength, a pale tongue with scanty fur, a relaxed, *i.e.*, on the verge of slow, forceless pulse

Treatment principles: Fortify the spleen and transform phlegm

Guiding formulas:
Liu Jun Zi Tang (Six Gentlemen Decoction)
Ren Shen (Radix Ginseng)
Bai Zhu (Rhizoma Atractylodis Macrocephalae)
Fu Ling (Poria)
Gan Cao (Radix Glycyrrhizae)
Chen Pi (Pericarpium Citri Reticulatae)
Ban Xia (Rhizoma Pinelliae)

Si Jun Zi Tang Jia Wei (Four Gentlemen Decoction with Added Flavors)
Dang Shen (Radix Codonopsitis)
Huang Qi (Radix Astragali)
Bai Zhu (Rhizoma Atractylodis Macrocephalae)
Fu Ling (Poria)
Gan Cao (Radix Glycyrrhizae)
Bai Guo (Semen Ginkgonis)
Zi Wan (Radix Asteris)

If cough is severe, add *Kuan Dong Hua* (Flos Farfarae) and *Che Qian Zi* (Semen Plantaginis). If there are chilled limbs, add *Fu Zi* (Radix Lateralis Praeparatus Aconiti Carmichaeli) and *Rou Gui* (Cortex Cinnamomi). If there is spontaneous perspiration, add *Wu Wei Zi* (Fructus Schisandrae) and calcined *Mu Li* (Concha Ostreae).

Ren Shen Wu Wei Zi Tang Jia Wei (Ginseng & Schisandra Decoction with Added Flavors)
Ren Shen (Radix Ginseng)
Huang Qi (Radix Astragali)
Bai Zhu (Rhizoma Atractylodis Macrocephalae)
Fu Ling (Poria)
Wu Wei Zi (Fructus Schisandrae)
Sang Bai Pi (Cortex Mori)
Chuan Bei Mu (Bulbus Fritillariae Cirrhosae)
Chen Pi (Pericarpium Citri Reticulatae)
Ban Xia (Rhizoma Pinelliae)
Mai Men Dong (Tuber Ophiopogonis)
Gan Cao (Radix Glycyrrhizae)

If there is diminished appetite and abdominal distention, add *Shen Qu* (Massa Medica Fermentata), *Mai Ya* (Fructus Germinatus Hordei), *Sha Ren* (Fructus Amomi), and *Shan Yao* (Radix Dioscoreae). If there is profuse, thin, watery phlegm with slimy, white tongue fur, use **Er Chen Tang Jia Wei (Two Aged [Ingredients] Decoction with Added Flavors):**
Ban Xia (Rhizoma Pinelliae)
Fu Ling (Poria)
Gan Cao (Radix Glycyrrhizae)
Chen Pi (Pericarpium Citri Reticulatae)
Chuan Bei Mu (Bulbus Fritillariae Cirrhosae)
Sang Bai Pi (Cortex Mori)

3. Kidney qi vacuity

Main symptoms: A somber or dull white facial complexion, a cold body and fear of chill, lack of warmth particularly in the feet and lower legs, lack of strength in the lower legs, exertion causing heart palpitations and rapid breathing, watery, loose stools, possible bed-wetting at night, a pale tongue with white fur, a fine, forceless pulse

Treatment principles: Supplement the kidneys and secure the root

Guiding formulas:
Jin Gui Shen Qi Wan Jia Wei (Kidney Qi Pills [from the book titled Essentials from] The Golden Cabinet with Added Flavors)
Fu Zi (Radix Lateralis Praeparatus Aconiti Carmichaeli)
Rou Gui (Cortex Cinnamomi)

Shu Di (cooked Radix Rehmanniae)
Shan Yao (Radix Dioscoreae)
Shan Zhu Yu (Fructus Corni)
Fu Ling (Poria)
Dan Pi (Cortex Moutan)
Ze Xie (Rhizoma Alismatis)
Ze He Che (Placenta Hominis)

Jin Gui Shen Qi Wan Jia Wei (Golden Cabinet Kidney Qi Pills with Added Flavors)

Shu Di (cooked Radix Rehmanniae)
Shan Yao (Radix Dioscoreae)
Shan Zhu Yu (Fructus Corni)
Fu Ling (Poria)
Dan Pi (Cortex Moutan)
Ze Xie (Rhizoma Alismatis)
Rou Gui (Cortex Cinnamomi)
Fu Zi (Radix Lateralis Praeparatus Aconiti Carmichaeli)
Yin Yang Huo (Herba Epimedii)
Ba Ji Tian (Radix Morindae)
Bu Gu Zhi (Fructus Psoraleae)

Jin Gui Shen Qi Wan Jia Jian (Golden Cabinet Kidney Qi Pills with Additions & Subtractions)

Fu Zi (Radix Lateralis Praeparatus Aconiti Carmichaeli)
Shu Di (cooked Radix Rehmanniae)
Shan Zhu Yu (Fructus Corni)
San Yao (Radix Dioscoreae)
Wu Wei Zi (Fructus Schisandrae)
Fu Ling (Poria)
Dan Pi (Cortex Moutan)
Hu Tao Ren (Semen Juglandis)
Dang Shen (Radix Codonopsitis)
Gan Cao (Radix Glycyrrhizae)

Gu Ben Pei Yuan Fen (Secure the Root & Bank Up the Origin Powder)

Zi He Che (Placenta Hominis)
Di Long (Pheretima)
Hai Ge Ke (Concha Cyclinae/Meretricis)
Cang Er Zi (Fructus Xanthii)
Gan Cao (Radix Glycyrrhizae)

If there is kidney yin vacuity, use *Mai Men Dong Ba Wei Wan Jia Jian* (Ophiopogon & Schisandra Eight Flavors Pills with Additions & Subtractions):

Mai Men Dong (Tuber Ophiopogonis)
Wu Wei Zi (Fructus Schisandrae)
Shu Di (cooked Radix Rehmanniae)
Shan Yao (Radix Dioscoreae)
Shan Zhu Yu (Fructus Corni)
Tian Dong (Tuber Asparagi)

4. Phlegm rheum lodged and deep-lying

Main symptoms: Chronic asthma during the remission stage due to deep-lying phlegm rheum, copious, white, watery phlegm, nasal obstruction, clear runny nose, slimy, white tongue fur

Treatment principles: Warm and transform recalcitrant phlegm

Guiding formula:
Wu Sheng Dan (Five Sages Elixir)
roasted *Tian Nan Xing* (Rhizoma Arisaematis)
Ban Xia (Rhizoma Pinelliae)
Chen Pi (Pericarpium Citri Reticulatae)
Xing Ren (Semen Armeniacae)
Gan Cao (Radix Glycyrrhizae)

Acupuncture & moxibustion

During the acute stage, needle *Ding Chuan* (M-BW-1), *Tian Tu* (CV 22), *Da Zhu* (Bl 11), *Nei Guan* (Per 6), and/or *Shan Zhong* (CV 17) once per day. During the remission stage, moxa *Shen Que* (CV 8) and *Guan Yuan* (CV 4) plus the back transport points of the lungs, spleen, and/or kidneys as appropriate.

Adjunctive treatments

During an acute episode of hot or cold asthma, one can use *gua sha*, cupping, or seven star hammer on the upper back. For heat and phlegm, anything which would increase heat in the body, such as hot, spicy foods, or anything which would increase phlegm, such as fatty, greasy foods, sugars and sweets, and dairy products, are contraindicated. Obviously, patients with the cold pattern of acute asthma should be kept warm and not be allowed to eat anything cold, frozen, or chilled. Nor should they eat sugar, sweets, and dairy products.

During the remission stage, because this disease is associated with an abnormal production of phlegm and because it is an allergic condition, proper diet is vitally important in this pattern. Children with asthma should stick to a clear, bland, hypoallergenic diet. They should also be encouraged to exercise more in order to build up their resistance and strength. Because of their cold nature, many Chinese doctors think that bananas should not be eaten too regularly by persons with a weak spleen, with asthma, or other lung problems. Moxibustion over the navel and the lower abdomen is a common adjunctive treatment and, in children less than six years of age, daily spinal pinch-pull massage can help strengthen the constitution.

If the asthma is cold-natured, one can apply blistering medicinals to the back transport points associated with the lungs during the hottest part of summer. One formula to use is:
　　Bai Jie Zi (Semen Sinapis), 30g
　　Yan Hu Suo (Rhizoma Corydalis), 30g
　　Xi Xin (Herba Asari), 15g
　　Gan Sui (Radix Euphorbiae Kansui), 15g

These are ground into powder and made into six medicinal cakes with ginger juice. Three grams of *Ding Xiang* (Flos Caryophylli) are placed in the center of these cakes and they are then applied to *Bai Lao* (M-HN-30), *Da Zhui* (GV 14), *Fei Shu* (Bl 13), and *Gao Huang Shu* (Bl 43). The cakes are kept on for two hours each time, and this repeated one time every 10 days in summer. If blisters develop and break open, they should be covered with sterile gauze and kept free from infection.

Comments

As one can see, the emphasis with asthma should be on prevention. Because this is an allergic condition, diet is vitally important. For more information on diet and allergies see the section on allergies below. It is also true that emotional stress plays its part in most cases of asthma as does a history of antibiotic use leading to chronic candidiasis. So many of my son's friends can't come to our house because they have allergic asthma triggered by animal hair and dander. These are the same children whose parents do not seem to care how much sugar, ice cream, and soda they consume and who run to the MD for antibiotics at the first sign of an ear infection or sore throat. Because my wife and I both suffered from pediatric asthma, our son should have a higher than normal likelihood of having this disease. Because of suffering from pediatric asthma and allergies myself as a child, I know what a pain this is, and I also know that much of this suffering is entirely unnecessary if one pays attention to proper diet and avoids antibiotics if at all possible.

The reader should note that many modern Chinese TCM practitioners use wind medicinals, such as *Di Long* (Pheretima), *Jiang Can* (Bombyx Batryticatus), *Quan Xie* (Scorpio), and *Wu Gong* (Scolopendra), for their antispasmodic effect in the treatment of acute asthma.

21. Swollen Glands (Tonsillitis & Strep)

In the back of the throat and under the jaws there are a number of salivary and lymph glands. These may become infected and/or enlarged. In some cases, if the child is taken to a Western MD or clinic and a throat culture is done, the Western medical diagnosis is a strep (short for streptococcus) infection. Unless the parent refuses, children who test positive for strep are given antibiotics. In my generation, children with recurrent sore throats and swollen glands or tonsillitis eventually had their tonsils removed. Happily today,

Western MDs do not seem to be so quick to recommend a tonsillectomy. In most cases of sore throat, swollen glands, and tonsillitis, antibiotics and surgery are not necessary and these conditions can be treated successfully by Chinese medicine, including Chinese herbal medicine and acupuncture.

Treatment based on pattern discrimination:

Acute tonsillitis

1. Wind heat

Main symptoms: Fever, no or slight chills, slight perspiration, sore throat, difficulty swallowing, headache, body aches, red, swollen tonsils, stuffed and/or runny nose, possible cough, a red tongue with thin, yellow fur, and a floating, rapid pulse

Treatment principles: Scatter wind and clear heat, disperse swelling and disinhibit the throat

Guiding formulas:
Yin Qiao San Jia Jian (Lonicerae & Forsythia Powder with Additions & Subtractions)
Jin Yin Hua (Flos Lonicerae)
Lian Qiao (Fructus Forsythiae)
Ye Ju Hua (Flos Chrysanthemi Indici)
Zi Hua Di Ding (Herba Violae)
Jing Jie (Herba Schizonepetae)
Jie Geng (Radix Platycodi)
Niu Bang Zi (Fructus Arctii)
Bo He (Herba Menthae Haplocalycis)
She Gan (Rhizoma Belamcandae)
Gan Cao (Radix Glycyrrhizae)

Xiao E Tang (Disperse the Tonsils Decoction)
Jing Jie (Herba Schizonepetae)
Fang Feng (Radix Saposhnikoviae)
Ju Hua (Flos Chrysanthemi)
Lian Qiao (Fructus Forsythiae)
Dan Pi (Cortex Moutan)
Xuan Shen (Radix Scrophulariae)
Jin Yin Hua (Flos Lonicerae)
Shi Gao (Gypsum Fibrosum)
Niu Bang Zi (Fructus Arctii)
She Gan (Rhizoma Belamcandae)
Ban Lan Gen (Radix Isatidis/Baphicacanthi)
Tian Hua Fen (Radix Trichosanthis)
Gan Cao (Radix Glycyrrhizae)

2. Lung-stomach heat

Main symptoms: High fever, severe sore throat, oral thirst, desire for cold drinks, constipation, yellowish red urination, a bitter taste in the mouth, very red and very swollen tonsils possibly covered by a yellowish white membrane, yellow tongue fur, a rapid pulse

Treatment principles: Clear heat, drain fire, and scatter nodulation

Guiding formulas:
Pu Ji Xiao Du Yin (Universal Benefit Disperse Toxins Beverage)
Ban Lan Gen (Radix Isatidis/Baphicacanthi)
Shi Gao (Gypsum Fibrosum)
Lian Qiao (Fructus Forsythiae)
Huang Qin (Radix Scutellariae)
Sang Ye (Folium Mori)
Zi Hua Di Ding (Herba Violae)
Ma Bo (Lasiosphaera/Calvatia)
Tian Hua Fen (Radix Trichosanthis)
Da Huang (Radix Et Rhizoma Rhei)
Lu Gen (Rhizoma Phragmitis)

Qing Yan Li Ge Tang (Clear the Throat & Disinhibit the Diaphragm Decoction)
Jin Yin Hua (Flos Lonicerae)
Lian Qiao (Fructus Forsythiae)
Zhi Zi (Fructus Gardeniae)
Huang Qin (Radix Scutellariae)
Niu Bang Zi (Fructus Arctii)
Jing Jie (Herba Schizonepetae)
Fang Feng (Radix Saposhnikoviae)
Xuan Shen (Radix Scrophulariae)
Bo He (Herba Menthae Haplocalycis)
Da Huang (Radix Et Rhizoma Rhei)
Mang Xiao (Natri Sulfas)
Huang Lian (Rhizoma Coptidis)
Jie Geng (Radix Platycodi)
Gan Cao (Radix Glycyrrhizae)

If the tonsils are red and swollen and covered by a white membrane, add *Dan Pi* (Cortex Moutan), *Chi Shao* (Radix Paeoniae Rubrae), and *She Gan* (Rhizoma Belamcandae). If there is profuse, thick, yellow phlegm, add *Jiang Can* (Bombyx Batryticatus), *Zhe Bei Mu* (Bulbus Fritillariae Thunbergii), and *Shan Dou Gen* (Radix Sophorae Subprostratae).

Chronic tonsillitis

1. Yin vacuity

Main symptoms: Slight sore throat, dry throat, better in the morning and worse in the evening, worse after speaking or eating acrid, peppery foods, thick phlegm, throat slightly red and swollen, tonsils covered by a dry membrane, a red tongue, a fine, rapid pulse

Treatment principles: Enrich yin, downbear fire, and disinhibit the throat

Guiding formula:
Zhi Bai Ba Wei Wan Jia Jian (Anemarrhena & Phellodendron Eight Flavors Pills with Additions & Subtractions)

Sheng Di (uncooked Radix Rehmanniae)
Shan Zhu Yu (Fructus Corni)
Shan Yao (Radix Dioscoreae)
Fu Ling (Poria)
Dan Pi (Cortex Moutan)
Zhi Mu (Rhizoma Anemarrhenae)
Huang Bai (Cortex Phellodendri)
Qing Guo (Fructus Canarii)
Jie Geng (Radix Platycodi)
Lu E Mei (Flos Mume)

2. Stone tonsils

Main symptoms: A dull, dark red throat, markedly swollen and distended tonsils, possible slight pain, dry hacking, discomfort within the throat, submaxillary swollen lymph nodes, a red tongue, a rapid pulse

Treatment principles: Quicken the blood and disinhibit the qi, scatter nodulation and disperse swelling

Guiding formula:
Qing Yan Shuang He Yin (Clear the Throat Double Harmony Beverage)

Dan Gui Wei (rootlets of Radix Angelicae Sinensis)
Chi Shao (Radix Paeoniae Rubrae)
Dan Pi (Cortex Moutan)
Jie Geng (Radix Platycodi)
Xuan Shen (Radix Scrophulariae)
Qian Hu (Radix Peucedani)
Jin Yin Hua (Flos Lonicerae)
Gan Cao (Radix Glycyrrhizae)

Acupuncture & moxibustion

For severe acute tonsillitis, bleed *Shao Shang* (Lu 11) and *Shang Yang* (LI 1). If there is fever, one can also bleed *Da Zhui* (GV 14). For less severe cases, needle *He Gu* (LI 4) and *Nei Ting* (St 44). For chronic tonsillitis due to yin vacuity, needle *Lie Que* (Lu 7) and *Zhao Hai* (Ki 6). For chronic tonsillitis involving blood stasis, needle *Xue Hai* (Sp 10) and *He Gu* (LI 4).

Adjunctive treatments

For wind heat acute tonsillitis, use alternating hot and cold compresses around the throat (15 minutes hot, 5 minutes cold) plus *gua sha*, cupping, or seven star hammer on the upper back and neck wind points. If there is fever, one can also rub down the spine several hundred times in a row. If there is lung-stomach heat with constipation, an enema can help speed recovery. If the tonsils are swollen and purulent, massaging the tonsils to express the pus can be very beneficial. Further, one can spray *Xi Gua Shuang* (Watermelon Frost) into the mouth and onto the tonsils. If the child is old enough to gargle, a gargle can be made from a decoction of *Jing Jie* (Herba Schizonepetae), *Fang Feng* (Radix Saposhnikoviae), *Gan Cao* (Radix Glycyrrhizae), *Jin Yin Hua* (Flos Lonicerae), *Lian Qiao* (Fructus Forsythiae), and *Bo He* (Herba Menthae Haplocalycis).

Comments

Chronic tonsillitis should not be confused with recurrent tonsillitis. In recurrent tonsillitis, there are repeated acute episodes separated by periods of apparent remission. For children with a history of recurrent tonsillitis who have been treated repeatedly with antibiotics and are facing an immanent tonsillectomy, a radical change to a clear, bland diet and the use of a preventive formula such as *Xiao Chai Hu Tang* (Minor Bupleurum Decoction) can break this cycle and save the tonsils. Usually I recommend the child taking such a formula till April of the current year and then starting again in late September and again taking it till April. It is my assumption that the body has evolved the tonsils for a good reason and that removing them unless absolutely necessary is not a good idea for the long-term health and immunity of the person.

Strep

When throat cultures are done and they come back positive for strep, then the parents face a dilemma. The Western clinician will say that antibiotics are absolutely necessary in order to avoid scarlatina or what used to be called scarlet fever. It is true that some strep infections, left untreated, may develop into scarlatina and that scarlatina, if left untreated or is poorly treated, may develop into rheumatic fever affecting the heart. No one, least of all myself, wants to see any child develop rheumatic heart disease which can weaken the heart for the rest of one's life. However, neither do I want to see children receive antibiotics unless absolutely necessary, since I have seen too many long-term negative repercussions from these, such as enduring food, respiratory, and skin allergies and eventual autoimmune conditions. So what is a parent to do?

The key is the word untreated. If a strep infection is left untreated, then yes, it may potentially, although by no means always, develop into scarlatina and even eventually into rheumatic fever affecting the heart. But there is more than one way to treat a strep infection of the throat. Antibiotics are one way. They effectively knock out the strep, but they also knock out all the good bacteria and lead to an imbalance in the bacteria and fungi in the guts which then may lead to chronic allergies which may lead to autoimmune disorders. Chinese herbal medicine is another way of treating strep infections — but a way without the negative side effects of antibiotics. A number of the Chinese medicinals which are used for treating throat infections, swollen glands, and tonsillitis have been proven to have broad spectrum antibiotic ability, in some cases even surpassing antibiotics in efficiency. In particular, a number of Chinese medicinals for these problems have been shown in laboratory tests that they do kill the streptococcus bacteria, such as *Ban Lan Gen* (Radix Isatidis/Baphicacanthi), *Huang Lian* (Rhizoma Coptidis), *Huang Qin* (Radix Scutellariae), *Yu Xing Cao* (Herba Hedyotis Diffusae), *Ma Bo* (Lasiosphaera/Calvatia), *Pu Gong Ying* (Herba Taraxaci), *Lian Qiao* (Fructus Forsythiae), and *Yin Hua* (Flos Lonicerae). In other words, Chinese herbal medicines can definitely treat strep infections without antibiotics. And since these Chinese medicinals are always administered as part of a balanced formula, they do not damage the spleen the way antibiotics do.

In like manner, Chinese medicine also treats scarlatina. In other words, even if a strep infection did progress to scarlet fever, it does not necessarily have to wind up damaging the heart. The issue is whether or not there is the effective treatment preventing the disease from going deeper into the body. If treatment effectively cures the disease without either short- or long-term side effects, then that is the best, and that can be accomplished with Chinese herbal medicine for these problems. On the other hand, if for some reason, the Chinese herbal medicine does not get an entirely satisfactory effect and the child's condition is getting worse, one can always fall back on antibiotics at that point, after one has given safer, less harmful treatments first. Thus the issue is not simply whether to give antibiotics, but when to give antibiotics.

In order to allay parents' fears about strep throat, I would like to quote Robert S. Mendelsohn, MD, from his excellent book, *How to Raise a Healthy Child, In Spite of Your Doctor*:

> First, you should be aware that sore throats, most of the time, are caused by viruses for which Modern Medicine has no cure . . .

> Secondly, you should know that taking a culture to determine the presences of "strep" is a waste of your money and the doctor's time. It will *not* prove beyond doubt that your child has, or does not have, a strep infection . . .

Third, the chances that your child will experience rheumatic fever, even if he has a strep infection, are extremely remote. During a quarter of a century in a pediatric practice that had more than 10,000 patient contacts a year, I saw only one case of rheumatic fever. In real life, the threat of rheumatic fever does not exist in most populations. The disease is rarely seen except among malnourished children living in the crowded conditions associated with desperate poverty.

22. Lack of Appetite

Sometimes children will lose their appetite for relatively long periods of time, even at times refusing to eat. This mostly occurs in children from 1-6 years of age. Although the child eats very little, they are, nevertheless, energetic and seem in good spirits. If lack of appetite and refusal to eat continues for a long time, it may affect the child's growth and development. There are four basic patterns which Chinese pediatric texts associate with pediatric anorexia or lack of appetite in children.

Treatment based on pattern discrimination:

1. Loss of fortification of spleen transportations (a.k.a. food stagnation)

Main symptoms: A lusterless facial complexion, no thought for food or drink, no taste in eating or drinking, refusal to eat or drink, a somewhat emaciated body, a distended abdomen, flatulence, possible bad breath, basically normal urination and defecation, thin, white, slimy tongue fur, a slippery, forceful pulse

Treatment principles: Harmonize the spleen and strengthen transportation

Guiding formulas:
Qu Mai Zhi Zhu Wan (Massa Medica, Hordeus, Aurantium & Atractylodes Pills)
Bai Zhu (Rhizoma Atractylodis Macrocephalae)
Zhi Shi (Fructus Immaturus Aurantii)
Shen Qu (Massa Medica Fermentata)
Mai Ya (Fructus Germinatus Hordei)

Xiao Ji Hua Zhi Tang (Disperse Accumulation & Transform Stagnation Decoction)
Shan Zha (Fructus Crataegi)
Bing Lang (Semen Arecae)
Zhi Shi (Fructus Immaturus Aurantii)
Lai Fu Zi (Semen Raphani)
Lian Qiao (Fructus Forsythiae)

Jian Pi Xiao Ji Tang (Fortify the Spleen & Disperse Accumulation Decoction)

Bai Zhu (Rhizoma Atractylodis Macrocephalae)
Fu Ling (Poria)
Ji Nei Jin (Endothelium Corneum Gigeriae Galli)
Mu Xiang (Radix Auklandiae)
Bai Shao (Radix Paeoniae Albae)
Yan Hu Suo (Rhizoma Corydalis)
Gan Cao (Radix Glycyrrhizae)

2. Dampness & turbidity encumbering the spleen

Main symptoms: Chest oppression, nausea, bodily fatigue, stools not crisp, abdomen relatively distended forcing the baby to feed resulting in vomiting, thick, slimy fur on the top of the tongue

Treatment principles: If the tongue is pale, supplement the spleen and transform dampness. If the tongue is red, clear heat and transform dampness.

Guiding formulas:

To supplement the spleen and transform dampness, use **Shen Ling Bai Zhu San Jia Jian (Ginseng, Poria & Atractylodes Powder with Additions & Subtractions)**

Ren Shen (Radix Ginseng)
Bai Zhu (Rhizoma Atractylodis Macrocephalae)
Fu Ling (Poria)
Yi Yi Ren (Semen Coicis)
Hou Po (Cortex Magnoliae)
Huo Xiang (Herba Pogostemonis)

To clear heat and transform dampness, use **Gan Lu Xiao Du Dan Jia Jian (Sweet Dew Disperse Toxins Elixir with Additions & Subtractions):**

Huo Xiang (Herba Pogostemonis)
Yin Chen Hao (Herba Artemisiae Scopariae)
Fu Ling (Poria)
Lian Qiao (Fructus Forsythiae)
Hou Po (Cortex Magnoliae)
Ban Xia (Rhizoma Pinelliae)
Shi Chang Pu (Rhizoma Acori Tatarinowii)
Yi Yi Ren (Semen Coicis)
Hua Shi (Talcum)

If the stools are not crisp, add *Zhi Shi* (Fructus Immaturus Aurantii).

3. Spleen-stomach qi vacuity

Main symptoms: A somewhat depressed spirit, a sallow yellow facial complexion, lack of appetite, refusal to eat, when the child eats, there tends to be loose stools soon afterwards with undigested food in the stools, easy perspiration, a pale tongue with thin, white fur, a forceless pulse. If the child is still an infant or young toddler, there will likely be a visible blue vein at the root of the nose.

Treatment principles: Fortify the spleen and boost the qi

Guiding formula:
Xiang Sha Liu Jun Zi Tang Jia Wei (Auklandia & Amomum Six Gentlemen Decoction with Added Flavors)
    Dang Shen (Radix Codonopsitis)
    Bai Zhu (Rhizoma Atractylodis Macrocephalae)
    Fu Ling (Poria)
    Ban Xia (Rhizoma Pinelliae)
    Chen Pi (Pericarpium Citri Reticulatae)
    Mu Xiang (Radix Auklandiae)
    Sha Ren (Fructus Amomi)
    Gan Cao (Radix Glycyrrhizae)
    Shan Yao (Radix Dioscoreae)

If there are loose stools, add *Bai Bian Dou* (Semen Dolichoris) and *Yi Yi Ren* (Semen Coicis). If there is abdominal distention, add *Gu Ya* (Fructus Germinatus Oryzae) and *Mai Ya* (Fructus Germinatus Hordei).

If spleen vacuity reaches the kidneys so that there are symptoms of spleen vacuity and kidney debility, such as torpid intake and diminished appetite, loose stools, and fatigue, but also slow growth and development and weak bones, use **Jian Pi Bu Shen Tang (Fortify the Spleen & Supplement the Kidneys Decoction):**
    Huang Qi (Radix Astragali)
    Dang Shen (Radix Codonopsitis)
    Bai Zhu (Rhizoma Atractylodis Macrocephalae)
    Fu Ling (Poria)
    Gan Cao (Radix Glycyrrhizae)
    Ji Nei Jin (Endothelium Corneum Gigeriae Galli)
    Shu Di (cooked Radix Rehmanniae)
    Gui Ban (Plastrum Testudinis)
    Dong Chong Xia Cao (Cordyceps)
    Jiang Can (Bombyx Batryticatus)

4. Stomach yin insufficiency

Main symptoms: A dry mouth and a tendency to drink a lot yet no desire to eat food, dry skin, dry stools, a mirror-like or shiny tongue with peeled fur or scarlet red tongue with a scanty coating and scanty fluids, a fine pulse

Note: This pattern typically manifests after a febrile disease, such as measles. In this case, the heat of the fever has consumed and dried up the healthy fluids of the stomach. If these fluids within the stomach are insufficient, the stomach cannot perform its function of receiving and taking in foods.

Treatment principles: Nourish the stomach and foster yin

Guiding formulas:
Yang Wei Zeng Jin Tang (Nourish the Stomach & Increase Fluids Decoction)
Shi Hu (Herba Dendrobii)
Wu Mei (Fructus Mume)
Bei Sha Shen (Radix Glehniae)
Yu Zhu (Rhizoma Polygonati Odorati)
Bai Shao (Radix Paeoniae Albae)
Gan Cao (Radix Glycyrrhizae)

If there is also spleen vacuity, add *Shan Yao* (Radix Dioscoreae).

Ye Shi Yang Wei Tang Jia Jian (Master Ye's Nourish the Stomach Decoction with Additions & Subtractions)
Tian Men Dong (Tuber Asparagi)
Mai Men Dong (Tuber Ophiopogonis)
Yu Zhu (Rhizoma Polygonati Odorati)
Bei Sha Shen (Radix Glehniae)
Shan Yao (Radix Dioscoreae)
Shi Hu (Herba Dendrobii)

If there is constipation, add *Dang Gui* (Radix Angelicae Sinensis). If there is severe heat in the hands, feet, and heart, add *Qing Hao* (Herba Artemesiae Annuae) and *Bai Wei* (Radix Cynanchi Atrati).

Acupuncture & moxibustion

For food stagnation, needle *He Gu* (LI 4) and *Nei Ting* (St 44) or needle *Si Feng* (M-UE-9). For damp turbidity, add *Zu San Li* (St 36). For spleen vacuity, needle *Zu San Li* (St 36), *Pi Shu* (Bl 20), and *Wei Shu* (Bl 21). For stomach yin vacuity, needle *Nei Ting* (St 44) and *San Yin Jiao* (Sp 6). If spleen vacuity reaches the kidneys, moxa *Shen Que* (CV 8), *Guan Yuan* (CV 4), *Pi Shu* (Bl 20), and *Shen Shu* (Bl 23).

Adjunctive treatments

For food stagnation, massaging the abdomen with small clockwise circles within the large circles can help transport and conduct the food through the intestines. An enema can also be helpful to open the bowels and lead away stagnation. However, it is important not to force the child to eat if they do not want to. After all, this condition is due to the child's overeating. For spleen vacuity lack of appetite, when the child does eat, they should not be allowed to eat raw, chilled, cold, or frozen foods or drinks on the one hand or sugars and sweets on the other. A simple Chinese herbal home remedy for this pattern of pediatric lack of appetite is to drink a tea made from 20 cloves and some black tea.

23. Cold Sores

Some children are plagued with cold sores which occur periodically on or around their mouths. These sores are red, inflamed, and blistery. Eventually, crusts and scabs are formed. According to Western medicine, these are due to infection by the *Herpes simplex* virus which becomes active when the person has a cold or flu. However, they may occur even when the child appears otherwise healthy. In Chinese medicine, such cold sores are called *re qi chuang* or hot qi sores. This underscores that their occurrence has something to do with an accumulation of evil heat in the body. In children, this heat is usually located in the stomach and intestines. This heat is due to overeating in general and to overeating greasy, fatty, fried or hot, spicy foods in particular. This heat then floats upward to accumulate in the lungs.

Treatment based on pattern discrimination:

1. Wind heat evils in the lungs & stomach

Main symptoms: Fever blisters on the lips or angles of the mouth typically occurring with other symptoms of a cold or flu, dry mouth, dry stools, vexation and agitation, a red tongue with thin, white or yellow fur, a wiry, slippery, rapid pulse

Treatment principles: Clear heat and dispel wind

Guiding formulas:
Xin Yi Qing Fei Yin (Magnolia Flower Clear the Lungs Beverage)
Shi Gao (Gypsum Fibrosum)
Ju Hua (Flos Chrysanthemi)
Jin Yin Hua (Flos Lonicerae)
Pi Pa Ye (Folium Eriobotryae)
Lian Qiao (Fructus Forsythiae)
Huang Qin (Radix Scutellariae)
Zhi Zi (Fructus Gardeniae)
Zhi Mu (Rhizoma Anemarrhenae)
Xin Yi (Flos Magnoliae)

Xin Yi Qing Fei Yin (Magnolia Flower Clear the Lungs Beverage)
Xin Yi (Flos Magnoliae)

Gan Cao (Radix Glycyrrhizae)
calcined *Shi Gao* (Gypsum Fibrosum)
Zhi Mu (Rhizoma Anemarrhenae)
Zhi Zi (Fructus Gardeniae)
Huang Qin (Radix Scutellariae)
Pi Pa Ye (Folium Eriobotryae)
Sheng Ma (Rhizoma Cimicifugae)
Bai He (Bulbus Lilii)
Mai Men Dong (Tuber Ophiopogonis)

2. Spleen-stomach accumulation & heat

Main symptoms: Recurrent blistery lesions on the lips and corners of the mouth, diminished appetite, dry stools or constipation, red lips, a red tongue with dry, yellow fur, a surging, rapid pulse

Treatment principles: Clear heat and disperse accumulation

Guiding formula:
***Zhu Ye Shi Gao Tang* (Lophaterum & Gypsum Decoction)**
Dan Zhu Ye (Herba Lophateri)
Shi Gao (Gypsum Fibrosum)
Ren Shen (Radix Ginseng)
Ban Xia (Rhizoma Pinelliae)
Geng Mi (Fructus Oryzae Sativae)
mix-fried *Gan Cao* (Radix Glycyrrhizae)

Acupuncture & moxibustion

Mainly needle *He Gu* (LI 4) and *Nei Ting* (St 44).

Adjunctive treatments

First of all, one should institute a clear, bland diet. Secondly, if there are hard stools or constipation, one may give an enema. Externally, one can apply **Jin Huang San (Golden Yellow Powder)** mixed with cold, boiled water:

Da Huang (Radix Et Rhizoma Rhei), 25g
Huang Bai (Cortex Phellodendri), 25g
Huang Jiang (Rhizoma Curcumae Longae), 25g
Bai Zhi (Radix Angelicae Dahuricae), 25g
Nan Xing (Rhizoma Arisaematis), 10g
Chen Pi (Pericarpium Citri Reticulatae), 10g
Cang Zhu (Rhizoma Atractylodis), 10g
Hou Po (Cortex Magnoliae), 10g
Gan Cao (Radix Glycyrrhizae), 10g
Tian Hua Fen (Radix Trichosanthis), 5g

24. Bed-wetting

Bed-wetting refers to the involuntary discharge of urine during sleep at night in children over three years of age. It is mainly due to the inherent immaturity of the kidneys in children. The kidneys control growth and development according to Chinese medicine. For instance, one's second or permanent teeth and puberty are both signs of the maturation of the Chinese concept of the kidneys. As in Western medicine, the kidneys are also responsible for urination. However, pediatric enuresis, as this condition is technically called, may also be due to spleen and lung vacuity or damp heat.

Treatment based on pattern discrimination:

1. Kidney vacuity (a.k.a. vacuity cold of the lower origin)

Main symptoms: Nighttime enuresis 1-2 or more times each night, frequent, clear urination, a pale facial complexion, a tendency to low back or knee soreness or weakness, possible chilled limbs and a fear of cold, a pale tongue with thin, white fur

Treatment principles: Warm and supplement kidney yang, secure and astringe the urination

Guiding formulas:
Jin Suo Gu Jing Wan (Golden Lock Secure the Essence Pills)
  Jin Ying Zi (Fructus Rosae Laevigatae)
  Suo Yang (Herba Cynomorii)
  Sha Yuan Zi (Semen Astragali Complanati)
  Qian Shi (Semen Euryalis)
  Lian Zi (Semen Nelumbinis)
  Lian Xu (Stamen Nelumbinis)
  Long Gu (Os Draconis)
  Mu Li (Concha Ostreae)

Sang Piao Xiao San Jia Jian (Mantis Egg-case Powder with Additions & Subtractions)
  Sang Piao Xiao (Ootheca Mantidis)
  Yi Zhi Ren (Fructus Alpiniae Oxyphyllae)
  Bu Gu Zhi (Fructus Psoraleae)
  Fu Pen Zi (Fructus Rubi)
  Huang Qi (Radix Astragali)
  Dang Shen (Radix Codonopsitis)
  Shi Chang Pu (Rhizoma Acori Tatarinowii)

Tu Si Zi San (Cuscuta Powder)
  Tu Si Zi (Semen Cuscutae)
  Rou Cong Rong (Herba Cistanchis)
  Fu Zi (Radix Lateralis Praeparatus Aconiti Carmichaeli)

Wu Wei Zi (Fructus Schisandrae)
Mu Li (Concha Ostreae)

Suo Quan San (Lock the Spring Powder)
Yi Zhi Ren (Fructus Alpiniae Oxyphyllae)
Wu Yao (Radix Linderae)
Shan Yao (Radix Dioscoreae)

If phlegm dampness brewing internally, add *Nan Xing* (Rhizoma Arisaematis), *Ban Xia* (Rhizoma Pinelliae), *Shi Chang Pu* (Rhizoma Acori Tatarinowii), and *Yuan Zhi* (Radix Polygalae). If there is torpid intake and loose stools, add *Dang Shen* (Radix Codonopsitis), *Bai Zhu* (Rhizoma Atractylodis Macrocephalae), *Fu Ling* (Poria), and *Shan Zha* (Fructus Crataegi).

Unnamed formula
Sang Piao Xiao (Ootheca Mantidis)
Lu Rong (Cornu Parvum Cervi)
Huang Qi (Radix Astragali)
calcined *Mu Li* (Concha Ostreae)
Chi Shi Zhi (Hallyositum Rubrum)
Ren Shen (Radix Ginseng)
Hou Po (Cortex Magnoliae)

Ma Huang Yi Zhi Tang (Ephedra & Alpinia Oxyphylla Decoction)
mix-fried *Ma Huang* (Herba Ephedrae)
Wu Wei Zi (Fructus Schisandrae)
Yi Zhi Ren (Fructus Alpiniae Oxyphyllae)

2. Spleen/lung qi vacuity

Main symptoms: Nighttime enuresis, shortness of breath, disinclination to speak, lassitude of the spirit, lack of strength, a somber white facial complexion, devitalized appetite, loose stools, spontaneous perspiration, a pale tongue with white fur, a pulse with diminished force

Treatment principles: Bank the origin and boost the qi, secure and astringe the urination

Guiding formulas:
Bu Zhong Yi Qi Tang (Supplement the Center & Boost the Qi Decoction) plus Suo Quan Wan (Lock the Spring Pills)
Ren Shen (Radix Ginseng)
Huang Qi (Radix Astragali)
Bai Zhu (Rhizoma Atractylodis Macrocephalae)
Shan Yao (Radix Dioscoreae)

mix-fried *Gan Cao* (Radix Glycyrrhizae)
Sheng Ma (Rhizoma Cimicifugae)
Chai Hu (Radix Bupleuri)
Dang Gui (Radix Angelicae Sinensis)
Yi Zhi Ren (Fructus Alpiniae Oxyphyllae)
Wu Yao (Radix Linderae)
Chen Pi (Pericarpium Citri Reticulatae)

If there are loose stools, add *Pao Jiang* (blast-fried Rhizoma Zingiberis). If there is difficulty arousing from sleep, add *Shi Chang Pu* (Rhizoma Acori Tatarinowii).

Bu Zhong Yi Qi Tang (Supplement the Center & Boost the Qi Decoction) plus *Suo Quan Wan* (Lock the Spring Pills) with additions and subtractions
Ren Shen (Radix Ginseng)
Huang Qi (Radix Astragali)
Bai Zhu (Rhizoma Atractylodis Macrocephalae)
Dang Gui (Radix Angelicae Sinensis)
Shan Yao (Radix Dioscoreae)
Yi Zhi Ren (Fructus Alpiniae Oxyphyllae)
Sheng Ma (Rhizoma Cimicifugae)
Wu Wei Zi (Fructus Schisandrae)
Jin Ying Zi (Fructus Rosae Laevigatae)

Bu Zhong Yi Qi Tang Jia Jian (Supplement the Center & Boost the Qi Decoction with Additions & Subtractions)
Ren Shen (Radix Ginseng)
Huang Qi (Radix Astragali)
Bai Zhu (Rhizoma Atractylodis Macrocephalae)
Dang Gui (Radix Angelicae Sinensis)
Shan Yao (Radix Dioscoreae)
Tu Si Zi (Semen Cuscutae)
Fu Pen Zi (Fructus Rubi)
Gou Qi Zi (Fructus Lycii)
Yi Zhi Ren (Fructus Alpiniae Oxyphyllae)

3. Liver channel damp heat

Main symptoms: Slippage of a small amount of urine which smells foul and is colored relatively yellow, emotional tension and agitation, talking in their sleep, bruxism during sleep, red lips, yellow tongue fur, a rapid, forceful pulse

Treatment principles: Drain the liver and clear heat

Guiding formulas:
Long Dan Xie Gan Tang Jia Jian (Gentiana Drain the Liver Decoction with Additions & Subtractions)

Long Dan Cao (Radix Gentianae)
Zhi Zi (Fructus Gardeniae)
Mu Tong (Caulis Akebiae)
Chai Hu (Radix Bupleuri)
Sheng Di (uncooked Radix Rehmanniae)
Huang Bai (Cortex Phellodendri)
Zhi Mu (Rhizoma Anemarrhenae)
Gan Cao (Radix Glycyrrhizae)

Long Dan Xie Gan Tang Jia Jian (Gentiana Drain the Liver Decoction with Additions & Subtractions)

Long Dan Cao (Radix Gentianae)
Zhi Zi (Fructus Gardeniae)
Mu Tong (Caulis Akebiae)
Chai Hu (Radix Bupleuri)
Sheng Di (uncooked Radix Rehmanniae)
Ze Xie (Rhizoma Alismatis)
Che Qian Zi (Semen Plantaginis)
Gan Cao (Radix Glycyrrizhae)

If damp heat endures and this disease is not cured, damp fire internally brewing may consume and damage kidney yin as evidenced by a red tongue. In that case, use **Zhi Bai Di Huang Wan (Anemarrhena & Phellodendron Rehmannia Pills):**

Zhi Mu (Rhizoma Anemarrhenae)
Huang Bai (Cortex Phellodendri)
Shu Di (cooked Radix Rehmanniae)
Shan Yao (Radix Dioscoreae)
Shan Zhu Yu (Fructus Corni)
Fu Ling (Poria)
Ze Xie (Rhizoma Alismatis)
Dan Pi (Cortex Moutan)

Acupuncture & moxibustion

Needle *Ye Niao Dian* (Nighttime Urination Point) located at the center of the second transverse crease on the palmar surface of the little finger. Or one may needle *San Yin Jiao* (Sp 6) and *Guan Yuan* (CV 4). If there is concomitant spleen vacuity, add *Zu San Li* (St 36).

Adjunctive treatments

For vacuity cold of the lower origin make a tea out of cinnamon and licorice and add 2 teaspoons of molasses. For either kidney vacuity or lung-spleen vacuity, do spinal pinch-pull several times each day to strengthen the bodily constitution. One can also grind a small amount of *Gong Ding Xiang* (Flos Caryophylli), *Bai Jie Zi* (Semen Sinapis), *Yi Zhi Ren* (Fructus Alpiniae Oxyphyllae), *Wu Yao* (Radix Linderae), and *Xi Xin* (Herba Asari) into powder. This is then mixed with vinegar and held in place with *Shang Shi Zhi Tong*

Gao (Injury [due to] Dampness, Stop Pain Plasters) at *Zhong Ji* (CV 3), *Da He* (Ki 12), and *San Yin Jiao* (Sp 6). These should be changed 1 time each day. And for both the vacuity and damp heat patterns, a clear, bland diet is very important. For vacuity cold cases, they should avoid anything which is chilled, cold, or frozen. For lung-spleen vacuity cases, they should avoid sugar and sweets as well as chilled and raw foods. In the case of the damp heat in the liver channel, it is also important to help the child develop stress-reducing and relaxation techniques as well as to identify and correct any causes of emotional tension and frustration.

Comments

In my clinical practice, the cases of pediatric enuresis I commonly see are due to kidney vacuity and lung-spleen qi vacuity. Quite frankly, such cases may only present with a scant few of the symptoms listed above. Happily, when due to kidney vacuity, *Jin Suo Gu Jing Wan* (Golden Lock Secure the Essence Pills), which comes as ready-made pills, are easy for young children to swallow and usually provide cheap, easy, and effective treatment. When due to lung-spleen vacuity, I usually prescribe a decoction which is then administered by an eyedropper.

Some parents both in China and the West try to shame their children into stopping their bed-wetting, but this is seldom the answer. If the child has weak kidneys, the fear of the parents anger or disdain will only further damage the kidneys according to Chinese medicine. While children with damp heat enuresis in part due to anger and frustration will obviously only get worse in response to their parents' anger and frustration.

Obviously, if a child is having trouble with bed-wetting, they should not be allowed to drink too much in the evening, and the parents should make sure the child empties their bladder before bed each evening. In addition, if due to kidney deficiency or lung-spleen deficiency, the child should not be allowed to become too fatigued before going to bed. Overfatigue only results in further weakening of the kidneys, spleen, and lungs.

25. Impetigo

Impetigo is a contagious, blistery, skin disease which is mostly seen in children. From the Western medical point of view, it is due to a bacterial infection. It is characterized by clusters of red, watery blisters mostly occurring on the arms, legs, and face. When the blisters break, they ooze a thin, honey-colored fluid which, when it dries, forms crusts around the lesions. Because of this yellow-colored exudate, impetigo is traditionally called "yellow fluid sores" or "pus-dripping sores" in Chinese. This disease mostly occurs in the summertime.

In Chinese medicine, this disease is mainly due to damp heat attacking and accumulating in the skin. Therefore, it typically occurs during seasons or in locales where there is a preponderance of dampness and heat, such as the summer. Although this disease is seen as an invasion of external dampness and heat, children with a propensity to be damp and hot internally are more susceptible to this condition, and dampness and heat accumulate internally in children primarily due to their weak spleens and faulty diet.

Internal treatments

Guiding formulas:
Qing Pi Chu Shi Yin (Clear the Spleen & Eliminate Dampness Beverage)

Fu Ling (Poria)
Sheng Di (uncooked Radix Rehmanniae)
Lian Qiao (Fructus Forsythiae)
Yin Chen Hao (Herba Artemisiae Scopariae)
Bai Zhu (Rhizoma Atractylodis Macrocephalae)
Cang Zhu (Rhizoma Atractylodis)
Mai Men Dong (Tuber Ophiopogonis)
Ze Xie (Rhizoma Alismatis)
Zhi Zi (Fructus Gardeniae)
Xiang Fu (Rhizoma Cyperi)
Huang Qi (Radix Astragali)

Er Miao San Jia Wei (Two Wonders Powder with Added Flavors)

Cang Zhu (Rhizoma Atractylodis)
Bai Zhu (Rhizoma Atractylodis Macrocephalae)
Huang Bai (Cortex Phellodendri)
Bing Lang (Semen Arecae)
Huang Qin (Radix Scutellariae)
Ku Shen (Radix Sophorae Flavescentis)
Di Fu Zi (Fructus Kochiae)
Ze Xie (Rhizoma Alismatis)

Qing Shu Tang Jia Jian (Clear Summerheat Decoction with Additions & Subtractions)

Qing Hao (Herba Artemisiae Annuae)
Huo Xiang (Herba Pogostemonis)
Pei Lan (Herba Eupatorii)
Jin Yin Hua (Flos Lonicerae)
Lian Qiao (Fructus Forsythiae)
Che Qian Zi (Semen Plantaginis)
Hua Shi (Talcum)
Gan Cao (Radix Glycyrrhizae)
Chi Shao (Radix Paeoniae Rubrae)
Zhi Zi (Fructus Gardeniae)
Pu Gong Ying (Herba Taraxaci)

External treatments

Guiding formulas:
Ku Shen Tang (Sophora Decoction)
   Ku Shen (Radix Sophora Flavescentis), 60g
   Ju Hua (Flos Chrysanthemi), 60g
   She Chuang Zi (Fructus Cnidii), 30g
   Jin Yin Hua (Flos Lonicerae), 30g
   Bai Zhi (Radix Angelicae Dahuricae), 15g
   Huang Bai (Cortex Phellodendri), 15g
   Di Fu Zi (Fructus Kochiae), 15g
   Shi Chang Pu (Rhizoma Acori Tatarinowii), 15g

Method of preparation & use: Decoct in water and wash the affected area.

San Huang Xi Ji (Three Yellows Washing Prescription)
   Da Huang (Radix Et Rhizoma Rhei)
   Huang Bai (Cortex Phellodendri)
   Huang Qin (Radix Scutellariae)
   Ku Shen (Radix Sophorae Flavescentis)

Method of preparation & use: Decoct equal amounts of the above medicinals in water and wash the affected area.

Qing Dai San (Indigo Powder)
   Qing Dai (Pulvis Indigonis), 20g
   Huang Bai (Cortex Phellodendri), 20g
   Shi Gao (Gypsum Fibrosum), 40g
   Hua Shi (Talcum), 40g

Method of preparation & use: Powder finely and mix with cold, boiled water to form a paste. Apply this paste to the lesions. Cover with gauze and replace 2-3 times per day.

Adjunctive treatments

In order to prevent impetigo, it is important to foster a healthy spleen and to promote a clear, bland diet. One can fortify the spleen by doing daily infant massage, while a clear, bland diet of primarily cooked foods low in fats and greases and low in sugars and sweets both fortifies the spleen *and* helps to prevent the accumulation of dampness and heat internally. During the summer, in order to prevent and treat impetigo and other damp heat conditions, one can also make porridges or soups out of either *Yi Yi Ren* (Semen Coicis), or *Lu Dou* (Semen Phaseoli Munginis).

Comments

If a child does catch impetigo, it is important that the lesions be lightly covered with a gauze bandage, since the lesions will spread wherever the yellowish fluid touches. This means that other children should not come in physical contact with either the lesions themselves or the suppurative fluid. It also means that the child must be kept from scratching these lesions. If the lesions are touched, one should immediately wash. Since impetigo often occurs secondary to scratching a small cut or insect bite with dirty hands, children should be taught to wash their hands frequently and also not to scratch small cuts and bites, since this may lead to infection.

26. Allergies

There is no chapter simply titled allergies in any Chinese pediatric text of which I know. Below I discuss the main allergic pediatric conditions—pediatric eczema, pediatric hives, and allergic rhinitis — and we have already discussed pediatric asthma above. However, before going into those individual diseases, it is important to understand the underlying disease mechanisms at work in most, if not all, allergic conditions. In my experience, allergies in children are due to two main causes. The first cause is dietary. Either solid foods were not introduced properly or the child has been allowed to eat the wrong diet. As discussed above, solid foods should only be introduced when the child is old enough to grab for them off their parents' plates. This typically corresponds to the first teething around five months or so. When introducing foods, it is important to only introduce one food at a time. That way, if there is a negative reaction due to the child's digestion not being ready to handle that food, it can be identified and withdrawn until the digestion has matured. If the food is continued to be fed to the child and they really are not digesting it, then the child will tend to become reactive to that food.

In addition, if the child is fed a diet high in sugars and sweets, this will weaken their spleen and cause an accumulation of dampness within the body. If this dampness lingers and accumulates, it will typically give rise to damp heat in the intestines. This damp hot environment then provides the perfect breeding ground for overgrowths of yeast and fungi. These move outside the intestines. As they do so, they cause the intestinal lining to become more permeable, and so large food molecules which should not enter the blood stream do, where they provoke immune or allergic responses. Also, when these yeast and fungi move outside the guts and into the body, they eventually die. When they die their proteins are also recognized as foreign and provoke immune or allergic responses.

The other main mechanism for causing allergic states in the body is antibiotics which also, in their own way, foster overgrowths of yeast and fungi. Whether due to faulty diet or to antibiotics, overgrowths of yeast and fungi are directly responsible for the body's becoming allergic or hypersensitive to things it should not ordinarily be allergic to. These may be airborne, upper respiratory allergies, such as hay fever or allergic asthma, these may be food allergies, or these may be types of allergic dermatitis, such as hives, eczema, and psoriasis.

All of these diseases can be treated according to their pattern discrimination with professionally prescribed Chinese herbal medicine. However, since diet is such an important part of such allergic conditions, if the parents adopt a clear, bland diet for the child, this will go a long way to solving any of these problems. And, in my experience, none of these problems can be lastingly cured with acupuncture and/or Chinese herbal medicine alone if the diet is not taken care of.

What is the clear, bland diet in terms of allergic diseases? I believe this is so important that I cannot overstate or explain this concept too often. It means eating cooked food at a warm temperature. Remember, for the spleen to do its work with maximum efficiency, all food in the stomach must be turned into 100 degree soup. It means eating a diet high in grains and complex carbohydrates. But these grains must be well-cooked and/or milled in order for them to be easily digestible. The main grain should be rice since it is so hypoallergenic. It means a diet high in beans and some nuts and seeds. It means a diet high in vegetables and fruits, but preferably cooked for infants and toddlers. It means a little bit of animal protein from time to time.

What should be minimized are sugars and sweets *from all sources.* In my experience, sugar from fruit juice or honey is just as bad as white or refined sugar. And a glass of fruit juice has as much or more sugar than a candy bar. It means only a very little of dairy products, like milk and yogurt, and when dairy products are eaten, they should be eaten warm or at least room temperature. It means a diet low in fats and oils. And it means a diet low or even free from foods made through fermentation or which are easily contaminated by yeasts and molds. This means that the child should not eat anything made with yeast, such as bread and cheese, anything with vinegar, or any food which gets moldy easily. Apples don't mold easily but peaches, strawberries, and most melons do, while the hazy outer layer of the grape skin is mold.

Such a clear, bland, hypoallergenic diet is a big change for many children and adults alike. But it is the key to curing so many chronic, otherwise knotty and difficult to treat diseases. When one switches to a diet like this, there may be an initial aggravation as many of the yeast and fungi in the body die off due to lack of nutrients (read sugar). By the end of the first week, there should be obvious improvement. However, although there can be startling improvement in only a few weeks, this diet must be preserved if it is going to have lasting effect. If it is not adhered to for at least three months, its effects will only be very short-lived. If one can keep it up for 6 months, there will be a much better foundation with less tendency to slip backwards. In actual fact, although one can eventually eat aggravating foods from time to time, this is the diet that is healthiest for the majority of people living in temperate climates. This diet has recently been promoted by the U.S. Department of Agriculture with their food pyramid. It is also very similar to the Pritikin diet, the Macrobiotic diet, and the Mediterranean diet at least in its broad outlines.

Adjunctive treatment

A simple treatment for all kinds of allergies is to do cupping over the navel. When cupping such as this is done over the navel, the cup is left in place for 5 minutes and then removed. This is repeated for 3-5 times per session and one session is done per day for several days. This treatment is not appropriate for tiny infants, but can be quite good for young children with all sorts of allergies.

27. Pediatric Eczema

Eczema refers to a superficial inflammation of the skin characterized by redness, swelling, blisters, oozing, crusting, scaling, and usually itching. This is different from tinea in that eczematous lesions do not have clearly defined borders. Pediatric eczema is divided into two main patterns in Chinese medicine. There is a damp heat brewing and steaming pattern and a spleen vacuity/blood depletion pattern. These two patterns can also be called wet or weeping eczema and dry, scaly eczema. The wet eczema tends to be acute, while the dry eczema tends to be more a subacute or chronic condition.

Treatment based on pattern discrimination:

1. Damp heat brewing & steaming

Main symptoms: Eczematous lesions which begin as a red rash. Over time, this rash develops blisters which eventually burst and weep. If these are scratched, a secondary infection may easily occur.

Treatment principles: Clear heat, disinhibit dampness, and dispel wind

Guiding formulas:
***Bei Xie Shen Shi Tang* (Dioscorea Hypoglauca Percolate Dampness Decoction)**
    Yi Yi Ren (Semen Coicis)
    Hua Shi (Talcum)
    Bei Xie (Rhizoma Dioscoreae Hypoglaucae)
    Fu Ling (Poria)
    Huang Bai (Cortex Phellodendri)
    Dan Pi (Cortex Moutan)
    Ze Xie (Rhizoma Alismatis)
    Tong Cao (Medulla Tetrapanacis)

***Bei Xie Shen Shi Tang Jia Jian* (Dioscorea Hypoglauca Percolate Dampness Decoction with Additions & Subtractions)**
    Bei Xie (Rhizoma Dioscoreae Hypoglaucae)
    Fu Ling (Poria)
    Ze Xie (Rhizoma Alismatis)

Huang Bai (Cortex Phellodendri)
Ku Shen (Radix Sophorae Flavescentis)
Long Dan Cao (Radix Gentianae)
Yi Yi Ren (Semen Coicis)
Hua Shi (Talcum)
Gan Cao (Radix Glycyrrhizae)
Tong Cao (Medulla Tetrapanacis)
Chan Yi (Periostracum Cicadae)

Er Miao San (Two Wonders Powder)

Cang Zhu (Rhizoma Atractylodis)
Huang Bai (Cortex Phellodendri)

If the lesions are on the upper body, add *Sang Ye* (Folium Mori), *Ju Hua* (Flos Chrysanthemi), and *Chan Yi* (Periostracum Cicadae). If the lesions are on the abdomen, add *Huang Lian* (Rhizoma Coptidis) and *Huang Qin* (Radix Scutellariae). If the lesions are on the lower limbs, add *Niu Xi* (Radix Achyranthis Bidentatae) and *Che Qian Zi* (Semen Plantaginis). If there is constipation, add *Da Huang* (Radix Et Rhizoma Rhei). If there is abdominal distention, bad breath, diminished appetite or other signs and symptoms of food stagnation and turbid dampness, add *Shan Zha* (Fructus Crataegi), *Shen Qu* (Massa Medica Fermentata), and *Huo Xiang* (Herba Pogostemonis).

Shu Feng Qu Shi Tang (Course Wind & Eliminate Dampness Decoction)

Ren Dong Teng (Caulis Lonicerae)
Huang Qin (Radix Scutellariae)
Chan Yi (Periostracum Cicadae)
Zhi Ke (Fructus Aurantii)
Chen Pi (Pericarpium Citri Reticulatae)
Jiang Can (Bombyx Batryticatus)
Bai Xian Pi (Cortex Dictamni)
Bai Zhu (Rhizoma Atractylodis Macrocephalae)
Huo Xiang (Herba Pogostemonis)

If heat is severe, add *Zhi Zi* (Fructus Gardeniae) and *Bai Mao Gen* (Rhizoma Imperatae). If wind is severe, add *Fang Feng* (Radix Saposhnikoviae) and *Sang Ye* (Folium Mori). If dampness is severe, add *Yi Yi Ren* (Semen Coicis). If bowel movements are inhibited and not smoothly flowing and if there is foul-smelling flatulence, add *Shan Zha* (Fructus Crataegi).

2. Spleen vacuity, blood depletion

Main symptoms: A red, swollen rash which is scaly and hard. Itching is relatively mild. There may be a yellow-colored, fatty exudate.

Treatment principles: Fortify the spleen and dry dampness, nourish the blood and dispel wind

Guiding formulas:
Ping Wei San (Level [or Calm] the Stomach Powder) plus *Si Wu Tang* (Four Materials Decoction) with additions and subtractions

    Cang Zhu (Rhizoma.Atractylodis)
    Hou Po (Cortex Magnoliae)
    Chen Pi (Pericarpium Citri Reticulatae)
    Gan Cao (Radix Glycyrrhizae)
    Dang Gui (Radix Angelicae Sinensis)
    Bai Shao (Radix Paeoniae Albae)
    Chi Shao (Radix Paeoniae Rubrae)
    Ku Shen (Radix Sophorae Flavescentis)
    Bai Xian Pi (Cortex Dictamni)
    Di Fu Zi (Fructus Kochiae)
    Huang Bai (Cortex Phellodendri)

Adjunctive treatments

Patients with eczema must avoid sugar and sweets, anything made through fermentation, and anything that molds easily, while they should eat a cooked, warm, clear, bland, anticandidal, hypoallergenic diet. Some simple Chinese herbal home remedies for damp heat eczema is a tea made out of Job's tears barley and mung beans; a tea made out of dandelion and corn silks; or a tea made out of aduki beans, Job's tears barley, and corn silk. Externally, one can wash the affected area with equal portions of salt and borax dissolved in warm water and applied 2-3 times per day. One may also use *San Huang Xi Ji* (Three Yellows Washing Prescription) described above under impetigo. Or one may use a poultice made from fresh, grated potato held in place by gauze and changed every 3 hours. For dry eczema, one can use *Qing Dai Gao* (Indigo Ointment). This is made by taking *Qing Dai San* (Indigo Powder) described above under impetigo and mixing it with roasted sesame oil. Apply this paste to the affected area. Do not use an oil-based application if there is weeping or this will make the condition worse by forcing the dampness into the surrounding tissues.

Comments

In both these patterns, the spleen plays the pivotal role. The presence of damp heat smoldering in the skin is due to poor spleen function. In Chinese medicine, the spleen is responsible for transforming and transporting body fluids. Damp heat occurs in infants and children because of weak spleen function compounded by faulty diet. Dampness accumulates and obstructs the free flow of warm qi which then backs up and turns into heat. This heat commingles with this dampness and thus there is damp heat. In the second pattern, spleen deficiency and weakness give rise to blood deficiency. In Chinese medicine, blood is made out of the essence of food and liquids digested and refined by the spleen. Because the blood nourishes and irrigates the skin, if there is blood deficiency, the skin may become dry, scaly, and itchy. Therefore, in both patterns, a spleen-strengthening, dampness eliminating diet is essential. This is the clear, bland diet described above with emphasis on avoiding sugars and sweets, fermented foods, and foods which mold easily. This then is an anticandidal, hypoallergenic diet as well.

28. Pediatric Hives

Hives, nettle rash, or urticaria are raised wheals on the skin. They can be large or small, red or white, all over the body or only in a very localized area. They develop quickly and can also disappear quickly. Most often they are a type of allergic response. Children are especially susceptible to hives because their skin is believed to be looser and less densely packed than adults'. Therefore, they are more easily invaded by evil winds. However, evil wind is only a poetic way of referring to an unseen pathogen. In Chinese pediatrics, there are three main patterns describing hives in children.

Treatment based on pattern discrimination:

1. Wind cold

Main symptoms: Pale-colored wheals which get worse on exposure to chill or wind. They also tend to be worse in the winter and better in the summer. The tongue has thin, white, possibly slimy fur, while the pulse is soggy and relaxed (*i.e.*, on the verge of slow).

Treatment principles: Dispel wind and scatter cold, regulate and harmonize the constructive and defensive

Guiding formulas:
Gui Zhi Tang Jia Jian (Cinnamon Twig Decoction with Additions & Subtractions)
   Gui Zhi (Ramulus Cinnamomi)
   Chi Shao (Radix Paeoniae Rubrae)
   Jing Jie (Herba Schizonepetae)
   Fang Feng (Radix Saposhnikoviae)
   Qiang Huo (Radix Et Rhizoma Notopterygii)
   Du Huo (Radix Angelicae Pubescentis)
   Fu Ping (Herba Lemnae/Spirodelae)
   Sheng Jiang (uncooked Rhizoma Zingiberis)
   Gan Cao (Radix Glycyrrhizae)
   Da Zao (Fructus Jujubae)

Jing Fang Bai Du San Jia Jian (Schizonepeta & Sapshnikovia Vanquish Toxins Powder with Additions & Subtractions)
   Jing Jie (Herba Schizonepetae)
   Fang Feng (Radix Saposhnikoviae)
   Gui Zhi (Ramulus Cinnamomi)
   Ma Huang (Herba Ephedrae)

Bai Shao (Radix Paeoniae Albae)
Qin Jiao (Radix Gentianae Macrophyllae)
Bai Xian Pi (Cortex Dictamni)
Sheng Jiang (uncooked Rhizoma Zingiberis)
Fu Ping (Herba Lemnae/Spirodelae)
Gan Cao (Radix Glycyrrhizae)

2. Wind heat

Main symptoms: Red-colored wheals which feel burning hot and which itch extraordinarily. They are worse on exposure to heat and are worse in the summer and better in the winter. The tongue has thin, yellow fur, and the pulse is floating and rapid.

Treatment principles: Dispel wind and clear heat, disinhibit dampness and stop itching

Guiding formulas:
Xiao Feng San Jia Jian (Dispersing Wind Powder with Additions & Subtractions)
Sang Ye (Folium Mori)
Chan Yi (Periostracum Cicadae)
Di Fu Zi (Fructus Kochiae)
Fu Ping (Herba Lemnae/Spirodelae)
Cang Zhu (Rhizoma Atractylodis)
Yi Yi Ren (Semen Coicis)
Zhi Zi (Fructus Gardeniae)
Ku Shen (Radix Sophorae Flavescentis)
Xu Chang Qing (Radix Cynanchi Paniculati)
Gan Cao (Radix Glycyrrhizae)

Zi Cao San (Lithospermum Powder)
Qing Dai (Pulvis Indigonis)
Zi Cao (Radix Lithospermi/Arnebiae)
Bai Zhi (Radix Angelicae Dahuricae)
Han Shui Shi (Calcitum)
Ru Xiang (Olibanum)

Jiang Can Jing Gong Yin (Bombyx, Schizonepeta & Scolopendra Beverage)
Jiang Can (Bombyx Batryticatus)
Jing Jie Sui (Herba Schizonepetae)
Wu Gong (Scolopendra)

Chu Feng Xiao Zhen Fang (Dispel Wind & Disperse Rash Formula)
Lu Lu Tong (Fructus Liquidambaris Taiwaniae)

Wu Mei (Fructus Mume)
Di Long (Pheretima)
Fang Feng (Radix Saposhnikoviae)
Chan Yi (Periostracum Cicadae)
Dan Pi (Cortex Moutan)
Gan Cao (Radix Glycyrrhizae)

Qu Feng Zhi Yang Tang (Dispel Wind & Stop Itching Decoction)
Chan Yi (Periostracum Cicadae)
Wu Shao She (Zaocys Dhumnades)
Jing Jie (Herba Schizonepetae)
Fang Feng (Radix Saposhnikoviae)
Fu Ping (Herba Lemnae/Spirodelae)
Bai Ji Li (Fructus Tribuli)
Dan Pi (Cortex Moutan)
Gan Cao (Radix Glycyrrhizae)

If the external defensive is vacuous, add *Huang Qi* (Radix Astragali) and *Bai Zhu* (Rhizoma Atractylodis Macrocephalae). If there is yin vacuity, add *Sheng Di* (uncooked Radix Rehmanniae) and *Mai Men Dong* (Tuber Ophiopogonis). If there is blood vacuity, add *Dang Gui* (Radix Angelicae Sinensis) and *He Shou Wu* (Radix Polygoni Multiflori). If there is blood heat, add *Sheng Di* (uncooked Radix Rehmanniae) and *Chi Shao* (Radix Paeoniae Rubrae). If dampness is severe, add *Cang Zhu* (Rhizoma Atractylodis), *Bai Xian Pi* (Cortex Dictamni), and *Di Fu Zi* (Fructus Kochiae). If there is food accumulation, add *Shan Zha* (Fructus Crataegi), *Shen Qu* (Massa Medica Fermentata), *Gu Ya* (Fructus Germinatus Oryzae), and/or *Mai Ya* (Fructus Germinatus Hordei). If heat is severe, add *Huang Qin* (Radix Scutellariae) and *Jin Yin Hua* (Flos Lonicerae). If there is abdominal pain, add *Bai Shao* (Radix Paeoniae Albae) and *Yan Hu Suo* (Rhizoma Corydalis).

3. Intestines & stomach damp heat

Main symptoms: Hives typically accompanied by abdominal pain and mostly due to loss of discipline in eating and drinking. In other words, these hives are clearly associated with a food allergy. In some cases, there may even be intestinal parasites. The tongue fur is slimy and possibly yellow, while the pulse is slippery and rapid.

Treatment principles: Dispel wind and discharge heat, disperse, lead away, and kill parasites

Guiding formulas:
Fang Feng Tong Shen San Jia Jian (Sapshnikovia Communicate with the Sages Powder with Additions & Subtractions)
Jing Jie (Herba Schizonepetae)
Fang Feng (Radix Saposhnikoviae)

    Zhi Zi (Fructus Gardeniae)
    processed *Da Huang* (Radix Et Rhizoma Rhei)
    Cang Zhu (Rhizoma Atractylodis)
    Ku Shen (Radix Sophorae Flavescentis)
    Hua Shi (Talcum)
    Gan Cao (Radix Glycyrrhizae)
    Shan Zha (Fructus Crataegi)
    Shen Qu (Massa Medica Fermentata)

Unnamed formula
    Lian Qiao (Fructus Forsythiae)
    Dang Gui (Radix Angelicae Sinensis)
    Chi Shao (Radix Paeoniae Rubrae)
    Fang Feng (Radix Saposhnikoviae)
    Mu Tong (Caulis Akebiae)
    Hua Shi (Talcum)
    Niu Bang Zi (Fructus Arctii)
    Wu Gong (Scolopendra)
    Qu Mai (Herba Dianthi)
    Shi Gao (Gypsum Fibrosum)
    Jing Jie (Herba Schizonepetae)
    Chai Hu (Radix Bupleuri)
    Huang Qin (Radix Scutellariae)
    Zhi Zi (Fructus Gardeniae)
    Che Qian Zi (Semen Plantaginis)
    Gan Cao (Radix Glycyrrhizae)

If food stagnation and abdominal distention are more prominent than signs of heat, use **Ping Wei San Jia Jian (Level the Stomach Powder with Additions & Subtractions):**
    Cang Zhu (Rhizoma Atractylodis)
    Bai Zhu (Rhizoma Atractylodis Macrocephalae)
    Hou Po (Cortex Magnoliae)
    Chen Pi (Pericarpium Citri Reticulatae)
    Fu Ling (Poria)
    Ze Xie (Rhizoma Alismatis)
    Fang Feng (Radix Saposhnikoviae)
    Cang Er Zi (Fructus Xanthii)
    Ku Shen (Radix Sophorae Flavescentis)
    Gan Cao (Radix Glycyrrhizae)

If food stagnation and abdominal distention are more prominent with no signs of heat, use **Zhi Zhu San Jia Jian (Aurantium & Atractylodes Powder with Additions & Subtractions):**
    Zhi Shi (Fructus Immaturus Aurantii)

Sha Ren (Fructus Amomi)
Chen Pi (Pericarpium Citri Reticulatae)
Jing Jie (Herba Schizonepetae)
Fang Feng (Radix Saposhnikoviae)
Bai Zhu (Rhizoma Atractylodis Macrocephalae)
Xiang Fu (Rhizoma Cyperi)
Wu Yao (Radix Linderae)
Mu Xiang (Radix Auklandiae)

Acupuncture & moxibustion

Bleed either the apex of the ear, *Shi Xuan* (M-UE-1), or *Qi Duan* (M-LE-12). Or one can needle *Qu Chi* (LI 11) and *He Gu* (LI 4).

Adjunctive treatments

In the case of wind cold urticaria, the child should not be allowed to eat or drink anything chilled, raw, frozen, or cold. In the case of wind heat, they should not be allowed to eat anything hot and spicy. And, in the case of damp heat in the intestines and stomach, they should not be allowed to eat anything fried, greasy, or fatty nor should they eat particular foods which are believed in Chinese medicine to be outwardly emitting, such as strawberries, shellfish, and chocolate — all foods which are associated with allergic reactions. Clearly in this pattern, it is important for the patient to eat a hypoallergenic, clear, bland diet. A simple Chinese herbal home remedy for both the wind heat and stomach and intestine damp heat patterns of hives is to make a tea out of corn silk and Job's tears barley and drink two times each day for at least 10 days. As an external treatment, one can wash the affected area with a decoction of whole mashed grapefruit for 10 minutes each time, three times each day.

Comments

Insect medicinals which enter the network vessels and track down wind are important if the hives are either recalcitrant to treatment or enduring.

29. Allergic Rhinitis

Allergic rhinitis is also commonly called hay fever. Exposure to certain airborne particles, such as dust, mold, pollen, and animal dander causes episodes of sneezing, nasal congestion, itchy eyes, itchy nose and upper palate, and clear runny nose. If severe, these symptoms may progress to an acute episode of allergic or bronchial asthma.

Children with allergic rhinitis suffer from spleen qi vacuity with retention of phlegm and dampness. Because their spleens are weak, this qi vacuity 1) allows for easy invasion by external wind evils and 2) results in failure to control the transportation and transformation of body fluids. Thus body fluids tend to accumulate in the lungs based on the saying,

"The spleen is the root of phlegm engenderment, while the lungs are the place where phlegm is stored." Treatment is based on whether the patient is having an acute attack or is in remission.

Treatment based on pattern discrimination:

1. Acute attack (a.k.a. wind cold assailing the lungs)

Main symptoms: Itchy nose, nasal congestion, clear runny nose with profuse watery snivel, if severe, fatigue, disinclination to speak, shortness of breath, a somber white facial complexion, pale white or greyish white nasal mucosa, a pale tongue with thin, white fur, a fine pulse

Treatment principles: Warm the lungs and scatter cold

Guiding formula: Wen Fei Zhi Liu Dan Jia Jian (Warm the Lungs & Stop Flow Elixir with Additions & Subtractions)

Xi Xin (Herba Asari)
Jing Jie (Herba Schizonepetae)
Ma Huang (Herba Ephedrae)
He Zi (Fructus Terminaliae)
Dang Shen (Radix Codonopsitis)
Gan Cao (Radix Glycyrrhizae)
Wu Mei (Fructus Mume)
Cang Er Zi (Fructus Xanthii)
Fang Feng (Radix Saposhnikoviae)
Wu Wei Zi (Fructus Schisandrae)

If there is shortness of breath and spontaneous perspiration, add *Huang Qi* (Radix Astragali) and *Bai Zhu* (Rhizoma Atractylodis Macrocephalae).

2. Remission stage (a.k.a. lung-spleen qi vacuity)

Main symptoms: Clear runny nose on exposure to cold, frequent catching of cold, a pale facial complexion, lack of strength, loose stools, a pale tongue with thin, white fur, a fine pulse

Treatment principles: Supplement the spleen and boost the qi, transform dampness and secure the exterior

Guiding formula:
Bu Zhong Yi Qi Tang Jia Wei (Supplement the Center & Boost the Qi Decoction with Added Flavors)

Huang Qi (Radix Astragali)
Ren Shen (Radix Ginseng)
Bai Zhu (Rhizoma Atractylodis Macrocephalae)

mix-fried *Gan Cao* (Radix Glycyrrhizae)
Ban Xia (Rhizoma Pinelliae)
Shi Chang Pu (Rhizoma Acori Tatarinowii)
Yuan Zhi (Radix Polygalae)
Mai Men Dong (Tuber Ophiopogonis)
Wu Wei Zi (Fructus Schisandrae)
Wu Mei (Fructus Mume)
Chen Pi (Pericarpium Citri Reticulatae)
Dang Gui (Radix Angelicae Sinensis)
Chai Hu (Radix Bupleuri)
Sheng Ma (Rhizoma Cimicifugae)

If there is a large appetite, oral thirst with a desire for cold drinks, or other signs of stomach heat, add *Huang Qin* (Radix Scutellariae).

Acupuncture & moxibustion

During acute attacks, one can needle *Ying Xiang* (LI 20), *Lie Que* (Lu 7), and *He Gu* (LI 4). If there are itchy eyes, add *Zan Zhu* (Bl 2). During periods of remission, moxa *Shen Que* (CV 8) and *Zu San Li* (St 36).

Adjunctive treatments

Because of the pivotal importance of the spleen in allergic rhinitis, a clear, bland diet is very important and especially avoiding sugars and sweets, cold, raw foods, and dairy products. During remission, cupping over the navel may be helpful as described above under allergies in general.

Comments

Some children grow out of their allergies and some retain them their whole lives. When children grow out of their hay fever, this is because their spleens have matured and their qi engenderment and transformation is robust and exuberant. However, when a person becomes run down and if they eat a spleen-damaging diet high in sugars and sweets, cold, raw foods, and dairy products, then they may find that they are once again susceptible to their allergies. The long-term treatment and prevention of allergies in Chinese medicine rests squarely on a well regulated clear, bland diet. Chinese ready-made medicines for rhinitis, such as *Bi Yan Pian* (Rhinitis Tablets), should be seen as nothing more than symptomatic palliatives.

30. Common & Plantar Warts

Warts are a type of viral infection. Children are more prone to getting warts because of their weak immune systems in turn due to the inherent immaturity of their organs. In Chinese medicine, warts are called *qian ri chuang* or thousand day sores because they often spontaneously disappear after 1,000 days or so. In children, warts are due to a combination of factors. Usually there is a combination of damp heat brewing and steaming with blood vacuity in turn due to a weak spleen. This damp heat causes obstruction to the flow of qi and blood which accumulates to form the wart. Because there is an accumulation of tissue, there is also an element of phlegm nodulation. Because the top of the wart is dry and scaly, there is typically an element of blood dryness and vacuity. If the wart is kept covered and becomes damp, it often becomes inflamed due to this aggravating the underlying damp heat. Likewise, if the wart is picked at by the child, it will easily become inflamed also due to the underlying damp heat.

In Chinese medicine, the treatments for warts are very similar to their modern Western medical treatment. Either caustic medicinals are applied on top of the wart in order to chemically burn it off or moxibustion is used to physically burn it off. Frankly, if and when warts need to come off, one should go to a Western MD to have them removed. For this kind of thing, Western medicine is safer, quicker, and more efficient. For multiple and recurring warts, one can also try taking **Zi Lan Fang Jia Wei (Lithospermum & Isatidis Formula with Added Flavors)** internally:

Ma Chi Xian (Herba Portulacae)
Ban Lan Gen (Radix Isatidis/Baphicacanthi)
Da Qing Ye (Folium Daqingye)
Yi Yi Ren (Semen Coicis)
Zi Cao (Radix Lithospermi/Arnebiae)
Chi Shao (Radix Paeoniae Rubrae)
Hong Hua (Flos Carthami)
Xia Ku Cao (Spica Prunellae)

If the warts are very dry and scaly, add *He Shou Wu* (Radix Polygoni Multiflori) and *Dang Gui* (Radix Angelicae Sinensis). If the warts are very hard and nodular, add *Mu Li* (Concha Ostreae) and *Long Gu* (Os Draconis). If there is spleen vacuity, add *Ren Shen* (Radix Ginseng) and *Bai Zhu* (Rhizoma Atractylodis Macrocephalae). And if there is retained heat in the lungs and stomach, add *Huang Qin* (Radix Scutellariae) and *Zhi Zi* (Fructus Gardeniae). Administer the above decoction for 7-10 days. If there is some improvement, continue. If there is no visible improvement, discontinue.

Comments

Because pediatric warts are again associated with the spleen and damp heat, a clear, bland diet is also a very important component in the treatment of this condition. When the child's spleen matures with age and if their diet improves, then the warts will tend to go away all by themselves.

31. Poison Ivy

Strictly speaking, poison ivy, which is a kind of contact dermatitis or inflammation of the skin, is not a pediatric disease. But kids being kids, they often go out to play in wooded areas, and kids being kids, they are not always knowledgeable or careful about what plants they come in contact with. In Chinese medicine, because the skin lesions caused by poison ivy and poison oak are red, hot, painful, itchy, and weep a watery fluid when the blisters break, they are seen as a type of damp heat condition. In the West, poison ivy is treated primarily by the topical application of calamine lotion, and calamina is also a topical ingredient for external application in Chinese medicine as well. However, in Chinese medicine there are also internal herbal decoctions which can be taken to more quickly reduce the itching, inflammation, and discomfort.

Internal treatments

Guiding formulas:
Wu Wei Xiao Du Yin (Five Flavors Disperse Toxins Beverage)
Jin Yin Hua (Flos Lonicerae)
Pu Gong Ying (Herba Taraxaci)
Zi Hua Di Ding (Herba Violae)
Ye Ju Hua (Flos Chrysanthemi Indici)
Zi Bei Tian Kui (Herba Begoniae Fimbristipulatae)

If there is redness, swelling, and burning pain, add *Dan Pi* (Cortex Moutan), *Sheng Di* (uncooked Radix Rehmanniae), and *Hong Hua* (Flos Carthami). If there is severe itching, add *Di Fu Zi* (Fructus Kochiae), *Bai Xian Pi* (Cortex Dictamni), and *Chan Yi* (Periostracum Cicadae). For ulcerated lesions, add *Yi Yi Ren* (Semen Coicis), *Fu Ling Pi* (Cortex Sclerotii Poriae), and *Dong Gua Pi* (Epicarpium Benincasae).

Er Miao San Jia Wei (Two Wonders Powder with Added Flavors)
Da Huang (Radix Et Rhizoma Rhei)
Huang Qin (Radix Scutellariae)
Huang Bai (Cortex Phellodendri)
Cang Zhu (Rhizoma Atractylodis)

If the lesions are on the lower limbs, add *Niu Xi* (Radix Achyranthis Bidentatae), *Mu Gua* (Fructus Chaenomelis), and *Bing Lang* (Semen Arecae).

External treatments

Guiding formulas:
If the lesions are weeping and ulcerated, use **Ku Shen Tang (Sophora Decoction)**
Ku Shen (Radix Sophorae Flavescentis), 60g
Ju Hua (Flos Chrysanthemi), 60g
She Chuang Zi (Fructus Cnidii), 30g
Jin Yin Hua (Flos Lonicerae), 30g
Bai Zhi (Radix Angelicae Dahuricae), 15g

Huang Bai (Cortex Phellodendri), 15g
Di Fu Zi (Fructus Kochiae), 15g
Shi Chang Pu (Rhizoma Acori Tatarinowii), 15g

Method of preparation & use: Decoct in water and use as a wash several times each day.

Qing Dai San (Indigo Powder)
Qing Dai (Pulvis Indigonis), 20g
Huang Bai (Cortex Phellodendri), 20g
Shi Gao (Gypsum Fibrosum), 40g
Hua Shi (Talcum), 40g

Method of preparation & use: Grind the above medicinals into powder, mix with cold, boiled water, and apply to the affected area 2-3 times each day. Hold in place with cotton gauze.

If there is simple redness and papular eruption, use **San Huang Xi Ji (Three Yellows Washing Prescription):**
Da Huang (Radix Et Rhizoma Rhei)
Huang Bai (Cortex Phellodendri)
Huang Qin (Radix Scutellariae)
Ku Shen (Radix Sophorae Flavescentis)

Method of preparation & use: Grind equal portions of the above medicinals into a fine powder. Mix 10ml of this powder with 100ml of distilled water and 1ml of carbolic acid and wash the affected area several times each day.

32. Nosebleed

It is not uncommon for children to develop nosebleeds for no apparent reason. Usually parents pay little or no attention to this unless the nosebleeds are frequent and severe. Nevertheless, although such nosebleeds are not life-threatening, they can give a clue about the constitutional imbalance of the child and, therefore, can help identify a better diet. In Chinese pediatrics, there are two main patterns of children's nosebleed. These are lung heat combined with an external invasion and spleen-stomach brewing or smoldering heat.

Treatment based on pattern discrimination:

1. Lung heat combined with external invasion

Main symptoms: Headache, aversion to wind, a dry mouth and nose, occasional bloody nose, fresh red colored blood, cough with scanty, yellow phlegm, a floating, rapid pulse

Note: There is a tendency for the lungs to already or habitually harbor heat. If the child then "catches cold" or is invaded by an external pathogen, this adds even more heat to the lungs and this heat causes the blood to move frenetically outside its pathways.

Treatment principles: Clear heat and resolve the exterior, cool the blood and stop bleeding

Guiding formulas:
Qing Liang Zhi Nu Tang (Clear & Cool Stop Nosebleed Decoction)
Bo He (Herba Menthae Haplocalycis)
Sang Ye (Folium Mori)
Lian Qiao (Fructus Forsythiae)
Jin Yin Hua (Flos Lonicerae)
Bai Mao Gen (Rhizoma Imperatae)
Zhi Mu (Rhizoma Anemarrhenae)
Mu Tong (Caulis Akebiae)
Geng Mi (Semen Oryzae)
Gan Cao (Radix Glycyrrhizae)

Unnamed formula
Sang Bai Pi (Cortex Mori)
Di Gu Pi (Cortex Lycii)
Gan Cao (Radix Glycyrrhizae)
Dan Pi (Cortex Moutan)
Ce Bai Ye (Cacumen Platycladi)
Bai Mao Gen (Rhizoma Imperatae)
Huang Qin (Radix Scutellariae)

2. Spleen-stomach brewing heat

Main symptoms: Blood occasionally flowing from the nose, a dry nose, bad breath, thirst and a preference for cold drinks, constipation, yellow tongue fur, a slippery, rapid pulse

Treatment principles: Clear the stomach and downbear fire

Guiding formulas:
Qing Re Liang Xue Yin (Clear Heat & Cool the Blood Beverage)
Shi Gao (Gypsum Fibrosum)
Bai Mao Gen (Rhizoma Imperatae)
Zhi Mu (Rhizoma Anemarrhenae)
Sheng Di (uncooked Radix Rehmanniae)
Chuan Niu Xi (Radix Cyathulae)
Bai Shao (Radix Paeoniae Albae)
Dan Pi (Cortex Moutan)
Zhi Zi (Fructus Gardeniae)
Geng Mi (Semen Oryzae)

Gan Cao (rootlets of Radix Glycyrrhizae)

Unnamed formula
Sheng Di (uncooked Radix Rehmanniae)
Huang Lian (Rhizoma Coptidis)
Dang Gui (Radix Angelicae Sinensis)
Dan Pi (Cortex Moutan)
Shi Gao (Gypsum Fibrosum)
Deng Xin Cao (Medulla Junci)
Ce Bai Ye (Cacumen Platycladi)
Bai Mao Gen (Rhizoma Imperatae)

Acupuncture & moxibustion

For lung heat epistaxis, needle *Chi Ze* (Lu 5) and *He Gu* (LI 4). For spleen/stomach brewing heat, needle *Nei Ting* (St 44) and *He Gu* (LI 4).

Adjunctive treatments

Because both of the above patterns involve evil heat, children with bloody noses should not eat acrid, hot, spicy foods. Children with spleen/stomach brewing dampness should also avoid greasy, fatty, fried foods. If bleeding is profuse, one can try wrapping a cord fairly tightly around the palm of the hand from *Hou Xi* (SI 3) to *San Jian* (LI 3) and then making a fist, thus squeezing this cord even tighter.

Comments

Epistaxis due to heat is often associated with constipation, dental caries, bleeding gums, canker sores, and other similar problems related to stomach heat. Therefore, keeping the bowels open and freely flowing is very important. When children with this pattern get sick, they tend to develop a fever quickly since they tend to have a lot of heat in their body. Therefore, when children with habitual stomach heat have a nosebleed, this is a signal to the parents to modify their child's diet for awhile, reverting to a clear, bland diet as far as possible.

33. Canker Sores

Canker sores refer to small sores on the gums and the inner walls of the cheeks. Children tend to get these from time to time. They rarely require any kind of medical attention and the child may make no mention of them. Mostly they are due to damp heat smoldering in the spleen and stomach, similar to the second pattern of nosebleed above. Avoidance of hot, spicy foods and greasy, fatty foods is usually important in this kind of pattern as is keeping the bowel movements open and free-flowing. If the canker sores require treatment or there are canker sores along with some other complaint, usually some modification of **Bai Hu Tang (White Tiger Decoction)** or **Gan Lu Yin (Sweet Dew**

Beverage) will clear heat and disinhibit dampness, thus restoring balance to the organism.

Guiding formulas:
Bai Hu Tang (White Tiger Decoction)
Shi Gao (Gypsum Fibrosum)
Zhi Mu (Rhizoma Anemarrhenae)
mix-fried *Gan Cao* (Radix Glycyrrhizae)
Geng Mi (Semen Oryzae)

If there is constipation, use **Bai Hu Cheng Qi Tang (White Tiger Order the Qi Decoction):**
Shi Gao (Gypsum Fibrosum)
Zhi Mu (Rhizoma Anemarrhenae)
mix-fried *Gan Cao* (Radix Glycyrrhizae)
Geng Mi (Semen Oryzae)
Da Huang (Radix Et Rhizoma Rhei)
Mang Xiao (Natri Sulfas)

If there is enduring damp heat which has consumed stomach fluids accompanied by a dry mouth and desire for cold drinks, use **Gan Lu Yin (Sweet Dew Beverage):**
Sheng Di (uncooked Radix Rehmanniae)
Mai Men Dong (Tuber Ophiopogonis)
Tian Men Dong (Tuber Asparagi)
Shi Hu (Herba Dendrobii)
Yin Chen Hao (Herba Artemisiae Scopariae)
Huang Qin (Radix Scutellariae)
Pi Pa Ye (Folium Eriobotryae)
Zhi Shi (Fructus Immaturus Aurantii)
Gan Cao (Radix Glycyrrhizae)

Adjunctive treatments

A simple remedy for treating canker sores is to boil 5g of fresh peppermint in 1 cup of water and add a little salt. Drink this as a tea frequently through the day. This can also help toothache and nosebleed due to heat in the stomach. Another remedy is to boil watercress and carrots into a soup and drink. For better results, a few *Fan Xie Ye* (Folium Sennae) may be added especially if there is constipation. Obviously, a clear, bland diet is important.

Comments

Canker sores are rarely severe enough to be a major complaint. However, they are a good barometer of how much damp heat the child has brewing internally. Therefore, if the child mentions that they have canker sores, this is an indication that stricter control of their diet is in order so as to prevent some other, more serious or enduring condition from developing.

34. Conjunctivitis

Conjunctivitis is also referred to as pink eye, especially in children. It is not listed as a pediatric disease in Chinese pediatric texts, but because children often develop this condition, I have included it for the sake of parents who may not know otherwise what to do about pink eye. Acute conjunctivitis means an acute inflammation of the conjunctiva of the eye. According to Western medicine, this may be due to viruses, bacteria, or allergies. In Chinese medicine, redness is typically associated with some sort of pathological heat in the body. There are five main patterns associated with conjunctivitis. These are an external invasion of wind heat, heat toxins, stomach heat hyperactive above, liver fire hyperactive above, and yin deficiency with internal heat. In children, the two most commonly encountered patterns are the wind heat external invasion and the stomach heat hyperactive above.

Treatment based on pattern discrimination:

1. Wind heat external invasion

Main symptoms: During the early stage, there may be sudden reddening of the whites of the eyes, hot tearing, photophobia, and a rough sensation in the eye(s). Concomitant symptoms may include aversion to cold, fever, headache, nasal congestion, thin, white tongue fur, and a floating, rapid pulse. In severe cases, pain in the eyeballs may render the patient restless.

Treatment principles: Course wind and clear heat

Guiding formula:
Qiang Huo Sheng Feng Tang Jia Jian (Qiang Huo Overcome Wind Decoction with Additions & Subtractions)
 Bo He (Herba Menthae Haplocalycis)
 Chai Hu (Radix Bupleuri)
 Huang Qin (Radix Scutellariae)
 Qiang Huo (Radix Et Rhizoma Notopterygii)
 Jing Jie (Herba Schizonepetae)
 Chuan Xiong (Rhizoma Chuanxiong)
 Fang Feng (Radix Saposhnikoviae)
 Man Jing Zi (Fructus Viticis)
 Bai Zhi (Radix Angelicae Dahuricae)
 Qian Hu (Radix Peucedani)
 Mu Zei Cao (Herba Equiseti)
 Sang Ye (Folium Mori)

If there is constipation, add Radix Et Rhizoma Rhei (*Da Huang*).

2. Stomach heat hyperactive above

Main symptoms: Frequent hunger, a desire for cold drinks, possible constipation or diarrhea, restlessness, a red tongue with yellow fur, a slippery, rapid pulse

Treatment principles: Drain the stomach and clear heat

Guiding formulas:
Liang Ge Lian Qiao San (Cool the Diaphragm Forsythia Powder)
    Lian Qiao (Fructus Forsythiae)
    Da Huang (Radix Et Rhizoma Rhei)
    Huang Lian (Rhizoma Coptidis)
    Bo He (Herba Menthae Haplocalycis)
    Zhi Zi (Fructus Gardeniae)
    Gan Cao (Radix Glycyrrhizae)
    Huang Qin (Radix Scutellariae)
    Mang Xiao (Natri Sulfas)

However, because wind heat can stir up and aggravate stomach heat, often these two mechanisms occur together in children, thus producing conjunctivitis. In that case, use
Ju Hua Tong Sheng San Jia Jian (Chrysanthemum Communicate with the Sages Powder with Additions & Subtractions):
    Ju Hua (Flos Chrysanthemi)
    Hua Shi (Talcum)
    Shi Gao (Gypsum Fibrosum)
    Huang Qin (Radix Scutellariae)
    Jie Geng (Radix Platycodi)
    Gan Cao (Radix Glycyrrhizae)
    Da Huang (Radix Et Rhizoma Rhei)
    Mang Xiao (Natri Sulfas)
    Huang Lian (Rhizoma Coptidis)
    Qiang Huo (Radix Et Rhizoma Notopterygii)
    Fang Feng (Radix Saposhnikoviae)
    Chuan Xiong (Rhizoma Chuanxiong)
    Dang Gui (Radix Angelicae Sinensis)
    Bai Shao (Radix Paeoniae Albae)
    Bo He (Herba Menthae Haplocalycis)
    Lian Qiao (Fructus Forsythiae)
    Ma Huang (Herba Ephedrae)
    Ji Li (Fructus Tribuli)
    Jing Jie Sui (Herba Schizonepetae)
    Bai Zhu (Rhizoma Atractylodis Macrocephalae)
    Zhi Zi (Fructus Gardeniae)

Sheng Jiang (uncooked Rhizoma Zingiberis)

One can also use **Qu Feng San Re Yin Zi Jia Jian (Dispel Wind & Scatter Heat Beverage with Additions & Subtractions):**
Lian Qiao (Fructus Forsythiae)
Jin Yin Hua (Flos Lonicerae)
Niu Bang Zi (Fructus Arctii)
Bo He (Herba Menthae Haplocalycis)
Zhi Zi (Fructus Gardeniae)
Qiang Huo (Radix Et Rhizoma Notopterygii)
Da Huang (Radix Et Rhizoma Rhei)
Chi Shao (Radix Paeoniae Rubrae)
Dang Gui (Radix Angelicae Sinensis)
Chuan Xiong (Rhizoma Chuanxiong)
Mu Zei Cao (Herba Equiseti)

Unnamed formula
Fang Feng (Radix Saposhnikoviae)
Huang Qin (Radix Scutellariae)
Jie Geng (Radix Platycodi)
Chi Shao (Radix Paeoniae Rubrae)
Da Huang (Radix Et Rhizoma Rhei)
Dan Pi (Cortex Moutan)
Long Dan Cao (Radix Gentianae)
Wu Gong (Scolopendra)
Jing Jie Sui (Herba Schizonepetae)

Acupuncture & moxibustion

In the case of wind heat, needle *He Gu* (LI 4) and *Feng Chi* (GB 20). For stomach heat, needle *He Gu* (LI 4) and *Nei Ting* (St 44).

Adjunctive treatments

In the case of conjunctivitis, a clear, bland diet is a necessity. A simple remedy for conjunctivitis due to stomach heat is to make a tea out of broccoli and carrots, both of which are cool by nature. For either wind heat or stomach heat, make tea out of *Ju Hua* (Flos Chrysanthemi). A variation of this remedy is to make a tea out of both chrysanthemum flowers and spinach. Further, the warm chrysanthemum flowers used to make this tea can be placed over the affected eye as a type of poultice. Yet another possibility is to make a tea out of *Pu Gong Ying* (Herba Taraxaci). And finally, one can grate cucumbers and make a poultice to apply to the affected eye.

35. Frequent Urination

Frequent urination or polyuria is a commonly seen pediatric urinary tract complaint. Clinically, it manifests as frequent urination and urinary urgency as its main symptoms. The rate of incidence of this condition is higher in female children than in male children. This disease category in children includes urinary tract infections or cystitis as well as chronic polyuria due to functional causes. In Chinese medicine, this condition is traditionally categorized as *lin* or strangury.

Treatment based on pattern discrimination:

1. Damp heat pouring downward (urinary bladder damp heat)

Main symptoms: The onset of disease is relatively sudden. The urination is frequent, numerous, short, and reddish. There is burning pain in the urinary tract. The urine may dribble or drip or is turbid. There is lower abdominal sagging and distention with low back soreness and pain. Infants may sometimes cry and be restless. Commonly there is accompanying fever, agitation and vexation, oral thirst, headache, body pain, and nausea and vomiting. The tongue is red with thin, slimy, slightly yellow or slimy, yellow fur. The pulse is rapid and forceful.

Treatment principles: Clear heat and disinhibit dampness

Guiding formulas:
Ba Zheng San (Eight [Ingredients] Correcting Powder)
   Mu Tong (Caulis Akebiae)
   Qu Mai (Herba Dianthi)
   Che Qian Zi (Semen Plantaginis)
   Bian Xu (Herba Polygoni Avicularis)
   Hua Shi (Talcum)
   Da Huang (Radix Et Rhizoma Rhei)
   Zhi Zi (Fructus Gardeniae)
   Gan Cao (Radix Glycyrrhizae)

Shi Wei Dao Chi San (Ten Flavors Abduct the Red Powder)
   Sheng Di (uncooked Radix Rehmanniae)
   Zhi Zi (Fructus Gardeniae)
   Dan Zhu Ye (Herba Lophateri)
   Huang Qin (Radix Scutellariae)
   Gan Cao (Radix Glycyrrhizae)
   Qu Mai (Herba Dianthi)
   Hua Shi (Talcum)
   Mu Tong (Caulis Akebiae)
   Zhu Ling (Polyporus)
   Yin Chen Hao (Herba Artemisiae Scopariae)

Wu Lin San Jia Wei (Five [Ingredients] Strangury Powder with Added Flavors)
  Yin Chen Hao (Herba Artemisiae Scopariae)
  Dan Zhu Ye (Herba Lophateri)
  Mu Tong (Caulis Akebiae)
  Hua Shi (Talcum)
  Gan Cao (Radix Glycyrrhizae)
  Zhi Zi (Fructus Gardeniae)
  Chi Shao (Radix Paeoniae Rubrae)
  Chi Fu Ling (red Poria)

Qing Re Li Niao Fang (Clear Heat & Disinhibit Urination Formula)
  Qing Dai (Pulvis Indigonis)
  Zi Cao (Radix Lithospermi/Arnebiae)
  Bai Ji (Rhizoma Bletillae)
  Ru Xiang (Olibanum)
  Hu Po (Succinum)
  Zhu Sha (Cinnabar)

Bai Mao Gen Tang (Imperata Decoction)
  Bai Mao Gen (Rhizoma Imperatae)
  Huang Bai (Cortex Phellodendri)
  Jin Yin Hua (Flos Lonicerae)
  Lian Qiao (Fructus Forsythiae)
  Huang Qin (Radix Scutellariae)
  Hua Shi (Talcum)
  Ma Chi Xian (Herba Portulacae)
  Gan Cao (Radix Glycyrrhizae)
  Ban Zhi Lian (Radix Scutellariae Barbatae)
  Ban Bian Lian (Herba Lobeliae)

Huang Bai Shi Wei Tang (Phellodendron & Pyrrosia Decoction)
  Huang Bai (Cortex Phellodendri)
  Shi Wei (Folium Pyrrosiae)
  Pu Gong Ying (Herba Taraxaci)
  Zi Hua Di Ding (Herba Violae)
  Bian Xu (Herba Polygoni Avicularis)
  Qu Mai (Herba Dianthi)
  Che Qian Zi (Semen Plantaginis)
  Gan Cao (Radix Glycyrrhizae)

Jin Sha San Jia Wei (Lygodium Powder with Added Flavors)
  Hai Jin Sha (Spora Lygodii)
  Yu Jin (Tuber Curcumae)
  Hua Shi (Talcum)

Gan Cao (Radix Glycyrrhizae)
Deng Xin Cao (Medulla Junci)
Mu Tong (Caulis Akebiae)

Hua Shi San (Talcum Powder)
Hua Shi (Talcum)
Huang Qin (Radix Scutellariae)
Dong Gua Zi (Semen Benincasae)
Che Qian Zi (Semen Plantaginis)
Mu Tong (Caulis Akebiae)

Huang Qin Hua Shi Tang (Scutellaria & Talcum Decoction)
Huang Qin (Radix Scutellariae)
Hua Shi (Talcum)
Fu Ling Pi (Cortex Sclerotii Poriae)
Zhu Ling (Polyporus)
Da Fu Pi (Semen Arecae)
Bai Dou Kou (Fructus Cardamomi)
Mu Tong (Caulis Akebiae)

2. Liver/gallbladder damp heat

Main symptoms: Frequent, urgent, short, red urination which may sometimes be astringent and painful, aversion to cold, fever, a bitter taste in the mouth, torpid intake, nausea, possible vomiting, abdominal distention and lateral costal pain, vexation and agitation, slimy, yellow tongue fur, a purplish finger vein, a wiry, rapid pulse

Treatment principles: Clear heat and discharge dampness, course the liver and disinhibit the gallbladder

Guiding formula:
Long Dan Xie Gan Tang Jia Jian (Gentiana Drain the Liver Decoction with Additions & Subtractions)
Long Dan Cao (Radix Gentianae)
Zhi Zi (Fructus Gardeniae)
Huang Bai (Cortex Phellodendri)
Chai Hu (Radix Bupleuri)
Bai Hua She She Cao (Herba Herba Hedyotis Diffusae)
Che Qian Zi (Semen Plantaginis)
Mu Tong (Caulis Akebiae)
Ze Xie (Rhizoma Alismatis)
Bai Mao Gen (Rhizoma Imperatae)

If there is vomiting, add *Zhu Ru* (Caulis Bambusae In Taeniis).

3. Vacuity heat

Main symptoms: Difficult, astringent, painful urination, incessant dribbling and dripping, sometimes suffering and sometimes stopping, possibly accompanied by a low-grade fever, night sweats, dry lips, dry throat, a flushed red face, a red tongue with diminished fur, a red finger vein, a fine, rapid pulse

Treatment principles: Mainly enrich and supplement kidney yin, assisted by clearing and disinhibiting dampness and heat

Guiding formulas:
Zhi Bai Ba Wei Wan Jia Jian (Anemarrhena & Phellodendron Eight Flavors Pills with Additions & Subtractions)

Sheng Di (uncooked Radix Rehmanniae)
Shan Yao (Radix Dioscoreae)
Zhi Mu (Rhizoma Anemarrhenae)
Huang Bai (Cortex Phellodendri)
Dan Pi (Cortex Moutan)
Fu Ling (Poria)
Ze Xie (Rhizoma Alismatis)
Gui Ban (Plastrum Testudinis)
Nu Zhen Zi (Fructus Ligustri Lucidi)
Shi Wei (Folium Pyrrosiae)

If there is turbid urine like rice-washing water with no obvious urinary astringency or pain and a thin body, this is kidney vacuity with qi transformation not moving. In that case, in order to secure and contain, add *Lian Xu* (Stamen Nelumbinis), *Qian Shi* (Semen Euryalis), and *Long Gu* (Os Draconis).

If there is kidney yin vacuity with spleen vacuity, one can use ***Niao Beng Fang* (Urinary Flooding Formula):**

processed *He Shou Wu* (Radix Polygoni Multiflori)
Hei Zhi Ma (black Semen Sesami)
Da Zao (Fructus Jujubae)
Hei Zao (blackened Fructus Jujubae)
Shan Yao (Radix Dioscoreae)

Or, one can use ***Niao Beng Ji Ben Fang Jia Jian* (Urinary Flooding Foundation Formula with Additions & Subtractions):**

Sheng Di (uncooked Radix Rehmanniae)
Shan Yao (Radix Dioscoreae)
Gui Ban (Plastrum Testudinis)
Dang Shen (Radix Codonopsitis)
Gan Cao (Radix Glycyrrhizae)
Huang Lian (Rhizoma Coptidis)

    Huang Bai (Cortex Phellodendri)
    Ling Yang Jiao (Cornu Caprae)

If there is extreme oral thirst, add *Shi Gao* (Gypsum Fibrosum), *Ge Gen* (Radix Puerariae), and *Lu Gen* (Rhizoma Phragmitis). If there is markedly frequent urination, add *Gou Qi Zi* (Fructus Lycii), *Wu Wei Zi* (Fructus Schisandrae), and *Sang Piao Xiao* (Ootheca Mantidis). If there is constipation, add *Huo Ma Ren* (Semen Cannabis) and uncooked *Da Huang* (Radix Et Rhizoma Rhei). If there is torpid intake, add *Yu Zhu* (Rhizoma Polygonati Odorati) and *Shan Zha* (Fructus Crataegi).

One can also use **Yu Quan Wan (Jade Spring Pills):**
    Mai Men Dong (Tuber Ophiopogonis)
    Ren Shen (Radix Ginseng)
    Fu Ling (Poria)
    Huang Qi (Radix Astragali)
    Wu Mei (Fructus Mume)
    Gan Cao (Radix Glycyrrhizae)
    Tian Hua Fen (Radix Trichosanthis)
    dry *Gan Ge* (Radix Puerariae)

If there is yin vacuity with heat in the lungs, use **Mai Men Dong Yin (Ophiopogon Beverage):**
    Mai Men Dong (Tuber Ophiopogonis)
    Huang Qin (Radix Scutellariae)
    Ge Gen (Radix Puerariae)
    Zhi Mu (Rhizoma Anemarrhenae)
    Dan Zhu Ye (Herba Lophateri)
    Wu Mei (Fructus Mume)
    Lu Gen (Rhizoma Phragmitis)
    Tian Hua Fen (Radix Trichosanthis)
    Bei Sha Shen (Radix Glehniae)

Er Zhi Zi Yin Yin **(Two Ultimates Enrich Yin Beverage)**
    Han Lian Cao (Herba Ecliptae)
    Nu Zhen Zi (Fructus Ligustri Lucidi)
    Mai Men Dong (Tuber Ophiopogonis)
    Nan Sha Shen (Radix Adenophorae)
    Yu Zhu (Rhizoma Polygonati Odorati)
    Shan Yao (Radix Dioscoreae)

For heat in the stomach with yin vacuity of the stomach and lungs, use **Ge Gen Sha Shen Tang (Pueraria & Glehnia Decoction):**
    Ge Gen (Radix Puerariae)
    Bei Sha Shen (Radix Glehniae)
    Mai Men Dong (Tuber Ophiopogonis)

Tian Hua Fen (Radix Trichosanthis)
Shi Gao (Gypsum Fibrosum)
Shi Hu (Herba Dendrobii)
Lu Gen (Rhizoma Phragmitis)
Dan Zhu Ye (Herba Lophateri)

4. Vacuity cold (a.k.a. spleen-kidney qi vacuity)

Main symptoms: Condition enduring for a long time, frequent, numerous urination, incessant dribbling and dripping, no heavy astringency or pain, urine not clear, listlessness of the essence spirit, a somber white facial complexion, devitalized eating and drinking, if severe, fear of cold and dread of chill, lack of warmth in the hands and feet, loose stools, faint edema of the eyelids, a pale tongue which may have the indentations of the teeth on its edges and thin, slimy fur, a fine pulse with diminished strength

Treatment principles: Boost the qi and supplement the kidneys

Guiding formulas:
Suo Quan Wan (Lock the Spring Pills)
Shan Yao (Radix Dioscoreae)
Yi Zhi Ren (Fructus Alpiniae Oxyphyllae)
Wu Yao (Radix Linderae)

If damp turbidity is not transformed, add *Fu Ling* (Poria) and *Che Qian Zi* (Semen Plantaginis).

Si Jun Zi Tang (Four Gentlemen Decoction) plus *Ji Sheng Shen Qi Wan* (Aid the Living Kidney Qi Pills) with additions and subtractions
Dang Shen (Radix Codonopsitis)
Bai Zhu (Rhizoma Atractylodis Macrocephalae)
Shan Yao (Radix Dioscoreae)
Fu Ling (Poria)
Shu Di (cooked Radix Rehmanniae)
Tu Si Zi (Semen Cuscutae)
Bu Gu Zhi (Fructus Psoraleae)
Niu Xi (Radix Achyranthis Bidentatae)
Che Qian Zi (Semen Plantaginis)
Ze Xie (Rhizoma Alismatis)
Chen Pi (Pericarpium Citri Reticulatae)

If there is listlessness of the essence spirit with the four limbs clear (*i.e.*, pale) and chilly, add *Rou Gui* (Cortex Cinnamomi), *Lu Jiao Shuang* (Cornu Degelatinum Cervi), and *Xiao Hui Xiang* (Fructus Foeniculi). If there is devitalized eating and drinking with thick, white tongue fur, add *Cang Zhu* (Rhizoma Atractylodis) and *Hou Po* (Cortex Magnoliae). If there is pronounced frequent urination, add *Fu Pen Zi* (Fructus Rubi) and *Sang Piao Xiao* (Ootheca Mantidis).

If there is mainly spleen qi vacuity with a sallow yellow facial complexion, devitalized eating and drinking, loose stools, a white tongue, and a soft pulse, use **Shen Ling Bai Zhu San (Ginseng, Poria, & Atractylodes Powder):**

Ren Shen (Radix Ginseng)
Lian Zi (Semen Nelumbinis)
Shan Yao (Radix Dioscoreae)
Bai Zhu (Rhizoma Atractylodis Macrocephalae)
Fu Ling (Poria)
Bai Bian Dou (Semen Dolichoris)
Yi Yi Ren (Semen Coicis)
Sha Ren (Fructus Amomi)
Jie Geng (Radix Platycodi)
mix-fried Gan Cao (Radix Glycyrrhizae)

If there is mainly kidney yang vacuity with a bright white facial complexion, fear of cold and dread of chill, lack of warmth in the hands and feet, lower limb edema, clear, long urination, frequent, numerous urination, thin tongue fur, and a weak pulse, use **Ji Sheng Shen Qi Wan (Aid the Living Kidney Qi Pills):**

Shu Di (cooked Radix Rehmanniae)
Shan Zhu Yu (Fructus Corni)
Shan Yao (Radix Dioscoreae)
Ze Xie (Rhizoma Alismatis)
Fu Ling (Poria)
Dan Pi (Cortex Moutan)
Rou Gui (Cortex Cinnamomi)
Fu Zi (Radix Lateralis Praeparatus Aconiti Carmichaeli)
Chuan Niu Xi (Radix Cyathulae)
Che Qian Zi (Semen Plantaginis)

Yi Qi Gu She Tang (Boost the Qi, Secure & Contain Decoction)

Sang Piao Xiao (Ootheca Mantidis)
Bu Gu Zhi (Fructus Psoraleae)
Yi Zhi Ren (Fructus Alpiniae Oxyphyllae)
Wu Yao (Radix Linderae)
Huang Qi (Radix Astragali)
Shan Yao (Radix Dioscoreae)
Wu Wei Zi (Fructus Schisandrae)
Bai Guo (Semen Ginkgonis)
mix-fried Ji Nei Jin (Endothelium Corneum Gigeriae Galli)

Acupuncture & moxibustion

For damp heat in the lower burner, needle *Yin Ling Quan* (Sp 9) and *Zhong Ji* (CV 3). For liver/gallbladder damp heat, needle *Yang Ling Quan* (GB 34) and *Zhong Ji* (CV 3). If there is yin vacuity, needle *San Yin Jiao* (Sp 6) and *Shen Shu* (Bl 23). If there is heat in the stomach, needle *Nei Ting* (St 44). If there is heat in the lungs, needle *Chi Ze* (Lu 5). If there is spleen-kidney vacuity, moxa *Shen Que* (CV 8) and *Guan Yuan* (CV 4) or *Pi Shu* (Bl 20), *Shen Shu* (Bl 23), and *Ming Men* (GV 4).

Adjunctive treatments

A clear, bland diet is important in both the damp heat patterns. In those cases, one should also drink more water and one can drink cranberry juice. In yin vacuity conditions, it is important to avoid acrid, hot, peppery foods, while in spleen-kidney vacuity conditions, it is important to avoid chilled, frozen, cold, and raw foods and drinks and to eat only cooked, warm foods.

Comments

In my experience, one should not jump to the conclusion that every child with frequent urination suffers from kidney vacuity. Practitioners should remember that the stomach is the sluice-gate of the kidneys. Often, children with chronic polyuria have weak spleens, retained heat in their lungs, and dry, hot stomachs, all conspiring together to make the urination excessively frequent. In this case, it is also possible to use modifications of *Xiao Chai Hu Tang* (Minor Bupleurum Decoction).

36. Juvenile Rheumatoid Arthritis

Rheumatoid arthritis (RA) beginning before 16 years of age is called juvenile rheumatoid arthritis. In Western medicine, it is divided into three types: systemic onset or Still's disease, pauciarticular onset, and polyarticular onset. In systemic onset, there is high fever, rash, splenomegaly, generalized adenopathy, serositis, and marked neutrophilic leukocytosis. These systemic symptoms may precede the onset of arthritis. Rheumatoid factor (RF) is usually absent. In pauciarticular onset, there are antinuclear antibodies and iridocyclitis. And in polyarticular onset, antinuclear antibodies are usually absent and the symptoms are similar to adult RA. Approximately 20% of children with RA suffer from systemic onset, 40%, mostly girls, have pauciarticular onset, and another 40% have polyarticular onset. Seventy-five percent of all those affected with juvenile rheumatoid arthritis go into complete remission. Those with positive RF in the polyarticular onset group, mostly teenage girls, have the worst prognosis. In Chinese medicine, rheumatoid arthritis is categorized as *bi* syndrome.

Treatment based on pattern discrimination:

1. Heat patterns

A. Yin vacuity, internal heat

Main symptoms: Elevated body temperature, red, swollen, painful joints made worse by heat and better by cold, afternoon tidal fever, spontaneous perspiration, night sweats, withered and shrunken muscles and flesh, oral thirst with a desire to drink, a red tongue with diminished fur

Treatment principles: Enrich yin and clear heat, open the network vessels and stop pain

Guiding formula:
Ding Shi Qing Luo Yin Jia Jian (Master Ding's Clear the Network Vessels Beverage with Additions & Subtractions)

Jin Yin Hua (Flos Lonicerae)
Di Gu Pi (Cortex Lycii)
Sheng Di (uncooked Radix Rehmanniae)
Shi Hu (Herba Dendrobii)
Bai Wei (Radix Cynanchi Atrati)
Dan Pi (Cortex Moutan)
Qin Jiao (Radix Gentianae Macrophyllae)
Wei Ling Xian (Radix Clematidis)
Di Long (Pheretima)

If there is a pronounced low-grade fever, add *Qing Hao* (Herba Artemisiae Annuae).

B. Damp heat internally exuberant

Main symptoms: Red, swollen, painful joints made worse by heat and better by cold, an elevated body temperature, fever, nausea or a not very marked desire to vomit, torpid intake, loose stools or diarrhea, a red tongue with thick, slimy fur

Treatment principles: Clear heat and disinhibit dampness

Guiding formula:
San Miao San Jia Wei (Three Wonders Powder with Added Flavors)

Cang Zhu (Rhizoma Atractylodis)
Huang Bai (Cortex Phellodendri)
Yi Yi Ren (Semen Coicis)
Lian Qiao (Fructus Forsythiae)
Hua Shi (Talcum)
Ren Dong Teng (Caulis Lonicerae)
Wan Can Sha (Feces Bombycis)
Qin Jiao (Radix Gentianae Macrophyllae)
Mu Gua (Fructus Chaenomelis)
Yin Chen Hao (Herba Artemisiae Scopariae)
Fu Ling (Poria)

If heat is heavy and dampness is light, there is oral thirst leading to drinking, and there is great discharge of sweat, add uncooked *Shi Gao* (Gypsum Fibrosum) and *Zhi Mu*

(Rhizoma Anemarrhenae) to clear heat from the qi division. If there is constipation, add *Da Huang* (Radix Et Rhizoma Rhei) to discharge heat and open the bowels.

2. Cold pattern

Main symptoms: Cold body, chilled limbs, fear of wind, easily catches cold, stiff, tense, aching and painful joints, no manifestations of redness or heat, diminishing of pain if heat is obtained, worsening of pain if cold is obtained, a pale tongue with thin, white fur

Treatment principles: Dispel wind, scatter cold, and eliminate dampness

Guiding formulas:
Shu Jin Chu Bi Tang Jia Jian (Soothe the Sinews & Eliminate Bi Decoction with Additions & Subtractions)

Huang Qi (Radix Astragali)
Gui Zhi (Ramulus Cinnamomi)
Fu Zi (Radix Lateralis Praeparatus Aconiti Carmichaeli)
Dang Gui (Radix Angelicae Sinensis)
Chi Shao (Radix Paeoniae Rubrae)
Qiang Huo (Radix Et Rhizoma Notopterygii)
Chuan Xiong (Rhizoma Chuanxiong)
processed *Ru Xiang* (Olibanum)
processed *Mo Yao* (Myrrha)
Fu Ling (Poria)
Yi Yi Ren (Semen Coicis)

If there is recurrent cold damp impediment and depressed evils transform into heat, there will be the external manifestations of swelling and enlargement of peripheral joints and pain will be accompanied by a hot sensation. However, there will not be any fever. In that case, use **Gui Zhi Shao Yao Zhi Mu Tang (Cinnamon Twig, Peony & Anemarrhena Decoction):**

Gui Zhi (Ramulus Cinnamomi)
Ma Huang (Herba Ephedrae)
Fu Zi (Radix Lateralis Praeparatus Aconiti Carmichaeli)
Zhi Mu (Rhizoma Anemarrhenae)
Bai Shao (Radix Paeoniae Albae)
Fang Feng (Radix Saposhnikoviae)
Sheng Jiang (uncooked Rhizoma Zingiberis)
Gan Cao (Radix Glycyrrhizae)

If there is a marked heavy sensation in the body, add *Bai Zhu*. If the symptoms get worse at night, substitute *Chi Shao* (Radix Paeoniae Rubrae) for *Bai Shao*. If there is obvious heat in the joints, increase the *Bai Shao* and *Zhi Mu* and add *Sang Zhi* (Ramulus Mori) and *Ren Dong Teng* (Caulis Lonicerae). If there is concomitant qi and yin vacuity, add *Sheng Di* (uncooked Radix Rehmanniae) and *Niu Xi* (Radix Achyranthis Bidentatae).

3. Qi & blood dual vacuity

Main symptoms: A bright white or sallow yellow facial complexion, relatively profuse sweating, shortness of breath, disinclination to speak, torpid intake, irregular bowel movements, swollen, distended, abnormally formed joints, a pale tongue with thin, white fur

Treatment principles: Supplement the qi and nourish the blood, transform dampness and open the network vessels

Guiding formula:
Ba Zhen Tang Jia Jian (Eight Pearls Decoction with Additions & Subtractions)

    Dang Shen (Radix Codonopsitis)
    Bai Zhu (Rhizoma Atractylodis Macrocephalae)
    Fu Ling (Poria)
    Dang Gui (Radix Angelicae Sinensis)
    Chi Shao (Radix Paeoniae Rubrae)
    Chuan Xiong (Rhizoma Chuanxiong)
    Shu Di (cooked Radix Rehmanniae)
    Huang Qi (Radix Astragali)
    Rou Cong Rong (Herba Cistanchis)
    Bai Jie Zi (Semen Sinapis)
    Gan Cao (Radix Glycyrrhizae)

Acupuncture & moxibustion

For pain relief and increased mobility of the joints, choose local points around the affected joints as well as distant points on the affected channels. For hot conditions, use needles. For cold and vacuity conditions, use direct, non-scarring small cones of moxa. If there are signs and symptoms of blood stasis, bleed any visible network vessels even if they are distant from the site of pain and discomfort. For yin vacuity, needle *San Yin Jiao* (Sp 6), *Tai Xi* (Ki 3), and *Shen Shu* (Bl 23). For vacuity cold, moxa *Guan Yuan* (CV 4), *Zu San Li* (St 36), *Shen Shu* (Bl 23), and *Ming Men* (GV 4). For qi and blood vacuity, needle *Zu San Li* (St 36), *San Yin Jiao* (Sp 6), *Xin Shu* (Bl 15), *Ge Shu* (Bl 17), and *Pi Shu* (Bl 20).

Adjunctive treatments

Because rheumatoid arthritis is an immune deficiency disease which tends to evolve from multiple and/or persistent allergies, a clear, bland, hypoallergenic, yeast-free diet is absolutely necessary in order to achieve lasting effects. *Yi Yi Ren* (Semen Coicis) makes an excellent beverage or background tea and the main cereal should be rice.

Comments

Rheumatoid arthritis is considered a difficult to treat, so-called knotty disease in Chinese medicine. In my experience, RA can be treated with Chinese medicine only if there is a proper diet supporting the medicinals and other therapies. This is because intestinal permeability, intestinal dysbiosis, and food allergies are a part of this condition. Most patients, therefore, do have a combination of damp heat with underlying spleen-kidney vacuity. The kidney vacuity may be yin vacuity or yang vacuity even if there is damp heat. In addition, because RA tends to be a chronic or enduring disease, one should remember that enduring diseases enter the network vessels. This means that blood stasis in the network vessels is often a complicating factor in persistent or enduring diseases and especially so in those involving pain and *bi*. In addition, in real life patients, it is typical to also find an element of liver depression complicating the case, all of which needs to be addressed *toute ensemble*.

37. Epilepsy

Epilepsy is a seizure disorder characterized by sudden episodes of loss of consciousness, sudden collapse, eyes staring upward, tremors and spasms of the four limbs, white, frothy saliva drooling from the mouth, urinary incontinence, and guttural noises likened in China to the bleating of a goat. Therefore, the traditional Chinese name for epilepsy is goat epileptic wind. After a seizure, the child may be drowsy or confused or may sleep for some time. Between episodes, the child may appear otherwise healthy. At first the episodes are mild and spaced far apart. As the disease worsens, the seizures typically become more severe and more often. In general, epilepsy is associated with phlegm and wind in TCM. As we have seen above, phlegm may evolve from faulty diet and feeding. Because internal wind is nothing other than frenetically stirring and counterflowing qi, frequently blood stasis complicates this condition. In some cases, epilepsy is due to fetal fright or fright sustained while in utero.

Treatment based on pattern discrimination:

1. Fright epilepsy

Main symptoms: Episodes of spasms and tremors, spirit clouding, exaggerated startle reflex, restlessness, excessive timidity, sudden crying, vomiting drool, green-colored, pasty or sticky stools, short, reddish urination, a sometimes red and sometimes white facial complexion, a red tongue with white fur, a sometimes large and sometimes small, wiry, tense pulse

Treatment principles: Settle fright and quiet the spirit assisted by clearing heat and transforming phlegm

Guiding formulas:
Ding Jing Wan Jia Jian (Settle Fright Pills with Additions & Subtractions)
Fu Shen (Sclerotium Pararadicis Poriae)
Zhi Sha (Cinnabar)

Yuan Zhi (Radix Polygalae)
　　Suan Zao Ren (Semen Zizyphi Spinosae)
　　Mai Men Dong (Tuber Ophiopogonis)
　　Shi Chang Pu (Rhizoma Acori Tatarinowii)
　　Huang Lian (Rhizoma Coptidis)
　　Gou Teng (Ramulus Uncariae Cum Uncis)
　　Jiang Can (Bombyx Batryticatus)
　　Dan Nan Xing (bile-processed Rhizoma Arisaematis)
　　Tian Zhu Huang (Concretio Silicea Bambusae)

If spasms and tremors of the four limbs are particularly frequent and pronounced, add *Quan Xie* (Scorpio) and *Wu Gong* (Scolopendra). If there is listlessness of the essence spirit with frequent yawning, add *Ren Shen* (Radix Ginseng) and *Gan Cao* (Radix Glycyrrhizae).

Ding Po Wan Jia Jian (Settle the Corporeal Soul Pills with Additions & Subtractions)
　　Dang Shen (Radix Codonopsitis)
　　Tian Men Dong (Tuber Asparagi)
　　Fu Shen (Sclerotium Pararadicis Poriae)
　　Tian Ma (Rhizoma Gastrodiae)
　　Shi Chang Pu (Rhizoma Acori Tatarinowii)
　　Yuan Zhi (Radix Polygalae)
　　Suan Zao Ren (Semen Zizyphi Spinosae)
　　Quan Xie (Scorpio)
　　Jiang Can (Bombyx Batryticatus)
　　Zhu Sha (Cinnabar)
　　Hu Po (Succinum)
　　Gan Cao (Radix Glycyrrhizae)

If there are fright palpitations and insomnia, one can also use **Wen Dan Tang (Warm the Gallbladder Decoction):**
　　Ban Xia (Rhizoma Pinelliae)
　　Chen Pi (Pericarpium Citri Reticulatae)
　　Fu Ling (Poria)
　　Gan Cao (Radix Glycyrrhizae)
　　Zhu Ru (Caulis Bambusae In Taeniis)
　　Zhi Shi (Fructus Immaturus Aurantii)
　　Da Zao (Fructus Jujubae)

If fright epilepsy endures for many days with frequent attacks, fright palpitations, and insomnia due to heart vacuity and diminished blood, one can use **Yang Xin Tang (Nourish the Heart Decoction):**
　　Dang Gui (Radix Angelicae Sinensis)
　　Sheng Di (uncooked Radix Rehmanniae)
　　Shu Di (cooked Radix Rehmanniae)

Fu Shen (Sclerotium Pararadicis Poriae)
Ren Shen (Radix Ginseng)
Mai Men Dong (Tuber Ophiopogonis)
Suan Zao Ren (Semen Zizyphi Spinosae)
Bai Zi Ren (Semen Platycladi)
mix-fried *Gan Cao* (Radix Glycyrrhizae)
Wu Wei Zi (Fructus Schisandrae)

If there is habitual lassitude of the spirit and lack of strength due to righteous qi vacuity weakness, one can use **Da Bu Yuan Jian (Great Supplement the Source Decoction):**

Shu Di (cooked Radix Rehmanniae)
Ren Shen (Radix Ginseng)
Shan Yao (Radix Dioscoreae)
Dang Gui (Radix Angelicae Sinensis)
Du Zhong (Cortex Eucommiae)
Shan Zhu Yu (Fructus Corni)
Gou Qi Zi (Fructus Lycii)
mix-fried *Gan Cao* (Radix Glycyrrhizae)

2. Food epilepsy

Main symptoms: Epileptic seizures and spasms and tremors accompanied by epigastric and abdominal distention and fullness, lack of appetite, bad breath, vomiting and diarrhea of sour, putrid substances, thick, slimy tongue fur, a purplish, stagnant finger vein

Treatment principles: Disperse food and abduct stagnation, transform phlegm and extinguish wind

Guiding formula:
Bao He Wan Jia Jian (Protect Harmony Pills with Additions & Subtractions)

Shan Zha (Fructus Crataegi)
Shen Qu (Massa Medica Fermentata)
Bing Lang (Semen Arecae)
Lian Qiao (Fructus Forsythiae)
Ju Hua (Flos Chrysanthemi)
Gou Teng (Ramulus Uncariae Uncis)
Ban Xia (Rhizoma Pinelliae)
Zhi Shi (Fructus Immaturus Aurantii)

If there is constipation, add *Da Huang* (Radix Et Rhizoma Rhei).

3. Wind epilepsy

Main symptoms: Sudden episodes of spirit-will clouding, clenched teeth, eyes staring upward, spasms and contractions of the hands and feet which are particularly severe, arched back rigidity, crying and shouting, vomiting drool, body hot, spontaneous perspiration, a red face, a wiry, rapid pulse

Treatment principles: Clear heat and extinguish wind

Guiding formulas:
Xie Qing Wan Jia Jian (Drain the Green Pills with Additions & Subtractions)

Long Dan Cao (Radix Gentianae)
Zhi Zi (Fructus Gardeniae)
Da Huang (Radix Et Rhizoma Rhei)
Gou Teng (Ramulus Uncariae Cum Uncis)
Bai Shao (Radix Paeoniae Albae)
Wu Gong (Scolopendra)
Quan Xie (Scorpio)
Dan Nan Xing (bile-processed Rhizoma Arisaematis)
Zhu Ru (Caulis Bambusae In Taeniis)

If vomiting of phlegmy drool is relatively profuse, add *Ban Xia* (Rhizoma Pinelliae) and *Ju Hong* (Exocarpium Citri Erythrocarpae). If there is crying and shouting and restlessness, add *Zhu Sha* (Cinnabar) and *Hu Po* (Succinum). If signs of heat are not marked and after a seizure there is listlessness of the essence spirit with a somber white facial complexion, and a wiry, fine pulse, subtract *Long Dan Cao*, *Zhi Zi*, and *Da Huang* and add mix-fried *Gan Cao* (Radix Glycyrrhizae), *Xiao Mai* (Fructus Levis Tritici), *Da Zao* (Fructus Jujubae), and *Dang Shen* (Radix Codonopsitis).

Qian Jin Long Dan Tang (Thousand [Pieces of] Gold Gentiana Decoction)

Long Dan Cao (Radix Gentianae)
Gou Teng (Ramulus Uncariae Cum Uncis)
Tian Ma (Rhizoma Gastrodiae)
Chai Hu (Radix Bupleuri)
Huang Qin (Radix Scutellariae)
Chi Shao (Radix Paeoniae Rubrae)
Dan Nan Xing (bile-processed Rhizoma Arisaematis)
Yuan Zhi (Radix Polygalae)
Di Long (Pheretima)
Gan Cao (Radix Glycyrrhizae)

4. Phlegm epilepsy

Main symptoms: Habitually there is profuse phlegm. During seizures there is crying and shouting, clouding and loss of consciousness or sudden torpor of the intelligence, lack of spirit, frothy saliva or vomiting phlegmy fluids, and the sound of phlegm in the throat. Spasms and contractions are not marked. The facial complexion is yellow and lusterless, and the tongue fur is thick, slimy, and white. The pulse is wiry and slippery.

Treatment principles: Flush phlegm and open the portals

Guiding formulas:
Di Tan Tang (Flush Phlegm Decoction)
Ju Hong (Exocarpium Citri Erythrocarpae)
Ban Xia (Rhizoma Pinelliae)
Dan Nan Xing (bile-processed Rhizoma Arisaematis)
Shi Chang Pu (Rhizoma Acori Tatarinowii)
Zhi Shi (Fructus Immaturus Aurantii)
Zhu Ru (Caulis Bambusae In Taeniis)

Ding Xian Wan (Stabilize Epilepsy Pills)
Tian Ma (Rhizoma Gastrodiae)
Shi Chang Pu (Rhizoma Acori Tatarinowii)
Quan Xie (Scorpio)
Jiang Can (Bombyx Batryticatus)
Hu Po (Succinum)
Zhu Sha (Cinnabar)
Fu Shen (Sclerotium Pararadicis Poriae)
Yuan Zhi (Radix Polygalae)
Chuan Bei Mu (Bulbus Fritillariae Cirrhosae)
Dan Nan Xing (bile-processed Rhizoma Arisaematis)
Ban Xia (Rhizoma Pinelliae)
Zhu Li (Succus Bambusae)

If there is spleen vacuity engendering phlegm with phlegm following qi counterflow, one can use **Liu Jun Zi Tang Jia Wei (Six Gentlemen Decoction with Added Flavors):**
Ren Shen (Radix Ginseng)
Bai Zhu (Rhizoma Atractylodis Macrocephalae)
Fu Ling (Poria)
Gan Cao (Radix Glycyrrhizae)
Ban Xia (Rhizoma Pinelliae)
Chen Pi (Pericarpium Citri Reticulatae)
Tian Ma (Rhizoma Gastrodiae)
Gou Teng (Ramulus Uncariae Cum Uncis)

5. Static blood epilepsy

Main symptoms: Habitual headache in a fixed location, crying and shouting, insomnia, restlessness, sudden onset of seizures, loss of consciousness of human affairs, spasms and contractions of the four limbs, skin colored bluish green and purple or the appearance of static macules, a purplish, dull or dark tongue, a deep, stagnant finger vein, a fine, choppy pulse

Treatment principles: Quicken the blood and transform stasis, open the portals and stabilize epilepsy

Guiding formulas:
Tong Qiao Huo Xue Tang (Open the Portals & Quicken the Blood Decoction)
Chuan Xiong (Rhizoma Chuanxiong)
Dang Gui (Radix Angelicae Sinensis)
Tao Ren (Semen Persicae)
Hong Hua (Flos Carthami)
She Xiang (Moschus)
Cong Bai (Bulbus Allii Fistulosi)

Tong Qiao Huo Xue Tang Jia Jian (Open the Portals & Quicken the Blood Decoction with Additions & Subtractions)
Chi Shao (Radix Paeoniae Rubrae)
Chuan Xiong (Rhizoma Chuanxiong)
Dan Shen (Radix Salviae Miltiorrhizae)
Tao Ren (Semen Persicae)
Hong Hua (Flos Carthami)
Quan Xie (Scorpio)
Di Long (Pheretima)
She Xiang (Moschus)
Cong Bai (Bulbus Allii Fistulosi)
Sheng Jiang (uncooked Rhizoma Zingiberis)
Da Zao (Fructus Jujubae)

If there is lassitude of the spirit with diminished eating, add *Dang Shen* (Radix Codonopsitis) and *Bai Zhu* (Rhizoma Atractylodis Macrocephalae). If the body is emaciated with a dark red tongue and a fine, rapid pulse, add *Sheng Di* (uncooked Radix Rehmanniae), *Shu Di* (cooked Radix Rehmanniae), and *Dang Gui* (Radix Angelicae Sinensis).

6. Vacuity detriment

Main symptoms: The epilepsy is chronic and enduring with repeated seizures. It has lasted for many days without healing. After each episode, there is listlessness of the essence spirit, diminished eating and drinking, lack of strength in the lower limbs, clouding of the head, a lusterless facial complexion, a pale red tongue, and a deep, fine pulse.

Treatment principles: Mainly supplement and boost the liver and kidney essence and blood, assisted by nourishing the heart and fortifying the spleen

Guiding formula:
He Che Ba Wei Wan Jia Jian (Placenta Eight Flavors Pills with Additions & Subtractions)
Zi He Che (Placenta Hominis)

Shan Yao (Radix Dioscoreae)
Shu Di (cooked Radix Rehmanniae)
Dan Pi (Cortex Moutan)
Fu Ling (Poria)
Mai Men Dong (Tuber Ophiopogonis)
Wu Wei Zi (Fructus Schisandrae)
Lu Jiao (Cornu Cervi)
Gui Ban (Plastrum Testudinis)
Dang Shen (Radix Codonopsitis)
Rou Gui (Cortex Cinnamomi)
Da Zao (Fructus Jujubae)

If there is restless sleep due to heart blood vacuity, add *Suan Zao Ren* (Semen Zizyphi Spinosae) and *Bai Zi Ren* (Semen Platycladi). If intake is torpid and eating is diminished or there is abdominal distention after eating, add *Mu Xiang* (Radix Auklandiae), *Sha Ren* (Fructus Amomi), and *Shen Qu* (Massa Medica Fermentata).

Acupuncture & moxibustion

During an acute seizure, needle *Ren Zhong* (GV 26), *He Gu* (LI 4), *Nei Guan* (Per 6), *Shi Xuan* (M-HN-1-5), and/or *Yong Quan* (Ki 1) depending upon the pattern. For instance, if there is food stagnation or pronounced phlegm, needle *Nei Guan*, while if there is obvious heat, needle *Shi Xuan*. After a seizure, needle *Da Zhui* (GV 14), *Shen Men* (Ht 7), and *Xin Shu* (Bl 15) and moxa *Bai Hui* (GV 20) and *Zu San Li* (St 36), three cones one time every other day.

Adjunctive treatments

Diet plays an important part in any pediatric epilepsy due to food stagnation or involving phlegm. In such cases, feeding should be well regulated and a child on solid foods should be fed a clear, bland diet, strictly avoiding foods which are mucus-producing such as cheese and nuts, cold milk, and yogurt.

Comments

Epilepsy due to fright experienced in utero or the mother's faulty diet during pregnancy, such as overconsumption of alcohol and greasy, spicy foods, is difficult to treat with complete success with Chinese medicine alone. In many cases, best results come from combining modern Western and traditional Chinese medicines. The severity of this disease, the duration of the seizures themselves, and the length of time between seizures are dependent upon the depth of the phlegm binding and the exuberance or debility of the righteous qi. As the disease goes on, phlegm binding becomes deeper and more recalcitrant and the righteous qi of the body becomes vacuous and weak. Thus the seizures tend to last longer and come at closer intervals the longer they remain unhealed. If this disease has endured for any length of time, the case is typically a complicated combination of vacuity and repletion, phlegm, wind, and blood stasis lodged in the network vessels. Therefore, its treatment should not be delayed.

38. Tourette's Syndrome

Tourette's syndrome in Chinese is called *chou dong yi hui yu zeng he zheng*. Literally, this translates as twitching and foul language syndrome. Like epilepsy above, Tourette's syndrome in Chinese medicine is mostly seen as a wind and phlegm disease. Clinical audits in China show that Chinese medicine can treat this condition if it is treated early in children. TCM treatment of adults is not effective. This is because, like epilepsy, the longer this disease remains unhealed, the deeper the phlegm binding goes and the more vacuity of righteous qi is mixed with repletion. TCM treatment of Tourette's syndrome is mainly aimed at the lungs, spleen, liver, and kidneys.

Treatment based on pattern discrimination:

1. Wind phlegm evils lingering in the lungs

Main symptoms: Squeezing of the brow, blinking of the eyes, stuffy nose, shrugging of the shoulders, itchy throat, repetitive strange noises, incessant cursing, endless twitching movement of the body and limbs

Treatment principles: Dispel and eliminate wind

Guiding formula:
Unnamed formula
   Xin Yi (Flos Magnoliae)
   Cang Er Zi (Fructus Xanthii)
   Xuan Shen (Radix Scrophulariae)
   Ban Lan Gen (Radix Isatidis/Baphicacanthi)
   Shan Dou Gen (Radix Sophorae Subprostratae)
   Ban Xia (Rhizoma Pinelliae)
   Gou Teng (Ramulus Uncariae Cum Uncis)

If twitching movement of the limbs is severe, add *Quan Xie* (Scorpio) and *Wu Gong* (Scolopendra).

2. Phlegm heat internally harassing, liver wind internally stirring

Main symptoms: Twitching of the brow, blinking of the eyes, erratic and uncontrollable movement of the head, twitching of the corners of the mouth, drooling, strange sounds uttered from the throat, heart vexation, emotional tension, occasional suffering from fright and jumpiness

Treatment principles: Sweep away phlegm and open the portals, soften the liver and extinguish wind

Guiding formulas:
Huo Tan Xi Feng Tang (Sweep Away Phlegm & Extinguish Wind Decoction)

Shi Chang Pu (Rhizoma Acori Tatarinowii)
Yu Jin (Tuber Curcumae)
Dan Shen (Radix Salviae Miltiorrhizae)
Meng Shi (Lapis Chloriti/Mica)
Huang Qin (Radix Scutellariae)
Ban Xia (Rhizoma Pinelliae)
processed *Da Huang* (Radix Et Rhizoma Rhei)
Shi Hu (Herba Dendrobii)
Gou Teng (Ramulus Uncariae Cum Uncis)
Quan Xie (Scorpio)
Shan Zha (Fructus Crataegi)
Shen Qu (Massa Medica Fermentata)
Mai Ya (Fructus Germinatus Hordei)

Ning Gan Xi Feng Tang *(Calm the Liver & Extinguish Wind Decoction)*

Hu Po (Succinum)
Long Dan Cao (Radix Gentianae)
Jiang Can (Bombyx Batryticatus)
Bai Ji Li (Fructus Tribuli)
Bai Shao (Radix Paeoniae Albae)
Zhi Zi (Fructus Gardeniae)
Chan Yi (Periostracum Cicadae)
Bing Lang (Semen Arecae)
Gou Teng (Ramulus Uncariae Cum Uncis)
Fu Ling (Poria)
Zao Xiu (Rhizoma Paradis Polyphyllae)

If there is internal stirring of liver wind without any signs of heat, use **Zhen Gan Xi Feng Tang (Settle the Liver & Extinguish Wind Decoction)**:

Bai Shao (Radix Paeoniae Albae)
Tian Men Dong (Tuber Asparagi)
Xuan Shen (Radix Scrophulariae)
Mu Li (Concha Ostreae)
Dai Zhe Shi (Haemititum)
Chuan Lian Zi (Fructus Toosendan)
Long Gu (Os Draconis)
Gou Teng (Ramulus Uncariae Cum Uncis)
Bai He (Bulbus Lilii)
Yu Jin (Tuber Curcumae)

Or one can use **Hua Tan Xi Feng Tang (Transform Phlegm & Extinguish Wind Decoction)**:

Ban Xia (Rhizoma Pinelliae)
Chen Pi (Pericarpium Citri Reticulatae)
Fu Ling (Poria)

Dan Nan Xing (bile-processed Rhizoma Arisaematis)
Zhu Ru (Caulis Bambusae In Taeniis)
Jiang Can (Bombyx Batryticatus)
Yu Jin (Tuber Curcumae)
He Huan Hua (Flos Albiziae)
Long Gu (Os Draconis)
Mu Li (Concha Ostreae)

3. Spleen vacuity, liver hyperactivity, vacuity wind stirring internally

Main symptoms: Twitching and cursing, blinking of the eyes, sometimes mild, sometimes severe, spasms and tremors of the limbs, deviated mouth, a weak, feeble voice, diminished intake, a yellow facial complexion

Treatment principles: Support the spleen and repress the liver

Guiding formula:
Fu Tu Yi Mu Tang (Support Earth & Repress Wood Decoction)
Dang Shen (Radix Codonopsitis)
Huang Qi (Radix Astragali)
Fu Ling (Poria)
Bai Zhu (Rhizoma Atractylodis Macrocephalae)
Bai Shao (Radix Paeoniae Albae)
mix-fried *Gan Cao* (Radix Glycyrrhizae)
Gou Teng (Ramulus Uncariae Cum Uncis)
Chen Pi (Pericarpium Citri Reticulatae)
Ban Xia (Rhizoma Pinelliae)
Mai Ya (Fructus Germinatus Hordei)
Shan Zha (Fructus Crataegi)
Shen Qu (Massa Medica Fermentata)
mix-fried *Ji Nei Jin* (Endothelium Corneum Gigeriae Galli)
stir-fried *Gu Ya* (Fructus Germinatus Oryzae)
Quan Xie (Scorpio)

4. Yin vacuity, wind stirring

Main symptoms: Twitching and cursing, blinking of the eyes, twitching of the muscles and flesh, sounds emitted from the throat, emotional tension and agitation, heat in the hands, feet, and heart

Treatment principles: Enrich yin and extinguish wind

Guiding formula:
San Jia Fu Mai Tang (Three Shells Restore the Pulse Decoction)
Gui Ban (Plastrum Testudinis)
Bie Jia (Carapax Trionycis)
Mu Li (Concha Ostreae)

mix-fried *Gan Cao* (Radix Glycyrrhizae)
Bai Shao (Radix Paeoniae Albae)
Mai Men Dong (Tuber Ophiopogonis)
Sheng Di (uncooked Radix Rehmanniae)
E Jiao (Gelatinum Corii Asini)

Acupuncture & moxibustion

Needle *Bai Hui* (GV 20), *Feng Chi* (GB 20), *Nei Guan* (Per 6), and *Feng Long* (St 40). If there is liver hyperactivity, add *Tai Chong* (Liv 3). If there is emotional tension and stress, add *Shen Men* (Ht 7). If there is spleen vacuity, add *Zu San Li* (St 36) and *Pi Shu* (Bl 20). If there is food stagnation, add *Nei Ting* (St 44) and *Liang Men* (St 21). If there is yin vacuity, add *San Yin Jiao* (Sp 6).

Adjunctive treatments

As with epilepsy, diet is very important in the treatment of pediatric Tourette's syndrome. Because phlegm plays an important part in this disease, mucus-forming foods and over-feeding in general should be avoided, while a clear, bland diet should be the norm.

Comments

Also as with epilepsy above, according to Chinese medicine, some children's Tourette's syndrome begins in utero due to fetal fright, congenital insufficiency, or the mother's faulty diet during pregnancy. It is difficult to completely cure such cases with Chinese medicine because the condition is so deep-seated.

39. Pediatric Hyperactivity

In Chinese medicine, pediatric hyperactivity mainly has to do with the Chinese concept of the spirit residing in the heart. Spirit here refers to the mind and to consciousness. If the spirit is healthy, then it is calm. If the spirit is calm, then the mind is not agitated nor the body restless. According to Chinese medicine, there are three basic causes which can disturb the spirit residing in the heart — either the spirit is not nourished sufficiently which causes the spirit to flutter around nervously, some sort of heat wafts upward and disturbs the spirit as if one's house were on fire, or phlegm blocks the portals or openings of the heart. In this latter case, the spirit's connection with the outside world is confused and hindered as if shutters had been put on all the doors and windows of the mind's house. In addition, blood stasis obstructing the channels causing malnourishment of the portals can complicate any of the three patterns. Further, because the spleen is weak and the liver has a surplus in children, there may be a combination of insufficient spirit (due to insufficient qi) with liver depression transforming wind due to malnourishment by the blood. In fact, this last pattern is the most commonly seen in clinical practice. These patterns also cover attention deficit disorder/attention deficit syndrome or ADD/ADS.

Treatment based on pattern discrimination:

1. Spleen vacuity, liver hyperactivity

Main symptoms: Uncontrollable fidgeting, emotional tension, easy anger, poor sleep, fatigue, diminished appetite, easily developing diarrhea in response to emotional stress, thin, white tongue fur, a wiry pulse

Treatment principles: Fortify the spleen and harmonize the liver

Guiding formulas:
Gui Zhi Tang (Cinnamon Twig Decoction)
   Gui Zhi (Ramulus Cinnamomi)
   Bai Shao (Radix Paeoniae Albae)
   mix-fried *Gan Cao* (Radix Glycyrrhizae)
   Sheng Jiang (uncooked Rhizoma Zingiberis)
   Da Zao (Fructus Jujubae)

Yi Gan San (Repress the Liver Powder)
   Chai Hu (Radix Bupleuri)
   Gou Teng (Ramulus Uncariae Cum Uncis)
   Dang Gui (Radix Angelicae Sinensis)
   Chuan Xiong (Rhizoma Chuanxiong)
   Bai Zhu (Rhizoma Atractylodis Macrocephalae)
   Fu Ling (Poria)
   mix-fried *Gan Cao* (Radix Glycyrrhizae)

2. Heart/spleen insufficiency

Main symptoms: A sallow yellow or somber white facial complexion, pale nails and pale lips, fatigue, insomnia, heart palpitations, shortness of breath, poor appetite, tendency to loose stools, poor memory, a fat, pale tongue with thin, white fur, a fine, weak pulse

Treatment principles: Fortify the spleen and supplement the heart, supplement the qi and nourish the blood

Guiding formulas:
Yang Xin Yi Pi Tang (Nourish the Heart & Boost the Spleen Decoction)
   Dang Gui (Radix Angelicae Sinensis)
   Bai Zi Ren (Semen Platycladi)
   Fu Ling (Poria)
   Fu Xiao Mai (Fructus Levis Tritici)
   Long Gu (Os Draconis)
   Huang Lian (Rhizoma Coptidis)
   Gan Cao (Radix Glycyrrhizae)

Gui Pi Tang (Return the Spleen Decoction) plus *Gan Mai Da Zao Tang* (Licorice, Triticus & Red Date Decoction) with additions and subtractions

Tai Zi Shen (Radix Pseudostellariae)
Fu Shen (Sclerotium Pararadicis Poriae)
Bai Zhu (Rhizoma Atractylodis Macrocephalae)
Dang Gui (Radix Angelicae Sinensis)
Huang Qi (Radix Astragali)
Yuan Zhi (Radix Polygalae)
Suan Zao Ren (Semen Zizyphi Spinosae)
Shi Chang Pu (Rhizoma Acori Tatarinowii)
Wu Wei Zi (Fructus Schisandrae)
Da Zao (Fructus Jujubae)
Fu Xiao Mai (Fructus Levis Tritici)
Gan Cao (Radix Glycyrrhizae)

If there is sleepwalking, profuse dreaming, or nightmares, add *Gou Teng* (Ramulus Uncariae Cum Uncis), *Long Chi* (Dens Draconis), and *Zhen Zhu Mu* (Concha Margaritiferae). If there is impaired memory, add *Yuan Zhi* (Radix Polygalae), *Long Gu* (Os Draconis), and *Shi Chang Pu* (Rhizoma Acori Tatarinowii).

3. Yin vacuity, yang hyperactivity

Main symptoms: Besides tending to be thin, children with this pattern also have a red tongue with diminished fur or a pale tongue with a red tip. Their pulses are fine and rapid and they tend to suffer from insomnia, heart palpitations, agitation, dizziness, ringing in the ears, possible low back pain, possible bed-wetting at night, flushed cheeks, and possible night sweats.

Treatment principles: Supplement the kidneys and enrich yin, subdue yang and quiet the spirit

Guiding formulas:
You Yin Qian Yang Wan (Foster Yin & Subdue Yang Pills)

Zhi Mu (Rhizoma Anemarrhenae)
Sheng Di (uncooked Radix Rehmanniae)
Gui Ban Jiao (Gelatinum Plastri Testudinis)
Wu Wei Zi (Fructus Schisandrae)
Long Gu (Os Draconis)
Mai Men Dong (Tuber Ophiopogonis)
Yuan Zhi (Radix Polygalae)
Shi Chang Pu (Rhizoma Acori Tatarinowii)
stir-fried *Suan Zao Ren* (Semen Zizyphi Spinosae)
Lu Jiao Jiao (Gelatinum Cornu Cervi)

Zuo Gui Wan Jia Jian (Restore the Left [Kidney] Pills with Additions & Subtractions)
Shu Di (cooked Radix Rehmanniae)
Shan Yao (Radix Dioscoreae)
Dan Pi (Cortex Moutan)
Gui Ban (Plastrum Testudinis)
Bai Shao (Radix Paeoniae Albae)
Long Gu (Os Draconis)
Mu Li (Concha Ostreae)
Yuan Zhi (Radix Polygalae)
Shi Chang Pu (Rhizoma Acori Tatarinowii)
Wu Wei Zi (Fructus Schisandrae)
Yi Zhi Ren (Fructus Alpiniae Oxyphyllae)
Gou Qi Zi (Fructus Lycii)
Gan Cao (Radix Glycyrrhizae)

If there is bed-wetting, add *Tu Si Zi* (Semen Cuscutae), *Sang Piao Xiao* (Ootheca Mantidis), and *Jin Ying Zi* (Fructus Rosae Laevigatae).

Qing Nao Yi Zhi Tang (Clear the Brain & Boost the Intelligence Decoction)
Yi Zhi Ren (Fructus Alpiniae Oxyphyllae)
Shu Di (cooked Radix Rehmanniae)
Sha Ren (Fructus Amomi)
Di Long (Pheretima)
Dan Shen (Radix Salviae Miltiorrhizae)
mix-fried *Gui Ban* (Plastrum Testudinis)
Shi Chang Pu (Rhizoma Acori Tatarinowii)
Gou Qi Zi (Fructus Lycii)
mix-fried *Yuan Zhi* (Radix Polygalae)

Sheng Mai Yin (Engender the Pulse [or Vessels] Beverage)
Hong Shen (red Radix Ginseng)
Wu Wei Zi (Fructus Schisandrae)
Mai Men Dong (Tuber Ophiopogonis)

Bu Shen Yi Zhi Tang (Supplement the Kidneys & Boost the Intelligence Decoction)
Lu Jiao (Cornu Cervi)
processed *He Shou Wu* (Radix Polygoni Multiflori)
Long Gu (Os Draconis)
Mu Li (Concha Ostreae)
Shi Chang Pu (Rhizoma Acori Tatarinowii)
Yu Jin (Tuber Curcumae)
Dan Shen (Radix Salviae Miltiorrhizae)

Yi Zhi Ren (Fructus Alpiniae Oxyphyllae)
Gou Qi Zi (Fructus Lycii)

Bu Shen Huo Xue Tang (Supplement the Kidneys & Quicken the Blood Decoction)

Shu Di (cooked Radix Rehmanniae)
Gou Qi Zi (Fructus Lycii)
He Shou Wu (Radix Polygoni Multiflori)
Dan Shen (Radix Salviae Miltiorrhizae)
Dang Gui (Radix Angelicae Sinensis)
Chi Shao (Radix Paeoniae Rubrae)
Fu Ling (Poria)
Gou Teng (Ramulus Uncariae Cum Uncis)
Long Gu (Os Draconis)
Mu Li (Concha Ostreae)

Bu Shen Er Xian Tang (Supplement the Kidneys Two Immortals Decoction)

Xian Mao (Rhizoma Curculiginis)
Xian Ling Pi (Herba Epimedii)
Ba Ji Tian (Radix Morindae)
Rou Cong Rong (Herba Cistanchis)
Dang Gui (Radix Angelicae Sinensis)
Shu Di (cooked Radix Rehmanniae)
Nu Zhen Zi (Fructus Ligustri Lucidi)
Shan Zhu Yu (Fructus Corni)
Lu Jiao Jiao (Gelatinum Cornu Cervi)
Gui Ban (Plastrum Testudinis)
stir-fried *Suan Zao Ren* (Semen Zizyphi Spinosae)
Yi Zhi Ren (Fructus Alpiniae Oxyphyllae)
mix-fried *Gan Cao* (Radix Glycyrrhizae)

Chang Pu Wu Wei San (Acorus & Schisandra Powder)

Shi Chang Pu (Rhizoma Acori Tatarinowii)
Wu Wei Zi (Fructus Schisandrae)
Yi Zhi Ren (Fructus Alpiniae Oxyphyllae)
Jiang Can (Bombyx Batryticatus)
Di Long (Pheretima)
Bai Zhi (Radix Angelicae Dahuricae)

4. Phlegm confounding the portals of the heart & heat harassing the heart spirit

Main symptoms: Easy anger or pronounced irritability, vexation and restlessness, possible nausea, possible profuse phlegm, chest fullness and oppression, a bitter taste in the mouth when waking up in the morning, a tongue with red edges and slimy, yellow fur, a wiry, slippery, rapid pulse

Guiding formulas:
Huang Lian Wen Dan Tang Jia Jian (Coptis Warm the Gallbladder Decoction with Additions & Subtractions)

Ban Xia (Rhizoma Pinelliae)
Chen Pi (Pericarpium Citri Reticulatae)
Fu Ling (Poria)
Hou Po (Cortex Magnoliae)
Yu Jin (Tuber Curcumae)
Shi Chang Pu (Rhizoma Acori Tatarinowii)
Hua Shi (Talcum)
Zhi Ke (Fructus Aurantii)
Lian Qiao (Fructus Forsythiae)
Huang Lian (Rhizoma Coptidis)
Gan Cao (Radix Glycyrrhizae)

If there is phlegm confounding the portals but with no or minor heat, use **Chang Zhi Long Mu Tang (Acorus, Polygala, Dragon Bone & Oyster Shell Decoction):**

Shi Chang Pu (Rhizoma Acori Tatarinowii)
mix-fried *Yuan Zhi* (Radix Polygalae)
Long Gu (Os Draconis)
Mu Li (Concha Ostreae)
Hu Po (Succinum)

If there is heat, add *Huang Lian* (Rhizoma Coptidis), *Long Dan Cao* (Radix Gentianae), and *Dan Zhu Ye* (Herba Lophateri). If there is yin vacuity, add *Shu Di* (cooked Radix Rehmanniae), *Bai He* (Bulbus Lilii), and *Shi Hu* (Herba Dendrobii). If there is yang vacuity, add *Fu Zi* (Radix Lateralis Praeparatus Aconiti Carmichaeli), *Lu Jiao* (Cornu Cervi), and *Huang Qi* (Radix Astragali).

5. Blood stasis obstructing the channels & (causing) malnourishment of the portals

Main symptoms: Hyperactivity plus a history of birth trauma with intracranial hemorrhage, a dull, dark facial complexion, easy anger over nothing, a dark red tongue, a choppy pulse

Treatment principles: Quicken the blood and dispel stasis

Guiding formula: Since this pattern merely complicates one of the four above patterns, one should choose from among the above formulas and then add *Chi Shao* (Radix Paeoniae Rubrae), *Dan Shen* (Radix Salviae Miltiorrhizae), and *Hong Hua* (Flos Carthami).

Acupuncture & moxibustion

Needle *Shen Men* (Ht 7) and *Nei Guan* (Per 6) in all five patterns. Add *Tai Chong* (Liv 3) and *Zu San Li* (St 36) for spleen vacuity, liver hyperactivity. Add *Xin Shu* (Bl 15) and *Pi Shu* (Bl 20) for heart blood, spleen qi vacuity. Add *Tai Chong* (Liv 3) and *Feng Long* (St 40) for phlegm obstructing the portals. Add *San Yin Jiao* (Sp 6) and *Shen Shu* (Bl 23) for yin vacuity with yang hyperactivity. And add *He Gu* (LI 4) and *Xue Hai* (Sp 10) for blood stasis.

Adjunctive treatments

In the case of heart blood, spleen qi vacuity and also in yin vacuity, yang hyperactivity, the diet should be a nourishing, cooked, warm, clear bland diet. By nourishing, I mean that there should be a little more animal protein in this child's diet in order to help manufacture sufficient blood. Soups made out of black beans, chicken or beef broth, and lots of root and leafy green vegetables are good. In phlegm confounding the portals, it is important to avoid foods which either weaken the spleen, such as chilled, cold, raw foods or sugar and sweets, or foods which cause dampness and phlegm to be generated in the body, such as sugar and sweets, dairy foods, and fatty, greasy, fried foods.

Comments

The reader will notice that phlegm-transforming, portal-opening medicinals are used in guiding formulas for all three major patterns of pediatric hyperactivity and not just for the pattern of phlegm heat. Likewise, one should not forget the use of insect medicinals which enter the network vessels and track down wind as well as quicken the blood and open the network vessels.

40. Measles

Measles, also called rubeola, is an acute, epidemic, infectious disease caused by the measles virus. It may strike at any age during childhood, and it may attack adults who have never had measles before. It mainly occurs during the spring. Once one has had measles, they then have a lifetime immunity. In the past, measles were often a life-threatening disease especially for children. Fortunately because of hereditary immunity built up over generations among most Westerners, measles is rarely fatal these days.

In Chinese medicine, measles is believed to be due to a combination of *tai du* or fetal toxins plus invasion by an external pathogen. In other words, there is a predisposing factor to measles and that is this concept of fetal toxins. Fetal toxins are toxins developed during pregnancy. Not every person develops the same or the same amount of fetal toxins. Some people, due to the mother's diet and lifestyle or due to the mother's health at the time of conception and during pregnancy, inherit or develop more fetal toxins than others. For instance, if the mother recently had a severe, acute febrile disease just before conception or during pregnancy, this may predispose the child to more fetal toxins. Or if the mother had a very bad diet, eating lots of greasy, fried, fatty foods and drinking lots of alcohol, this might also result in the accumulation of more fetal toxins. Once generated, these toxins lie dormant in the body until they are provoked by some external factor. Thus they are also referred to as *fu wen xie* or deep-lying warm evils.

Chinese medicine divides the progression of measles into two basic types and three basic stages. First of all, there are those cases of measles that follow the normal progression of this disease and those that follow an abnormal progression. Basically, Chinese doctors want to see the measles rash "come out" fully on the body. This is then taken for a sign that the righteous or healthy energy of the body is sufficient to fight the evil or disease energy and that, in fact, the righteous energy is kicking this evil energy out of the body. Since this evil energy was generated during pregnancy, once it is gone, it is gone for good. If, on the other hand, the righteous energy of the body is not sufficiently strong to out-thrust these toxins from the body, then they sink back into the body and can cause a variety of diseases at a later date.

The three stages of measles are the pre-eruptive stage before the rash appears, the eruptive stage when the rash has discharged uniformly, and the rash-receding or resolution stage when the rash disappears. Further, there are several post-measles conditions which are also discussed in the Chinese pediatric literature.

The following chart gives some idea about the healthy or correct progression of this disease and an abnormal or unhealthy progression.

Stage	Favorable symptoms			Unfavorable symptoms
	Before rash appears	Rash appears	Rash fades	
Fever	Chills & fever	Continuous fever	Fever subsides	Fever too high or not high enough, high fever does not abate in the last stage
Cough	Mild	Worse	Better	Persistent, severe cough, shortness of breath, flaring of the wings of the nose
Spirit	Normal	Restless	Normal	Restlessness, mental cloudiness, delerium
Sweating	Mild	Mild	Mild	No sweating, dry heat sensation of the skin or profuse sweating with cold limbs
Order of eruption	Hairlines behind ear, neck, face, back, chest, four limbs, nose, hands, feet			Delayed eruption or untimely fading of the rash
Distribution	Even			Sparse and indistinct or dense and joining up into larger areas, absence of rash on the face and nose in severe cases
Color	Bright red and moist-looking			Pale and dull or dark purple

Treatment based on pattern discrimination:

Normal progression

1. Pre-eruptive stage

Main symptoms: A mild cough, watery, red eyes and photophobia, puffy, swollen eyelids, mental dullness and a wan, dispirited affect, possibly vomiting and diarrhea, a sore throat, greyish white spots in the mouth with red borders, known as Koplik's spots, thin, white or thin, yellow tongue fur, a floating, rapid pulse

Note: This is essentially a wind heat pattern with spleen complications.

Treatment principles: Use acrid, cool medicinals to out-thrust the exterior or, in other words, promote the expression of the rash

Guiding formulas:
Sheng Ma Ge Gen Tang (Cimicifuga & Pueraria Decoction)
    Sheng Ma (Rhizoma Cimicifugae)
    Ge Gen (Radix Puerariae)
    mix-fried *Gan Cao* (Radix Glycyrrhizae)
    Chi Shao (Radix Paeoniae Rubrae)

If exterior heat is marked, add *Bo He* (Herba Menthae Haplocalycis), *Chan Yi* (Periostracum Cicadae), *Niu Bang Zi* (Fructus Arctii), and *Jin Yin Hua* (Flos Lonicerae). If there is a sore, swollen throat, add *Jie Geng* (Radix Platycodi), *Xuan Shen* (Radix Scrophulariae), and *Ma Bo* (Lasiosphaera). If the rash is dark red, add *Zi Cao* (Radix Lithospermi/Arnebiae) and *Dan Pi* (Cortex Moutan). If there is cough with profuse phlegm, add *Xing Ren* (Semen Armeniaca), *Jie Geng* (Radix Platycodi), and *Qian Hu* (Radix Peucedani). If there is vomiting, add *Zhu Ru* (Caulis Bambusae In Taeniis).

Xuan Du Fa Biao Tang (Diffuse Toxins & Effuse the Exterior Decoction)
    Sheng Ma (Rhizoma Cimicifugae)
    Ge Gen (Radix Pueraria)
    Zhi Ke (Fructus Aurantii)
    Fang Feng (Radix Saposhnikoviae)
    Jing Jie (Herba Schizonepetae)
    Bo He (Herba Menthae Haplocalycis)
    Mu Tong (Caulis Akebiae)
    Lian Qiao (Fructus Forsythiae)
    Niu Bang Zi (Fructus Arctii)
    Dan Zhu Ye (Herba Lophateri)
    Gan Cao (Radix Glycyrrhizae)
    Qian Hu (Radix Peucedani)
    Jie Geng (Radix Platycodi)

If there is high fever, add *Jin Yin Hua* (Flos Lonicerae) and *Da Qing Ye* (Folium Daqingye) to clear heat and resolve toxins. If there is no sweating, add *Fu Ping* (Herba Lemnae/Spirodelae) and *Ma Huang* (Herba Ephedrae) to out-thrust the exterior and effuse sweat. If there is sore throat, add *Ma Bo* (Lasiosphaera) and *She Gan* (Rhizoma Belamcandae) to clear the throat and resolve toxins.

Xuan Du Fa Biao Tang Jia Jian (Diffuse Toxins & Effuse the Exterior Decoction with Additions & Subtractions)

Ge Gen (Radix Peurariae)
Sheng Ma (Rhizoma Cimicifugae)
Jin Yin Hua (Flos Lonicerae)
Bo He (Herba Menthae Haplocalycis)
Jing Jie (Herba Schizonepetae)
Lian Qiao (Fructus Forsythiae)
Dan Zhu Ye (Herba Lophateri)
Jie Geng (Radix Platycodi)
Niu Bang Zi (Fructus Arctii)
Gan Cao (Radix Glycyrrhizae)

If there is fatigue, lack of strength, a pale facial complexion, and cold limbs with retarded eruption of the rash, add *Huang Qi* (Radix Astragali), *Dang Shen* (Radix Codonopsitis), and *Huang Jing* (Rhizoma Polygonati).

Yin Qiao San Jia Jian (Lonicera & Forsythia Powder with Additions & Subtractions)

Lian Qiao (Fructus Forsythiae)
Jin Yin Hua (Flos Lonicerae)
Gan Cao (Radix Glycyrrhizae)
Jie Geng (Radix Platycodi)
Niu Bang Zi (Fructus Arctii)
Jing Jie (Herba Schizonepetae)
Chan Tui (Periostracum Cicadae)

Li Ma Tou Fa Tang (Support the Measles, Out-thrusting & Emitting Decoction)

Ge Gen (Radix Puerariae)
Bai Mao Gen (Rhizoma Imperatae)
Dan Zhu Ye (Herba Lophateri)
Zi Cao (Radix Lithospermi/Arnebiae)
Sheng Ma (Rhizoma Cimicifugae)
Bo He (Herba Menthae Haplocalycis)
Gan Cao (Radix Glycyrrhizae)

Xi Liang Tou Biao Tang (Acridly & Coolly Out-thrust the Exterior Decoction)

Lu Gen (Rhizoma Phragmitis)

Bai Mao Gen (Rhizoma Imperatae)
Bo He (Herba Menthae Haplocalycis)
Jing Jie Sui (Herba Schizonepetae)
Niu Bang Zi (Fructus Arctii)
Xing Ren (Semen Armeniacae)
Lian Qiao (Fructus Forsythiae)

Jing Jie Tou Zhen Tang (Schizonepeta Out-thrust the Rash Decoction)
Jing Jie (Herba Schizonepetae)
Niu Bang Zi (Fructus Arctii)
Chan Tui (Periostracum Cicadae)
Lian Qiao (Fructus Forsythiae)
Sang Ye (Folium Mori)
Ban Lan Gen (Radix Isatidis/Baphicacanthi)
Bo He (Herba Menthae Haplocalycis)

2. Eruptive stage

Main symptoms: A high fever which does not abate, thirst with a desire to drink, severe cough, a continued dull affect, gummed-up eyes, irritability and restlessness, possible delirium during high fever, possible twitching or convulsions due to high fever, a raised, red maculopapular rash starting first behind the ears and then spreading to the neck, face, head, chest, back, and limbs. The rash is bright red in color and may exude a watery fluid. Later the rash spreads and joins into larger areas and its color becomes darker. The tongue is red with yellow fur, and the pulse is surging and rapid.

Treatment principles: Clear heat, resolve toxins, and out-thrust the rash

Guiding formulas:
Qing Jie Tou Biao Tang (Clear, Resolve & Out-thrust the Exterior Decoction)
Xi He Liu (Ramulus Et Folium Tamaricis)
Chan Tui (Periostracum Cicadae)
Ge Gen (Radix Puerariae)
Sheng Ma (Rhizoma Cimicifugae)
Lian Qiao (Fructus Forsythiae)
Jin Yin Hua (Flos Lonicerae)
Zi Cao (Radix Lithospermi/Arnebiae)
Sang Ye (Folium Mori)
Gan Cao (Radix Glycyrrhizae)
Fu Ping (Herba Lemnae/Spirodelae)
Jing Jie (Herba Schizonepetae)

Dang Gui Hong Hua Yin (Dang Gui & Carthamus Beverage)
Dang Gui (Radix Angelicae Sinensis)

Hong Hua (Flos Carthami)
Ge Gen (Radix Puerariae)
Gan Cao (Radix Glycyrrhizae)
Huang Lian (Rhizoma Coptidis)
Zi Cao (Radix Lithospermi/Arnebiae)
Lian Qiao (Fructus Forsythiae)
Da Qing Ye (Folium Daqingye)
Niu Bang Zi (Fructus Arctii)

If the mouth is dry and the throat is sore with dry, chapped lips due to internal heat steaming and burning the lungs and stomach, add *Xuan Shen* (Radix Scrophulariae), *Huang Qin* (Radix Scutellariae), *Tian Hua Fen* (Radix Trichosanthis), *Ju Hua* (Flos Chrysanthemi), *Shan Dou Gen* (Radix Sophorae Subprostratae), and *She Gan* (Rhizoma Belamcandae).

Qing Re Jie Du Tang (Clear Heat & Resolve Toxins Decoction)
Jin Yin Hua (Flos Lonicerae)
Lian Qiao (Fructus Forsythiae)
Niu Bang Zi (Fructus Arctii)
Chan Tui (Periostracum Cicadae)
Sang Ye (Folium Mori)

If there is fever, cough, tearing eyes, heart vexation, delirious speech, and the rash does not erupt easily, use **Jia Jian Sheng Jiang San (Added Flavors Upbearing & Downbearing Powder):**
Chan Tui (Periostracum Cicadae)
Lu Gen (Rhizoma Phragmitis)
Gou Teng (Ramulus Uncariae Cum Uncis)
Jiang Can (Bombyx Batryticatus)
Jiang Huang (Rhizoma Curcumae Longae)

3. Resolution stage

Main symptoms: After the rash has covered the entire body, it begins to fade in the same order of progression with which it appeared. This may be accompanied by desquamation and a brown discoloration of the skin, receding of the fever, improvement of the spirit and appetite, a dry cough with scanty phlegm, yellowish urine, a red tongue with diminished fur, and a fine, rapid pulse.

Treatment principles: Support the righteous and nourish yin, clear any remaining heat

Guiding formulas:
Sha Shen Mai Dong Tang (Glehnia & Ophiopogon Decoction)
Bei Sha Shen (Radix Glehniae)
Mai Men Dong (Tuber Ophiopogonis)

Sang Ye (Folium Mori)
Tian Hua Fen (Radix Trichosanthis)
Yu Zhu (Rhizoma Polygonati Odorati)
Bai Bian Dou (Semen Dolichoris)
Gan Cao (Radix Glycyrrhizae)

Sha Shen Mai Dong Tang Jia Jian (Glehnia & Ophiopogon Decoction with Additions & Subtractions)
Bei Sha Shen (Radix Glehniae)
Mai Men Dong (Tuber Ophiopogonis)
Sang Ye (Folium Mori)
Tian Hua Fen (Radix Trichosanthis)
Qing Hao (Herba Artemisiae Annuae)
Bai Wei (Radix Cynanchi Atrati)
Bai Bian Dou (Semen Dolichoris)
Lu Gen (Rhizoma Phragmitis)

If the appetite is devitalized, add *Ji Nei Jin* (Endothelium Corneum Gigeriae Galli), *Gu Ya* (Fructus Germinatus Oryzae), and *Mai Ya* (Fructus Germinatus Hordei).

Sha Shen Mai Dong Tang Jia Jian (Glehnia & Ophiopogon Decoction with Additions & Subtractions)
Bei Sha Shen (Radix Glehniae)
Mai Men Dong (Tuber Ophiopogonis)
Yu Zhu (Rhizoma Polygonati Odorati)
Tian Hua Fen (Radix Trichosanthis)
Shan Zha (Fructus Crataegi)
Bai Bian Dou (Semen Dolichoris)
Gan Cao (Radix Glycyrrhizae)

If there is fatigue due to qi vacuity, add *Dang Shen* (Radix Codonopsitis). If fever does not recede, add *Di Gu Pi* (Cortex Lycii) and *Yin Chai Hu* (Radix Stellariae). If there is constipation due to fluid dryness, add *Gua Lou Ren* (Semen Trichosanthis) and *Huo Ma Ren* (Semen Cannabis).

Yang Yin Jie Du Tang (Nourish Yin & Resolve Toxins Decoction)
Xuan Shen (Radix Scrophulariae)
Shi Hu (Herba Dendrobii)
Mai Men Dong (Tuber Ophiopogonis)
Zi Hua Di Ding (Herba Violae)
Jin Yin Hua (Flos Lonicerae)
Lian Qiao (Fructus Forsythiae)
Zhi Zi (Fructus Gardeniae)
Dan Zhu Ye (Herba Lophateri)

Abnormal progression

1. Internal heat blazing & exuberant, measles blocked & not out-thrust

Main symptoms: Heat is extreme, *i.e.*, there is high fever, for 5-6 days. The measles rash wants to be discharged but cannot be. There is diminished, reddish urine and a red tongue.

Treatment principles: Drain fire and clear the lungs

Guiding formula:
Dao Chi San Jia Wei (Abduct the Red Powder with Added Flavors)
Sheng Di (uncooked Radix Rehmanniae)
Mu Tong (Caulis Akebiae)
Dan Zhu Ye (Herba Lophateri)
Gan Cao (Radix Glycyrrhizae)
Shi Gao (Gypsum Fibrosum)
Lian Qiao (Fructus Forsythiae)
Bo He (Herba Menthae Haplocalycis)
Xuan Shen (Radix Scrophulariae)

2. Measles toxins blocking the lungs (a.k.a. extreme heat suffering cold, measles toxins falling into the lungs)

Main symptoms: The rash is a dark, purplish color or is indistinct and not fully out-thrust. There is high fever which does not recede, severe cough, panting or asthma, flaring of the nasal wings when breathing, the sound of phlegm in the throat, heart vexation, oral thirst, lack of warmth in the four limbs, a bluish grey facial complexion and cyanotic lips, diminished, reddish urination, a scarlet red tongue with yellow, coarse fur, a bluish green, purplish finger vein, and a slippery, rapid pulse.

Note: This pattern describes measles complicated by pneumonia.

Treatment principles: Diffuse the lungs and transform phlegm, clear heat and resolve toxins

Guiding formulas:
Ma Xing Shi Gan Tang Jia Wei (Ephedra, Armeniaca, Gypsum & Licorice Decoction with Added Flavors)
Ma Huang (Herba Ephedrae)
Xing Ren (Semen Armeniacae)
Shi Gao (Gypsum Fibrosum)
Gan Cao (Radix Glycyrrhizae)
Yu Xing Cao (Herba Hedyotis Diffusae)
Huang Qin (Radix Scutellariae)

Ma Xing Shi Gan Tang Jia Wei (Ephedra, Armeniaca, Gypsum & Licorice Decoction with Added Flavors)

Ma Huang (Herba Ephedrae)
Xing Ren (Semen Armeniacae)
Shi Gao (Gypsum Fibrosum)
Gan Cao (Radix Glycyrrhizae)
Jin Yin Hua (Flos Lonicerae)
Lian Qiao (Fructus Forsythiae)
Zi Cao (Radix Lithospermi/Arnebiae)
Ban Lan Gen (Radix Isatidis/Baphicacanthi)
Ting Li Zi (Semen Lepidii/Descurainiae)
Qian Hu (Radix Peucedani)
Sang Bai Pi (Cortex Mori)

If there is coughing and panting with profuse phlegm, add *Tian Zhu Huang* (Concretio Silicea Bambusae) and *Zhu Li* (Succus Bambusae) or *Jie Geng* (Radix Platycodi) and *Bai Jie Zi* (Semen Sinapis). If there are cyanotic lips and chilled limbs, add *Ren Shen* (Radix Ginseng).

Ma Xing Shi Gan Tang Jia Wei (Ephedra, Armeniaca, Gypsum & Licorice Decoction with Added Flavors)

Ma Huang (Herba Ephedrae)
Xing Ren (Semen Armeniacae)
Shi Gao (Gypsum Fibrosum)
Gan Cao (Radix Glycyrrhizae)
Huang Qin (Radix Scutellariae)
Lian Qiao (Fructus Forsythiae)
Jie Geng (Radix Platycodi)
Qian Hu (Radix Peucedani)
Fu Ping (Herba Lemnae/Spirodelae)
Xi He Liu (Ramulus Et Folium Tamaricis)

3. Measles toxins entering the constructive, internally falling into the heart wrapper

Main symptoms: Densely distributed skin rashes which coalesce and which are dark purple in color, high fever, the body is burning hot, sweating but no abating of the fever, vexatious thirst, restlessness, delirious speech, spirit clouding, if severe, convulsions, spasms, and tremors, a dry, scarlet red tongue with thorns and/or coarse, yellow fur, a wiry, rapid or slippery, rapid pulse

Note: This pattern describes infantile convulsions due to high fever associated with measles.

Treatment principles: Clear the constructive and cool the blood, resolve toxins, extinguish wind, and open the portals

Guiding formulas:
Qing Ying Tang Jia Jian (Clear the Constructive Decoction with Additions & Subtractions)
   Shui Niu Jiao (Cornu Bubali)
   Sheng Di (uncooked Radix Rehmanniae)
   Xuan Shen (Radix Scrophulariae)
   Dan Pi (Cortex Moutan)
   Zhi Mu (Rhizoma Anemarrhenae)
   Shi Gao (Gypsum Fibrosum)
   Zi Cao (Radix Lithospermi/Arnebiae)
   Chi Shao (Radix Paeoniae Rubrae)
   Jin Yin Hua (Flos Lonicerae)
   Lian Qiao (Fructus Forsythiae)
   Dan Zhu Ye (Herba Lophateri)

Plus **An Gong Niu Huang Wan (Quiet the Palace Bezoar Pills, a Chinese ready-made medicine)**

Qing Ying Bai Du Yin (Clear the Constructive & Vanquish Toxins Beverage)
   Shui Niu Jiao (Cornu Bubali)
   Da Qing Ye (Folium Daqingye)
   Xuan Shen (Radix Scrophulariae)
   blast-fried *Chuan Shan Jia* (Squama Manitis)
   Sheng Ma (Rhizoma Cimicifugae)
   Dang Gui Wei (rootlets of Radix Angelicae Sinensis)
   Bai Shao (Radix Paeoniae Albae)
   Chai Hu (Radix Bupleuri)

Ling Jiao Gou Teng Tang Jia Jian (Antelope Horn & Uncaria Decoction with Additions & Subtractions)
   Shan Yang Jiao (Cornu Caprae)
   Gou Teng (Ramulus Uncariae Cum Uncis)
   Ju Hua (Flos Chrysanthemi)
   Sheng Di (uncooked Radix Rehmanniae)
   Bai Shao (Radix Paeoniae Albae)
   Dan Zhu Ye (Herba Lophateri)
   Dan Pi (Cortex Moutan)
   Fu Shen (Sclerotium Pararadicis Poriae)
   Gan Cao (Radix Glycyrrhizae)

Ling Jiao Gou Teng Tang Jia Jian (Antelope Horn & Uncaria Decoction with Additions & Subtractions)
   Shan Yang Jiao (Cornu Caprae)
   Gou Teng (Ramulus Uncariae Cum Uncis)

Sheng Di (uncooked Radix Rehmanniae)
Bai Shao (Radix Paeoniae Albae)
Dan Pi (Cortex Moutan)
Gan Cao (Radix Glycyrrhizae)
Yu Jin (Tuber Curcumae)
Shi Chang Pu (Rhizoma Acori Tatarinowii)
Chuan Bei Mu (Bulbus Fritillariae Cirrhosae)

With either of the two above formulas, if there is high fever and loss of consciousness, add **An Gong Niu Huang Wan (Quiet the Palace Bezoar Pills)**.

4. Toxic evils deep-lying & retained, measles toxins falling inward

Main symptoms: After the rash has been discharged uniformly, there is generalized fever which endures and does not improve. There is also tidal fever, vexatious heat, a dry mouth, and sore throat.

Treatment principles: Harmonize the blood and open the network vessels, resolve toxins and clear heat

Guiding formula:
Unnamed formula
Chai Hu (Radix Bupleuri)
Bai Shao (Radix Paeoniae Albae)
Dang Gui (Radix Angelicae Sinensis)
Sheng Di (uncooked Radix Rehmanniae)
Ren Shen (Radix Ginseng)
Chuan Xiong (Rhizoma Chuanxiong)
Di Gu Pi (Cortex Lycii)
Zhi Mu (Rhizoma Anemarrhenae)
wine-processed *Huang Qin* (Radix Scutellariae)
Mai Men Dong (Tuber Ophiopogonis)
Dan Zhu Ye (Herba Lophateri)
Sheng Jiang (uncooked Rhizoma Zingiberis)
Da Zao (Fructus Jujubae)

5. Extreme heat damaging yin, measles body producing maculae

Main symptoms: High fever, vexatious thirst, the rash is a dull purple in color and macular and lumpy in form, a dry, scarlet tongue with thorns

Treatment principles: Clear heat and resolve toxins, cool and quicken the blood

Guiding formulas: Xi Jiao Di Huang Tang Jia Jian (Rhinoceros Horn & Rehmannia Decoction with Additions & Subtractions)
Shui Niu Jiao (Cornu Bubali)

Sheng Di (uncooked Radix Rehmanniae)
Bai Shao (Radix Paeoniae Albae)
Dan Pi (Cortex Moutan)
Xi Hong Hua (Stamen Croci)
wine-processed *Huang Lian* (Rhizoma Coptidis)
Da Qing Ye (Folium Daqingye)
Zi Cao (Radix Lithospermi/Arnebiae)

Hua Ban Tang (Transform Macules Decoction) plus Xi Jiao Di Huang Tang (Rhinoceros Horn & Rehmannia Decoction) with additions and subtractions

Shui Niu Jiao (Cornu Bubali)
Shi Gao (Gypsum Fibrosum)
Zhi Mu (Rhizoma Anemarrhenae)
Gan Cao (Radix Glycyrrhizae)
Xuan Shen (Radix Scrophulariae)
Geng Mi (Semen Oryzae)
Sheng Di (uncooked Radix Rehmanniae)
Chi Shao (Radix Paeoniae Rubrae)
Dan Pi (Cortex Moutan)

6. Toxins attacking the throat

Main symptoms: Measles rash appears but the dots are not out-thrust. There is generalized fever, heart vexation, a red, swollen throat, and pain when swallowing. There is a hoarse voice, difficult, asthmatic breathing and wheezing, bluish grey facial complexion, a red tongue with thick, yellow fur, and a rapid, possibly slippery pulse.

Treatment principles: Clear heat and resolve toxins, disinhibit the throat and disperse swelling

Guiding formulas:
Qing Yan Xia Tan Tang (Clear the Throat & Descend Phlegm Decoction)

Xuan Shen (Radix Scrophulariae)
Niu Bang Zi (Fructus Arctii)
Gan Cao (Radix Glycyrrhizae)
Jie Geng (Radix Platycodi)
Jin Yin Hua (Flos Lonicerae)
Chuan Bei Mu (Bulbus Fritillariae Cirrhosae)
Shan Dou Gen (Radix Sophorae Subprostratae)
Gua Lou (Fructus Trichosanthis)

To increase this formula's effect, also administer **Liu Shen Wan (Six Spirits Pills, a Chinese ready-made medicine).**

Qing Yan Xia Tan Tang Jia Jian (Clear the Throat & Descend Phlegm Decoction with Additions & Subtractions)
   Xuan Shen (Radix Scrophulariae)
   Jie Geng (Radix Platycodi)
   Gan Cao (Radix Glycyrrhizae)
   Bo He (Herba Menthae Haplocalycis)
   Niu Bang Zi (Fructus Arctii)
   She Gan (Rhizoma Belamcandae)
   Chuan Bei Mu (Bulbus Fritillariae Cirrhosae)
   Gua Lou Pi (Pericarpium Trichosanthis)
   Ban Lan Gen (Radix Isatidis/Baphicacanthi)
   Zi Cao (Radix Lithospermi/Arnebiae)

Plus *Liu Shen Wan* (Six Spirits Pills)

If coughing leads to vomiting and there is a markedly hoarse voice, add *Da Ping Hai* (Fructus Sterculiae), *Yu Mu Die* (Semen Oroxyli), and *Zhu Ru* (Caulis Bambusae In Taeniis).

She Gan Xiao Du Yin (Belamcanda Disperse Toxins Beverage)
   She Gan (Rhizoma Belamcandae)
   Niu Bang Zi (Fructus Arctii)
   Jie Geng (Radix Platycodi)
   Lian Qiao (Fructus Forsythiae)
   Huang Qin (Radix Scutellariae)
   Chi Shao (Radix Paeoniae Rubrae)
   Ban Lan Gen (Radix Isatidis/Baphicacanthi)
   Chan Tui (Periostracum Cicadae)
   Xuan Shen (Radix Scrophulariae)
   Gan Cao (Radix Glycyrrhizae)

If there is constipation, add *Da Huang* (Radix Et Rhizoma Rhei) and *Mang Xiao* (Natri Sulfas).

Jia Wei Jie Geng Tang (Added Flavors Platycodon Decoction)
   Jie Geng (Radix Platycodi)
   Ren Dong Teng (Caulis Lonicerae)
   Lian Qiao (Fructus Forsythiae)
   Niu Bang Zi (Fructus Arctii)
   Ma Dou Ling (Fructus Aristolochiae)
   Jin Deng Long (Bulbus Shancigu)

7. Heat toxins attacking above, gum ulceration

Main symptoms: Oral *gan*, tongue sores, bleeding gums during any stage of measles

Treatment principles: Clear heat and resolve toxins

Guiding formula:
Unnamed formula
Sheng Di (uncooked Radix Rehmanniae)
Sheng Ma (Rhizoma Cimicifugae)
Shi Gao (Gypsum Fibrosum)
Lian Qiao (Fructus Forsythiae)
Dan Pi (Cortex Moutan)
Dang Gui (Radix Angelicae Sinensis)
Huang Lian (Rhizoma Coptidis)
Shui Niu Jiao (Cornu Bubali)
Gan Cao (Radix Glycyrrhizae)

8. Righteous vacuity, toxins blocked

Main symptoms: The measles spots are few and sparse. They are level or sunken and do not arise intensely. Their color is dull and pale. There is cough, shortness of breath, lack of warmth in the hands and feet, listlessness of the essence spirit, loose stools, a somber white facial complexion with no measles spots, cyanotic lips, a pale tongue with white fur, a pale finger vein, and a fine, weak pulse.

Treatment principles: Support the righteous and support (the expulsion of) toxins

Guiding formulas:
Bu Zhong Yi Qi Tang Jia Jian (Supplement the Center & Boost the Qi Decoction with Additions & Subtractions)
Ren Shen (Radix Ginseng)
mix-fried *Huang Qi* (Radix Astragali)
Bai Zhu (Rhizoma Atractylodis Macrocephalae)
mix-fried *Gan Cao* (Radix Glycyrrhizae)
Fu Ling (Poria)
Dang Gui (Radix Angelicae Sinensis)
Chi Shao (Radix Paeoniae Rubrae)
Sheng Ma (Rhizoma Cimicifugae)
Ge Gen (Radix Puerariae)

If the pulse is faint and weak and there is inversion chilling of the four limbs, add *Fu Zi* (Radix Lateralis Praeparatus Aconiti Carmichaeli), *Gan Jiang* (dry Rhizoma Zingiberis), calcined *Long Gu* (Os Draconis), and *Mu Li* (Concha Ostreae) in order to secure yang and stem counterflow.

Hui Yang Jiu Ji Tang Jia Jian (Return Yang & Stem Emergency Decoction with Additions & Subtractions)
Fu Zi (Radix Lateralis Praeparatus Aconiti Carmichaeli)
Gan Jiang (dry Rhizoma Zingiberis)

Gui Xin (Cortex Cinnamomi)
Dang Shen (Radix Codonopsitis)
Huang Qi (Radix Astragali)
Bai Zhu (Rhizoma Atractylodis Macrocephalae)
Fu Ling (Poria)
Dang Gui (Radix Angelicae Sinensis)
Ban Xia (Rhizoma Pinelliae)
Gan Cao (Radix Glycyrrhizae)
Hong Hua (Flos Carthami)
Chen Pi (Pericarpium Citri Reticulatae)

Post-measles Conditions

1. Post-measles tidal fever

Main symptoms: After the measles rash has dispersed and receded, there is still tidal fever which is not cleared, night sweats, bodily emaciation, cough with little phlegm, diminished and small eating and drinking, stools sometimes dry and sometimes loose, a red tongue with diminished fur, a pale red finger vein, and a fine, rapid pulse

Treatment principles: Nourish yin and clear heat

Guiding formula:
Di Gu Pi Yin Jia Jian (Cortex Lycii Beverage with Additions & Subtractions)
  Di Gu Pi (Cortex Lycii)
  Yin Chai Hu (Radix Stellariae)
  Zhi Mu (Rhizoma Anemarrhenae)
  Bie Jia (Carapax Trionycis)
  Chuan Bei Mu (Bulbus Fritillariae Cirrhosae)
  Bei Sha Shen (Radix Glehniae)
  Mai Men Dong (Tuber Ophiopogonis)
  Shan Yao (Radix Dioscoreae)
  Bai Bian Dou (Semen Dolichoris)

2. Post-measles dysentery

Main symptoms: There is no measles rash but the bodily heat does not abate. The stools are gluey and sticky and there is pus and blood. Each day there are five or six movements. If severe, there can be as many as 10 or more movements per day. There is abdominal pain, tenesmus after movements, no thought for food or drink, listlessness of the essence spirit, thick, yellow fur, and a slippery, rapid pulse.

Treatment principles: Clear heat and resolve toxins, transform dampness and harmonize the center

Guiding formulas:
Bai Tou Weng Tang Jia Jian (Pulsatilla Decoction with Additions & Subtractions)
- Bai Tou Weng (Radix Pulsatillae)
- Huang Lian (Rhizoma Coptidis)
- Huang Bai (Cortex Phellodendri)
- Shan Yao (Radix Dioscoreae)
- Chi Shao (Radix Paeoniae Rubrae)
- Bai Shao (Radix Paeoniae Albae)
- Jin Yin Hua (Flos Lonicerae)
- Mu Xiang (Radix Auklandiae)
- Gan Cao (Radix Glycyrrhizae)

If there is much blood and only a little pus in the stools, add *Di Yu* (Radix Sanguisorbae) and *San Qi* (Radix Notoginseng). If there is more pus and less blood, add *Cang Zhu* (Rhizoma Atractylodis) and *Yi Yi Ren* (Semen Coicis).

Ge Gen Qin Lian Tang Jia Wei (Pueraria, Scutellaria & Coptis Decoction with Added Flavors)
- Ge Gen (Radix Puerariae)
- Huang Qin (Radix Scutellariae)
- Huang Lian (Rhizoma Coptidis)
- Gan Cao (Radix Glycyrrhizae)
- Xi He Liu (Ramulus Et Folium Tamaricis)
- Fu Ping (Herba Lemnae/Spirodelae)
- Chan Yi (Periostracum Cicadae)
- Fang Feng (Radix Saposhnikoviae)

3. Post-measles night blindness

Main symptoms: After the measles rash has receded, both eyes feel dry and rough and at night the child cannot see clearly. The tongue is red with diminished fur, while the pulse is fine and rapid.

Treatment principles: Nourish the liver and brighten the eyes

Guiding formula:
Qi Ju Di Huang Wan Jia Jian (Lycium & Chrysanthemum Rehmannia Pills with Additions & Subtractions)
- Gou Qi Zi (Fructus Lycii)
- Ju Hua (Flos Chrysanthemi)
- Sheng Di (uncooked Radix Rehmanniae)
- Shan Zhu Yu (Fructus Corni)
- Shan Yao (Radix Dioscoreae)
- Dan Pi (Cortex Moutan)

Fu Ling (Poria)
Mu Zei Cao (Herba Equiseti)
Mi Meng Hua (Flos Buddleiae)
Chan Tui (Periostracum Cicadae)

4. Post-measles sand *lai*

Main symptoms: After there are no more lurking measles rashes, the skin itches incessantly and there is the appearance of sand *lai*. Their form is like a scab. There is also heart vexation and restlessness, difficulty going to sleep at night, slightly yellow tongue fur, a pale purplish finger vein, and a floating, slightly rapid pulse.

Treatment principles: Nourish the blood and resolve toxins, dispel wind and stop itching

Guiding formula:
Si Wu Tang (Four Materials Decoction) plus *Jia Wei Xiao Du Yin* (Added Flavors Disperse Toxins Beverage) with additions and subtractions

Sheng Di (uncooked Radix Rehmanniae)
Chi Shao (Radix Paeoniae Rubrae)
Dang Gui (Radix Angelicae Sinensis)
He Shou Qu (Radix Polygoni Multiflori)
Xuan Shen (Radix Scrophulariae)
Fang Feng (Radix Saposhnikoviae)
Niu Bang Zi (Fructus Arctii)
Ci Ji Li (Fructus Tribuli)
Gan Cao (Radix Glycyrrhizae)
Lian Qiao (Fructus Forsythiae)
Bai Wei (Radix Cynanchi Atrati)

5. Post-measles cough

Main symptoms: The measles rash is discharged uniformly, the fever recedes, but cough does not heal. There is profuse phlegm and panting or asthma.

Treatment principles: Transform phlegm and disinhibit the qi (*i.e.*, breathing), level asthma and stop coughing

Guiding formula:
Er Chen Tang (Two Aged [Ingredients] Decoction) plus *Si Wu Tang* (Four Materials Decoction) with additions and subtractions

Chen Pi (Pericarpium Citri Reticulatae)
Ban Xia (Rhizoma Pinelliae)
Fu Ling (Poria)
Dang Gui (Radix Angelicae Sinensis)

Bai Shao (Radix Paeoniae Albae)
Chuan Xiong (Rhizoma Chuanxiong)
Sheng Di (uncooked Radix Rehmanniae)
Zhi Ke (Fructus Aurantii)
Gua Lou Ren (Semen Trichosanthis)
Xing Ren (Semen Armeniacae)
Sang Bai Pi (Cortex Mori)
mix-fried *Gan Cao* (Radix Glycyrrhizae)

Acupuncture & moxibustion

During the pre-eruptive stage, needle *He Gu* (LI 4), *Lie Que* (Lu 7), and *Wai Guan* (TB 5). If there is high fever, add *Da Zhui* (GV 14) and *Qu Chi* (LI 11). During the eruption stage, needle *He Gu* (LI 4), *Qu Chi* (LI 11), and *Da Zhui* (GV 14). If there is heart vexation and restlessness, needle *Lao Gong* (Per 8). If there are convulsions, bleed *Shi Xuan* (M-UE-1-5). During the resolution stage, needle *Zu San Li* (St 36), *San Yin Jiao* (Sp 6), and *Qu Chi* (LI 11). If there is post-measles tidal fever, needle *Tai Xi* (Ki 3) and *Guan Yuan* (CV 4). If there is post-measles dysentery, needle *Tian Shu* (St 25), *Nei Ting* (St 44), and *Qu Chi* (LI 11). For post-measles night blindness, needle *Gan Shu* (Bl 18), *Shen Shu* (Bl 23), and *Guang Ming* (GB 37). And if there are post-measles sand *lai*, needle *Qu Chi* (LI 11), *Xue Huai* (Sp 10), and *Wei Zhong* (Bl 40).

Adjunctive treatments

During the initial stage, one should not use cold baths or cold water sponge baths to try to bring down the fever. Such external application of cold will only close the pores of the skin firmly shut, thus preventing the expulsion of the rash. In order to help the rash express itself quickly and completely, there are several Chinese herbal home remedies. First, one can boil 250-500g of fresh coriander (also called cilantro or Chinese parsley). After allowing this to cool to body temperature, one can wash the upper body with this simple and readily available herbal decoction. Secondly, one can crush five grams of sunflower seeds and make these into tea. Administer this tea two times each day. Third, cook carrots, parsley, and water chestnuts together and give this to the child to eat. Or fourth, one can boil nine grams of cherry seeds in one cup of water and drink the liquid. At the same time, boil 150g of cherry seeds in four cups of water and use the liquid to bathe the body.

Comments

Traditionally, parents would hold "measles parties" so that children would become infected when they were still young. In other words, if a child came down with a case of measles, parents of other children would bring those children to the house of the infected child specifically so that their children would catch the measles too. The idea is that it is better for children to get this disease when they are still young and to get it out of the way, and there is some sense to this practice since this disease is typically worse in older patients.

41. Rubella

We used to call rubella German measles when I was a kid. Rubella is a mild infectious disease marked by mild fever, cough, and a sand-like, light red rash which appears and then fades quickly. According to Western medicine, it is due to a virus. It most commonly affects children under five years of age and most commonly occurs in the winter and spring. In Chinese medicine, rubella is seen as a wind heat invasion of the lungs and defensive level of the qi. If severe, it may also manifest as an evil heat blazing and exuberant pattern.

Treatment based on pattern discrimination:

1. Evils depressed in the lung defensive

Main symptoms: Fever, aversion to wind, cough, runny nose, a rash over the entire body for one to two days which is pale red or bright red in color and is accompanied by an itching sensation, and a floating, moderately rapid pulse

Treatment principles: Course wind and clear heat

Guiding formulas:
Yin Qiao San Jia Jian **(Lonicera & Forsythia Powder with Additions & Subtractions)**
    Jin Yin Hua (Flos Lonicerae)
    Niu Bang Zi (Fructus Arctii)
    Lian Qiao (Fructus Forsythiae)
    Ge Gen (Radix Puerariae)
    Jing Jie Sui (Herba Schizonepetae)
    Chan Tui (Periostracum Cicadae)
    Bo He (Herba Menthae Haplocalycis)
    Gan Cao (Radix Glycyrrhizae)

Yin Qiao San Jia Jian **(Lonicera & Forsythia Powder with Additions & Subtractions)**
    Jin Yin Hua (Flos Lonicerae)
    Lian Qiao (Fructus Forsythiae)
    Bo He (Herba Menthae Haplocalycis)
    Niu Bang Zi (Fructus Arctii)
    Jing Jie Sui (Herba Schizonepetae)
    Dan Zhu Ye (Herba Lophateri)
    Jie Geng (Radix Platycodi)
    Gan Cao (Radix Glycyrrhizae)
    Sang Ye (Folium Mori)
    Chan Tui (Periostracum Cicadae)

Unnamed formula
    Bo He (Herba Menthae Haplocalycis)

Chan Tui (Periostracum Cicadae)
Qian Hu (Radix Peucedani)
Gua Lou Ke (Fructus Trichosanthis)
Niu Bang Zi (Fructus Arctii)
Dan Dou Chi (Semen Praeparatus Sojae)
Lian Qiao (Fructus Forsythiae)
Da Qing Ye (Folium Daqingye)

If there is cough and rapid dyspneic breathing, lung heat is severe. In that case, add *Huang Qin* (Radix Scutellariae) and *Zhi Mu* (Rhizoma Anemarrhenae). If the tongue fur is dry and yellow with oral thirst and a desire to drink, stomach heat is severe. In that case, add *Shi Gao* (Gypsum Fibrosum) and *Tian Hua Fen* (Radix Trichosanthis). If the lips and tongue are dry and parched, fluids and humors are debilitated. In that case, add *Xuan Shen* (Radix Scrophulariae) and *Mai Men Dong* (Tuber Ophiopogonis). If the throat is swollen and red, add *Ma Bo* (Lasiosphaera) and *She Gan* (Rhizoma Belamcandae). If cough is severe, add *Jie Geng* (Radix Platycodi) and *Mai Men Dong* (Tuber Ophiopogonis). If the rash is relatively red with dark red lips, this is blood division heat. In that case, add *Chi Shao* (Radix Paeoniae Rubrae) and *Dan Pi* (Cortex Moutan). If there is no desire to eat or drink with chest and diaphragmatic fullness and oppression, add *Shan Zha* (Fructus Crataegi), *Shen Qu* (Massa Medica Fermentata), and *Hou Po* (Cortex Magnoliae).

Jia Wei Xiao Du Yin (Added Flavors Disperse Toxins Beverage)

Jing Jie Sui (Herba Schizonepetae)
Fang Feng (Radix Saposhnikoviae)
Chan Tui (Periostracum Cicadae)
Xia Ku Cao (Spica Prunellae)
Niu Bang Zi (Fructus Arctii)
Jin Yin Hua (Flos Lonicerae)
Lian Qiao (Fructus Forsythiae)
Chi Shao (Radix Paeoniae Rubrae)
Bo He (Herba Menthae Haplocalycis)
Gan Cao (Radix Glycyrrhizae)

If there is food stagnation, add *Shen Qu* (Massa Medica Fermentata), *Shan Zha* (Fructus Crataegi), and *Mai Ya* (Fructus Germinatus Hordei). If the lymph nodes are markedly swollen and are painful when pressed, add more *Xia Ku Cao* and add *Mu Li* (Concha Ostreae).

Yin Hua Zi Cao Tang (Lonicera & Lithospermum Decoction)

Jin Yin Hua (Flos Lonicerae)
Zi Cao (Radix Lithospermi/Arnebiae)
Xuan Shen (Radix Scrophulariae)
Chan Tui (Periostracum Cicadae)
Bo He (Herba Menthae Haplocalycis)
Shi Gao (Gypsum Fibrosum)

2. Evil heat blazing & exuberant (a.k.a. blood heat or qi & constructive division pattern)

Main symptoms: High fever, oral thirst, vexation and agitation, restlessness, dry lips, red face, short, reddish urination, fresh red or dull purplish colored rash, incessant itching, constipation, no thought for food or drink, a red tongue with thick, yellow fur, a purple finger vein in the qi bar, a slippery rapid pulse

Treatment principles: Cool the blood and resolve toxins, clear heat and out-thrust evils

Guiding formulas:
Qiao He Tang (Forsythia & Mint Decoction)
Lian Qiao (Fructus Forsythiae)
Bo He (Herba Menthae Haplocalycis)
Jin Yin Hua (Flos Lonicerae)
Niu Bang Zi (Fructus Arctii)
Chi Shao (Radix Paeoniae Rubrae)
Zi Hua Di Ding (Herba Violae)
Zi Cao (Radix Lithospermi/Arnebiae)
Gan Cao (Radix Glycyrrhizae)
Zhi Zi (Fructus Gardeniae)
Huang Lian (Rhizoma Coptidis)

Tou Zhen Liang Jie Tang Jia Jian (Out-thrust the Rash, Cooling & Resolving Decoction with Additions & Subtractions)
Jin Yin Hua (Flos Lonicerae)
Sang Ye (Folium Mori)
Chi Shao (Radix Paeoniae Rubrae)
Dan Pi (Cortex Moutan)
Zi Cao (Radix Lithospermi/Arnebiae)
Dan Zhu Ye (Herba Lophateri)
Lian Qiao (Fructus Forsythiae)
Zi Hua Di Ding (Herba Violae)
Bo He (Herba Menthae Haplocalycis)
Ye Ju Hua (Flos Chrysanthemi Indici)
Chan Tui (Periostracum Cicadae)
Niu Bang Zi (Fructus Arctii)
Gan Cao (Radix Glycyrrhizae)

If there is severe thirst, add *Tian Hua Fen* (Radix Trichosanthis) and *Lu Gen* (Rhizoma Phragmitis). If there is constipation, add *Da Huang* (Radix Et Rhizoma Rhei) and *Gua Lou* (Fructus Trichosanthis).

Tou Zhen Liang Jie Tang Jia Jian (Out-thrust the Rash, Cooling & Resolving Decoction with Additions & Subtractions)
Sheng Di (uncooked Radix Rehmanniae)

Chi Shao (Radix Paeoniae Rubrae)
Dan Pi (Cortex Moutan)
Zi Cao (Radix Lithospermi/Arnebiae)
Jin Yin Hua (Flos Lonicerae)
Lian Qiao (Fructus Forsythiae)
Zi Hua Di Ding (Herba Violae)
Sang Ye (Folium Mori)
Bo He (Herba Menthae Haplocalycis)
Niu Bang Zi (Fructus Arctii)
Chan Yi (Periostracum Cicadae)

If there is constipation, add *Zhi Shi* (Fructus Immaturus Aurantii) and uncooked *Da Huang* (Radix Et Rhizoma Rhei).

Zhi Feng Zhen Fang (Treat Wind Rash Formula)
Sheng Di (uncooked Radix Rehmanniae)
Gu Sui Bu (Radix Drynariae)
Ci Ji Li (Fructus Tribuli)
Qiang Huo (Radix Et Rhizoma Notopterygii)
Chan Tui (Periostracum Cicadae)
Huo Ma Ren (Semen Cannabis)
Di Gu Pi (Cortex Lycii)
Dan Pi (Cortex Moutan)
Feng Fang (Nidus Vespae)
He Ye (Folium Nelumbinis)
Fu Zi Di (Fructus Kochiae)

Acupuncture & moxibustion

For wind heat, needle *He Gu* (LI 4), *Chi Ze* (Lu 5), *Feng Men* (Bl 12), and *Fei Shu* (Bl 13). If there is high fever, add *Qu Chi* (LI 11) and *Da Zhui* (GV 14). For blood heat, needle *Xue Hai* (Sp 10) and bleed *Shi Xuan* (M-UE-1-5) and *Wei Zhong* (Bl 40).

Adjunctive treatments

If there is relatively severe itching of the skin, decoct 30 grams each of *Di Fu Zi* (Fructus Kochiae) and *Ku Shen* (Radix Sophorae Flavescentis) and 15 grams each of *Feng Fang* (Nidus Vespae) and *Jing Jie* (Herba Schizonepetae), Remove the dregs and use the resulting liquid to fumigate and wash the affected area two times per day. For very severe itching, decoct in water 24 grams each of *Cang Er Zi* (Fructus Xanthii) and *Ku Shen* (Radix Sophorae Flavescentis), six grams of *Chuan Jiao* (Fructus Zanthoxyli), and *Zi Cao* (Radix Lithospermi/Arnebiae). Remove the dregs and use this several times each day to fumigate and wash the affected area. Because this is a hot condition, hot, acrid, peppery foods and greasy, fried, fatty foods should not be eaten.

Comments

Usually rubella is a mild disease and recovery is rapid and uncomplicated. It is better for a child to catch this disease when still young. If a woman catches this disease during the early stage of pregnancy, it can cause birth defects. Therefore, especially if one's child is a girl, if one does not intend to immunize against this disease, then a German measles party is a good idea.

42. Chicken Pox

Chicken pox is also known as varicella. It too is an acute, epidemic, viral infection which is very common in young children. Children under 15 years of age are the most susceptible and it mostly occurs in the winter and spring. It is a highly communicable disease and its symptoms are usually mild with a favorable and complete recovery. The Chinese name for this disease is *shui dou* or water pox since it is characterized by the eruption of watery blisters all over the body. Like rubella, Chinese medicine divides most cases of chicken pox into two basic patterns, a mild and a more severe pattern.

Treatment based on pattern discrimination:

1. Mild condition (a.k.a. wind heat mixed with dampness)

Main symptoms: Fever, headache, nasal congestion, runny nose, cough, and a moist, red rash made up of water blisters filled with a clear fluid. These blisters appear first on the scalp, face, and torso. Urination and defecation are normal, the tongue has thin, white fur, and the pulse is floating and rapid.

Treatment principles: Course wind, clear heat, and percolate dampness

Guiding formulas: *Yin Qiao San Jia Jian* (Lonicera & Forsythia Powder with Additions & Subtractions)
  Jin Yin Hua (Flos Lonicerae)
  Lian Qiao (Fructus Forsythiae)
  Dan Zhu Ye (Herba Lophateri)
  Bo He (Herba Menthae Haplocalycis)
  Niu Bang Zi (Fructus Arctii)
  Jie Geng (Radix Platycodi)
  Gan Cao (Radix Glycyrrhizae)
  Hua Shi (Talcum)

Yin Qiao San Jia Jian (Lonicera & Forsythia Powder with Additions & Subtractions)
  Jin Yin Hua (Flos Lonicerae)
  Lian Qiao (Fructus Forsythiae)

Niu Bang Zi (Fructus Arctii)
Bo He (Herba Menthae Haplocalycis)
Fang Feng (Radix Saposhnikoviae)
Hua Shi (Talcum)
Mu Tong (Caulis Akebiae)
Gan Cao (Radix Glycyrrhizae)

Yin Qiao San Jia Jian (Lonicera & Forsythia Powder with Additions & Subtractions)

Jin Yin Hua (Flos Lonicerae)
Lian Qiao (Fructus Forsythiae)
Ban Lan Gen (Radix Isatidis/Baphicacanthi)
Dan Zhu Ye (Herba Lophateri)
Chan Tui (Periostracum Cicadae)
Jing Jie Sui (Herba Schizonepetae)
Bo He (Herba Menthae Haplocalycis)
Jie Geng (Radix Platycodi)
Hua Shi (Talcum)
Fu Ling (Poria)

If there is high fever, flushed cheeks, and yellow tongue fur, add *Shi Gao* (Gypsum Fibrosum) and *Zhi Mu* (Rhizoma Anemarrhenae). If there is itching, add *Jiang Can* (Bombyx Batryticatus) and *Ci Ji Li* (Fructus Tribuli).

Yin Qiao San Jia Jian (Lonicera & Forsythia Powder with Additions & Subtractions)

Jin Yin Hua (Flos Lonicerae)
Lian Qiao (Fructus Forsythiae)
Jie Geng (Radix Platycodi)
Bo He (Herba Menthae Haplocalycis)
Niu Bang Zi (Fructus Arctii)
Dan Zhu Ye (Herba Lophateri)
Jing Jie (Herba Schizonepetae)
Gan Cao (Radix Glycyrrhizae)
Zi Hua Di Ding (Herba Violae)
Chi Shao (Radix Paeoniae Rubrae)
Mu Tong (Caulis Akebiae)

Yin Qiao Er Ding Tang (Lonicera & Forsythia Two Dings Decoction)

Jin Yin Hua (Flos Lonicerae)
Lian Qiao (Fructus Forsythiae)
Hua Shi (Talcum)
Gan Cao (Radix Glycyrrhizae)
Che Qian Zi (Semen Plantaginis)
Zi Hua Di Ding (Herba Violae)
Pu Gong Ying (Herba Taraxaci)

If dampness is exuberant as evidenced by densely packed pox with clear fluids and thick, white tongue fur, use **Shui Dou Fang (Water Pox, *i.e.*, Chicken pox, Formula):**

Chai Hu (Radix Bupleuri)
Fu Ling (Poria)
Jie Geng (Radix Platycodi)
Huang Qin (Radix Scutellariae)
uncooked *Gan Cao* (Radix Glycyrrhizae)
Dan Zhu Ye (Herba Lophateri)
Deng Xin Cao (Medulla Junci)

If damp heat is exuberant with itchy pox which are a dull purple in color and drip a turbid fluid when they burst, a red tongue with thick, yellow fur, and a slippery, rapid pulse, use **Yin Shi Tang (Lonicera & Gypsum Decoction):**

Jin Yin Hua (Flos Lonicerae)
Shi Gao (Gypsum Fibrosum)
Xuan Shen (Radix Scrophulariae)
Zi Cao (Radix Lithospermi/Arnebiae)
Ze Xie (Rhizoma Alismatis)
Bo He (Herba Menthae Haplocalycis)
Jing Jie Sui (Herba Schizonepetae)

If the water blisters have already come out, use the following **unnamed formula:**

Fang Feng (Radix Saposhnikoviae)
Chai Hu (Radix Bupleuri)
Jing Jie Sui (Herba Schizonepetae)
Zhi Zi (Fructus Gardeniae)
Huang Qin (Radix Scutellariae)
Lian Qiao (Fructus Forsythiae)
Chan Tui (Periostracum Cicadae)
Niu Bang Zi (Fructus Arctii)
Hua Shi (Talcum)
Che Qian Zi (Semen Plantaginis)
Chi Shao (Radix Paeoniae Rubrae)
Mu Tong (Caulis Akebiae)
Dang Gui Wei (rootlets of Radix Angelicae Sinensis)
Gan Cao (Radix Glycyrrhizae)

2. Severe condition (a.k.a. severe heat toxin condition or internal heat blazing & exuberant)

Main symptoms: High fever, vexation and agitation, dry mouth, red lips, red face, short, reddish urination, densely packed pox which are dull purple in color filled with turbid fluid, possible pox on the oral mucosa, small ulcerations when the pox rupture, thick, dry, yellow tongue fur, a rapid, surging, large pulse. If the pox are large in size and the skin surrounding them is markedly red, this is called water red pox and is due to heat toxins being relatively exuberant.

Treatment principles: Clear heat and cool the blood, resolve toxins and disinhibit dampness

Guiding formulas:
To the second ***Yin Qiao San Jia Jian* (Lonicera & Forsythia Powder with Additions & Subtractions)** above, add *Ban Lan Gen* (Radix Isatidis/Baphicacanthis), *Pu Gong Ying* (Herba Taraxaci), *Huang Lian* (Rhizoma Coptidis), and *Zi Hua Di Ding* (Herba Violae). If the water blisters are especially large, add *Zhu Ling* (Polyporus), *Fu Ling* (Poria), and *Yi Yi Ren* (Semen Coicis). If itching is severe, add *Jiang Can* (Bombyx Batryticatus) and *Chan Tui* (Periostracum Cicadae). If there is constructive division heat with heart vexation and restlessness, add *Sheng Di* (uncooked Radix Rehmanniae) and *Dan Pi* (Cortex Moutan).

Lai Mei Jie Du Tang (Humulus Resolve Toxins Decoction)
Lai Mei Hua (Flos Humuli)
Jin Yin Hua (Flos Lonicerae)
Lian Qiao (Fructus Forsythiae)
Ju Hua (Flos Chrysanthemi)
Ban Lan Gen (Radix Isatidis/Baphicacanthi)
Chi Shao (Radix Paeoniae Rubrae)
Gan Cao (Radix Glycyrrhizae)
Huang Lian (Rhizoma Coptidis)
Mu Tong (Caulis Akebiae)
Zi Hua Di Ding (Herba Violae)

If the pox have already burst, use ***Lai Mei Jie Du Tang Jia Jian* (Humulus Resolve Toxins Decoction with Additions & Subtractions):**
Lai Mei Hua (Flos Humuli)
Lian Qiao (Fructus Forsythiae)
Jin Yin Hua (Flos Lonicerae)
Ju Hua (Flos Chrysanthemi)
Niu Bang Zi (Fructus Arctii)
Che Qian Zi (Semen Plantaginis)
Chi Shao (Radix Paeoniae Rubrae)
Fang Feng (Radix Saposhnikoviae)
Gan Cao (Radix Glycyrrhizae)
Huang Lian (Rhizoma Coptidis)
Yi Yi Ren (Semen Coicis)

Jia Wei Xiao Du Yin (Added Flavors Disperse Toxins Beverage) plus *Qing Wei Jie Du Tang* (Clear the Stomach & Resolve Toxins Decoction) with additions and subtractions
Jin Yin Hua (Flos Lonicerae)
Lian Qiao (Fructus Forsythiae)
Zi Cao (Radix Lithospermi/Arnebiae)

Sheng Di (uncooked Radix Rehmanniae)
   Dan Pi (Cortex Moutan)
   Chi Shao (Radix Paeoniae Rubrae)
   Shi Gao (Gypsum Fibrosum)
   Zhi Mu (Rhizoma Anemarrhenae)
   Hua Shi (Talcum)
   Yi Yi Ren (Semen Coicis)
   Fu Ling (Poria)
   Gan Cao (Radix Glycyrrhizae)

Qing Li Jie Du Tang (Clear the Interior & Resolve Toxins Decoction)
   Huang Qin (Radix Scutellariae)
   Huang Lian (Rhizoma Coptidis)
   Shi Gao (Gypsum Fibrosum)
   Sheng Di (uncooked Radix Rehmanniae)
   Dan Pi (Cortex Moutan)

Qing Ying Tang Jia Jian (Clear the Constructive Decoction with Additions & Subtractions)
   Shi Gao (Gypsum Fibrosum)
   Jin Yin Hua (Flos Lonicerae)
   Xuan Shen (Radix Scrophulariae)
   Dan Pi (Cortex Moutan)
   Zhi Mu (Rhizoma Anemarrhenae)
   Zi Cao (Radix Lithospermi/Arnebiae)
   Lian Qiao (Fructus Forsythiae)
   Chi Shao (Radix Paeoniae Rubrae)
   Hua Shi (Talcum)
   Mu Tong (Caulis Akebiae)
   Gan Cao (Radix Glycyrrhizae)

If there is a dry mouth and dry lips due to consumption of fluids and humors, add *Mai Men Dong* (Tuber Ophiopogonis) and *Lu Gen* (Rhizoma Phragmitis). If there are sores on the tongue, constipation, and a red tongue with thick, yellow fur, add *Da Huang* (Radix Et Rhizoma Rhei) and *Zhi Shi* (Fructus Immaturus Aurantii).

Unnamed formula
   Jin Yin Hua (Flos Lonicerae)
   Lian Qiao (Fructus Forsythiae)
   Zi Hua Di Ding (Herba Violae)
   Da Qing Ye (Folium Daqingye)
   Sheng Di (uncooked Radix Rehmanniae)
   Chi Shao (Radix Paeoniae Rubrae)
   Zhi Zi (Fructus Gardeniae)

If there is a red, swollen, sore throat, add *She Gan* (Rhizoma Belamcandae) and *Shan Dou Gen* (Radix Sophorae Subprostratae). If there is vexation and agitation, add *Huang Lian* (Rhizoma Coptidis). If there is constipation, add *Da Huang* (Radix Et Rhizoma Rhei). If there is a dry mouth with a scarlet tongue and diminished fluids, add *Tian Hua Fen* (Radix Trichosanthis), *Mai Men Dong* (Tuber Ophiopogonis), and *Bei Sha Shen* (Radix Glehniae).

Huang Lian Jie Du Tang Jia Wei (Coptis Resolve Toxins Decoction with Added Flavors)

Huang Lian (Rhizoma Coptidis)
Huang Bai (Cortex Phellodendri)
Huang Qin (Radix Scutellariae)
Zhi Zi (Fructus Gardeniae)
Ye Ju Hua (Flos Chrysanthemi Indici)
Jin Yin Hua (Flos Lonicerae)
Pu Gong Ying (Herba Taraxaci)
Zi Hua Di Ding (Herba Violae)
Tian Kui Zi (Semen Semiaquilegiae)

Jie Du Xie Re Yin (Resolve Toxins & Drain Heat Beverage)

Jing Jie (Herba Schizonepetae)
Bo He (Herba Menthae Haplocalycis)
Jie Geng (Radix Platycodi)
Dang Gui Wei (rootlets of Radix Angelicae Sinensis)
Dan Pi (Cortex Moutan)
Huang Qin (Radix Scutellariae)
Huang Lian (Rhizoma Coptidis)
Lian Qiao (Fructus Forsythiae)
Mu Tong (Caulis Akebiae)
Sang Ye (Folium Mori)
Gan Cao (Radix Glycyrrhizae)

Acupuncture & moxibustion

For wind heat with dampness, needle *He Gu* (LI 4), *Chi Ze* (Lu 5), and *Yin Ling Quan* (Sp 9). For internal heat blazing and exuberant, needle *Qu Chi* (LI 11) and *Nei Ting* (St 44) and bleed *Da Zhui* (GV 14). If there is a dull purple color around the base of the pox, bleed *Wei Zhong* (Bl 40).

Adjunctive treatments

First of all, the child should be fed a clear, bland diet and they should most definitely avoid acrid, hot, peppery and greasy, fried, fatty foods. As a beverage, one can decoct and make a tea out of *Jin Yin Hua* (Flos Lonicerae) and *Gan Cao* (Radix Glycyrrhizae); *Ren Dong Teng* (Caulis Lonicerae) and *Gan Cao* (Radix Glycyrrhizae); *Lu Gen* (Rhizoma

Phragmitis) and *Ye Ju Hua* (Flos Chrysanthemi Indici); or mung beans. As an external wash for itching, one can decoct a suitable amount of *Lu Gan Shi* (Smithsonitum) and bathe the affected area several times per day.

Comments

The child's skin should be kept clean and they should be kept from scratching the pustules as much as possible since this can cause scarring and even infection. The child should definitely be kept from playing with other children or going to school, unless the parents of those other children want their children to catch chicken pox and get it over with. Likewise, the child should be isolated from any adults who have not already had chicken pox or been immunized against it. Chinese medicine does treat chicken pox very well, meaning that it reduces the suffering and prevents complications.

43. Scarlatina

We have talked briefly about scarlatina or scarlet fever above under strep throat. Scarlatina is another acute, infectious disease marked by fever, swelling, sore throat, and a diffuse, bright red skin rash all over the body. However, unlike the several preceding diseases which are due to viruses of one sort or another, scarlatina is a bacterial infection. It, like so many other acute, infectious diseases, is most common in the winter and spring, and it most commonly affects children between 2-8 years of age. Scarlatina may develop into rheumatic fever and damage the heart or develop into acute nephritis. However, this is not its most likely course. In most mild cases, the diagnosis is not confirmed until after the rash has disappeared, the fever abated, and the skin begun to peel from the palms of the hands and soles of the feet. Chinese medicine treats scarlatina by dividing its manifestations into three main patterns.

Treatment based on pattern discrimination:

1. Evils assailing & entering the lung defensive (a.k.a. evils in the lungs & stomach)

Main symptoms: Fever which goes from low to high, slight aversion to chill, oral thirst, headache, vomiting, cough, a swollen, sore throat, possible membranous, ulcerative tonsillitis, flushed red skin, an indistinct, bright red rash, a red tongue with thin, white or yellow fur, a blue-green purplish finger vein, a floating, rapid pulse

Treatment principles: Diffuse the lungs and out-thrust the rash by using acrid, cool herbs, clear heat and disinhibit the throat

Guiding formulas:
Yin Qiao Ma Bo She Gan Tang Jia Jian (Lonicera, Forsythia, Lasiosphaera & Belamcanda Decoction with Additions & Subtractions)
Jin Yin Hua (Flos Lonicerae)

Lian Qiao (Fructus Forsythiae)
She Gan (Rhizoma Belamcandae)
Jie Geng (Radix Platycodi)
Da Qing Ye (Folium Daqingye)
Chi Shao (Radix Paeoniae Rubrae)
Bo He (Herba Menthae Haplocalycis)
Chan Tui (Periostracum Cicadae)
Zhu Ru (Caulis Bambusae In Taeniis)
Gan Cao (Radix Glycyrrhizae)

Yin Qiao Ma Bo She Gan Tang Jia Jian (Lonicera, Forsythia, Lasiosphaera & Belamcanda Decoction with Additions & Subtractions)

Jin Yin Hua (Flos Lonicerae)
Lian Qiao (Fructus Forsythiae)
Niu Bang Zi (Fructus Arctii)
Ma Bo (Lasiosphaera/Calvatia)
She Gan (Rhizoma Belamcandae)
Bo He (Herba Menthae Haplocalycis)
Jie Geng (Radix Platycodi)
Zhi Zi (Fructus Gardeniae)
Lu Dou Pi (Testa Glycinis)
Gan Cao (Radix Glycyrrhizae)
Zhu Ru (Caulis Bambusae In Taeniis)

If the tongue fur is yellow and there is a high fever, add *Lu Gen* (Rhizoma Phragmitis) and *Huang Qin* (Radix Scutellariae). If the stools are dry, add *Xuan Shen* (Radix Scrophulariae) and *Mai Men Dong* (Tuber Ophiopogonis). If the throat is very painful, add more Platycodon and *Tian Hua Fen* (Radix Trichosanthis). If there is chest and diaphragmatic glomus and oppression with thick, slimy, white tongue fur, add *Huo Xiang* (Herba Pogostemonis) and *Shen Qu* (Massa Medica Fermentata).

Yin Qiao Ma Bo She Gan Tang Jia Wei (Lonicera, Forsythia, Lasiosphaera & Belamcanda Decoction with Added Flavors)

Jin Yin Hua (Flos Lonicerae)
Lian Qiao (Fructus Forsythiae)
Dan Dou Chi (Semen Praeparatus Sojae)
Niu Bang Zi (Fructus Arctii)
Jing Jie Sui (Herba Schizonepetae)
Jie Geng (Radix Platycodi)
She Gan (Rhizoma Belamcandae)
Ma Bo (Lasiosphaera/Calvatia)
Gan Cao (Radix Glycyrrhizae)
Da Qing Ye (Folium Daqingye)
Ban Lan Gen (Radix Isatidis/Baphicacanthi)

Yin Qiao San Jia Jian (Lonicera & Forsythia Powder with Additions & Subtractions)

Jin Yin Hua (Flos Lonicerae)
Lian Qiao (Fructus Forsythiae)
Niu Bang Zi (Fructus Arctii)
Bo He (Herba Menthae Haplocalycis)
Dan Dou Chi (Semen Praeparatus Sojae)
Gan Cao (Radix Glycyrrhizae)
Jie Geng (Radix Platycodi)
Chan Yi (Periostracum Cicadae)
Ge Gen (Radix Puerariae)

Jie Ji Tou Sha Tang (Resolve the Muscles & Out-thrust Sha Decoction)

Jing Jie Sui (Herba Schizonepetae)
Chan Tui (Periostracum Cicadae)
She Gan (Rhizoma Belamcandae)
Gan Cao (Radix Glycyrrhizae)
Ge Gen (Radix Puerariae)
Niu Bang Zi (Fructus Arctii)
Ma Bo (Lasiosphaera)
Jie Geng (Radix Platycodi)
Qian Hu (Radix Peucedani)
Lian Qiao (Fructus Forsythiae)
Jiang Chan (Bombyx Batryticatus)
Dan Dou Chi (Semen Praeparatus Sojae)
Zhu Ru (Caulis Bambusae In Taeniis)
Fu Ping (Herba Lemnae/Spirodelae)

2. Evil toxins entering the qi & constructive (division)

Main symptoms: High fever which does not resolve, a flushed, red face, oral thirst with a desire to drink, swelling, pain, erosion, and ulceration of the throat, a densely packed, bright red or purple rash, dry stools, diminished, reddish yellow urination, if severe, spirit clouding and delirious speech, a dark red or scarlet red tongue with thorns and deep yellow, coarse tongue fur, a rapid, forceful pulse

> **Note:** Some few Chinese pediatric texts divide this pattern into two: evil toxins entering the qi and constructive and evil toxins falling internally into the constructive and blood. In the latter case, there is spirit clouding and delirious speech.

Treatment principles: Clear the qi and cool the constructive (divisions), drain fire and resolve toxins

Guiding formulas:
Liang Ying Qing Qi Tang Jia Jian (Cool the Constructive & Clear the Qi Decoction with Additions & Subtractions)
   Shui Niu Jiao (Cornu Bubali)
   Sheng Di (uncooked Radix Rehmanniae)
   Dan Pi (Cortex Moutan)
   Lian Qiao (Fructus Forsythiae)
   Shi Gao (Gypsum Fibrosum)
   Zhi Zi (Fructus Gardeniae)
   Huang Lian (Rhizoma Coptidis)
   Gan Cao (Radix Glycyrrhizae)
   Xuan Shen (Radix Scrophulariae)

Qing Wen Bai Du Yin Jia Jian (Clear the Scourge & Vanquish Toxins Beverage with Additions & Subtractions)
   Shui Niu Jiao (Cornu Bubali)
   Sheng Di (uncooked Radix Rehmanniae)
   Jin Yin Hua (Flos Lonicerae)
   Lian Qiao (Fructus Forsythiae)
   Dan Pi (Cortex Moutan)
   Chi Shao (Radix Paeoniae Rubrae)
   Dan Zhu Ye (Herba Lophateri)
   Huang Lian (Rhizoma Coptidis)
   Zi Cao (Radix Lithospermi/Arnebiae)
   Bai Mao Gen (Rhizoma Imperatae)
   Lu Gen (Rhizoma Phragmitis)

If there is high fever, in order to prevent or treat convulsions, add **An Gong Niu Huang Wan** (Quiet the Palace Bezoar Pills, a Chinese ready-made medicine).

Qing Wen Bai Du Yin Jia Jian (Clear the Scourge & Vanquish Toxins Beverage with Additions & Subtractions)
   Shui Niu Jiao (Cornu Bubali)
   Sheng Di (uncooked Radix Rehmanniae)
   Dan Pi (Cortex Moutan)
   Chi Shao (Radix Paeoniae Rubrae)
   Lian Qiao (Fructus Forsythiae)
   Huang Qin (Radix Scutellariae)
   Shi Gao (Gypsum Fibrosum)
   Dan Zhu Ye (Herba Lophateri)
   Zhi Zi (Fructus Gardeniae)
   Xuan Shen (Radix Scrophulariae)
   Lu Gen (Rhizoma Phragmitis)

If the rash is not completely discharged and there is a high fever with no sweating, add

Fu Ping (Herba Lemnae/Spirodelae) and *Chan Yi* (Periostracum Cicadae) and omit Gypsum. If there is ulceration of the throat with coarse, yellow tongue fur and constipation, add *Da Huang* (Radix Et Rhizoma Rhei) and *Mang Xiao* (Natri Sulfas).

Qing Wen Bai Du Yin Jia Jian (Clear the Scourge & Vanquish Toxins Beverage with Additions & Subtractions)

Shui Niu Jiao (Cornu Bubali)
Sheng Di (uncooked Radix Rehmanniae)
Chi Shao (Radix Paeoniae Rubrae)
Dan Pi (Cortex Moutan)
Xuan Shen (Radix Scrophulariae)
Lian Qiao (Fructus Forsythiae)
Shi Hu (Herba Dendrobii)
Lu Gen (Rhizoma Phragmitis)
Bai Mao Gen (Rhizoma Imperatae)
Huang Lian (Rhizoma Coptidis)
Zhi Zi (Fructus Gardeniae)
Bo He (Herba Menthae Haplocalycis)
Gan Cao (Radix Glycyrrhizae)
Shi Gao (Gypsum Fibrosum)

Qing Ying Tang Jia Jian (Clear the Constructive Decoction with Additions & Subtractions)

Shui Niu Jiao (Cornu Bubali)
Sheng Di (uncooked Radix Rehmanniae)
Jin Yin Hua (Flos Lonicerae)
Lian Qiao (Fructus Forsythiae)
Dan Pi (Cortex Moutan)
Chi Shao (Radix Paeoniae Rubrae)
Dan Zhu Ye (Herba Lophateri)
Huang Lian (Rhizoma Coptidis)
Zi Cao (Radix Lithospermi/Arnebiae)
Bai Mao Gen (Rhizoma Imperatae)
Lu Gen (Rhizoma Phragmitis)

Unnamed formula

Shui Niu Jiao (Cornu Bubali)
Sheng Di (uncooked Radix Rehmanniae)
Xuan Shen (Radix Scrophulariae)
Mai Men Dong (Tuber Ophiopogonis)
Dan Shen (Radix Salviae Miltiorrhizae)
Jin Yin Hua (Flos Lonicerae)
Lian Qiao (Fructus Forsythiae)
Dan Zhu Ye (Herba Lophateri)
Huang Lian (Rhizoma Coptidis)

3. Yin vacuity with lingering heat

Main symptoms: If high fever has gone on for some time, this may consume and exhaust the healthy yin fluids of the body. Therefore, towards the tail end or recuperative phase of this disease, there may be a gradual diminishing of high fever or a lingering low-grade fever, gradual dispersion of the skin rash, dry skin with scaling and peeling, diminished sore throat, thirst, dry lips, dry cough, constipation, a red tongue with scanty fluids, and a fine, rapid pulse.

Treatment principles: Nourish yin and engender fluids, clear heat and moisten the throat

Guiding formulas:
Sha Shen Mai Dong Tang Jia Jian (Glehnia & Ophiopogon Decoction with Additions & Subtractions)
  Bei Sha Shen (Radix Glehniae)
  Mai Men Dong (Tuber Ophiopogonis)
  Yu Zhu (Rhizoma Polygonati Odorati)
  Tian Hua Fen (Radix Trichosanthis)
  Shi Hu (Herba Dendrobii)
  Gan Cao (Radix Glycyrrhizae)
  Sang Ye (Folium Mori)

Sha Shen Mai Dong Tang Jia Jian (Glehnia & Ophiopogon Decoction with Additions & Subtractions)
  Bei Sha Shen (Radix Glehniae)
  Mai Men Dong (Tuber Ophiopogonis)
  Tai Zi Shen (Radix Pseudostellariae)
  Tian Hua Fen (Radix Trichosanthis)
  Sheng Di (uncooked Radix Rehmanniae)
  Bai Bian Dou (Semen Dolichoris)
  Bai Shao (Radix Paeoniae Albae)
  Zhi Mu (Rhizoma Anemarrhenae)
  Gan Cao (Radix Glycyrrhizae)

If there are dry stools, add Huo Ma Ren (Semen Cannabis) and Gua Lou Ren (Semen Trichosanthis). If there is a lingering dry cough, add Chuan Bei Mu (Bulbus Fritillariae Cirrhosae) and Xing Ren (Semen Armeniacae).

Yang Yin Qing Fei Tang (Nourish Yin & Clear the Lungs Decoction)
  Sheng Di (uncooked Radix Rehmanniae)
  Xuan Shen (Radix Scrophulariae)
  Mai Men Dong (Tuber Ophiopogonis)
  Chuan Bei Mu (Bulbus Fritillariae Cirrhosae)
  Bai Shao (Radix Paeoniae Albae)
  Dan Pi (Cortex Moutan)

Bo He (Herba Menthae Haplocalycis)
  Gan Cao (Radix Glycyrrhizae)

If there is inability to sleep at night with heart palpitations and restlessness, a red face and lips, a red tongue with diminished fur, a bound or regularly interrupted pulse, and a purplish, stagnant finger vein, use the following **unnamed formula:**
  Bai Shao (Radix Paeoniae Albae)
  mix-fried *Gan Cao* (Radix Glycyrrhizae)
  Sheng Di (uncooked Radix Rehmanniae)
  Mai Men Dong (Tuber Ophiopogonis)
  E Jiao (Gelatinum Corii Asini)
  Bai Zi Ren (Semen Platycladi)
  Wu Wei Zi (Fructus Schisandrae)

If there are swollen lymph nodes in the neck region, use the following **unnamed formula:**
  Xuan Shen (Radix Scrophulariae)
  Zhe Bei Mu (Bulbus Fritillariae Thunbergii)
  Niu Bang Zi (Fructus Arctii)
  Xia Ku Cao (Spica Prunellae)
  Lian Qiao (Fructus Forsythiae)
  Mu Li (Concha Ostreae)

If there is swelling and pain of the joints, use **San Miao San Jia Wei (Three Wonders Powder with Added Flavors):**
  Cang Zhu (Rhizoma Atractylodis Macrocephalae)
  Huang Bai (Cortex Phellodendri)
  Niu Xi (Radix Achyranthis Bidentatae)
  Han Fang Ji (Radix Stephaniae Tetrandrae)
  Qin Jiao (Radix Gentianae Macrophyllae)
  Jiang Huang (Rhizoma Curcumae Longae)
  Hai Tong Pi (Cortex Erythrinae)
  Yi Yi Ren (Semen Coicis)

Acupuncture & moxibustion

Bleed *Jin Jin* (M-HN-20a) and *Yu Ye* (M-HN-20b). Needle or bleed *Da Zhui* (GV 14). Needle *Feng Chi* (GB 20). If there is high fever and convulsions or spirit clouding and delirious speech, bleed *Shi Xuan* (M-UE-1-5). During the resolution phase with yin vacuity signs and symptoms, needle *Qu Chi* (LI 11) and *San Yin Jiao* (Sp 6).

Adjunctive treatments

If a child has been exposed to someone with this disease, in order to prevent contraction of it, one can administer a tea made by decocting *Jin Yin Hua* (Flos Lonicerae), 15g, *Ban Lan Gen*

(Radix Isatidis/Baphicacanthi), 12g, and *Lian Qiao* (Fructus Forsythiae), 12g. Continue giving this for three days. If there is swollen, ulcerated tonsils, spray *Xi Gua Shuang* (Water Melon Frost, a Chinese ready-made medicine) or *Bing Peng San* (Borneol & Borax Powder) into the throat 3-4 times each day. The latter is made by powdering and mixing *Peng Sha* (Borax), 15g, *Mang Xiao* (Natri Sulfas), 15g, *Zhu Sha* (Cinnabar), 1.8g, and *Bing Pian* (Borneol), 1.5g. The patient should not be allowed to eat any acrid, hot, peppery or fatty, greasy, fried foods. During the last or yin vacuity stage, one can eat cooked pears, applesauce, and a little sugar and warm, boiled milk to enrich yin and engender fluids.

Comments

There are three traditional prohibitions when treating scarlatina in TCM:

1) Acrid, warm medicinals to resolve the exterior are forbidden so as not to plunder yin fluids.
2) Bitter, cold medicinals too early in the disease course is also forbidden so as not to suppress the out-thrusting of the rash.
3) Attacking and precipitating medicinals draining heat downward are forbidden so as not to lead the evils deeper into the body.

In terms of complications or adverse developments, there are also three to be careful of:

1) Enduring damage to qi and yin fluids may result in heart palpitations and a bound pulse.
2) If evils are retained, they may attack the joints and sinews causing redness, swelling, and pain of the joints.
3) If evils are retained and invade the triple burner causing impairment to the qi mechanism, generalized edema may result.

Formulas have been given above for the treatment of heart palpitations and arthritis as a complication of scarlatina. Edema should be treated as water swelling according to the pattern of its manifestations.

Two to three weeks after recuperation from a bout of scarlet fever, the child's heart and urine should be examined by a physician to rule out damage to the heart or kidneys. The severity of scarlet fever varies considerably from individual to individual. My own son had scarlet fever which was not treated by antibiotics but only by Chinese herbs. Eventually, all the skin on his palms and soles of his feet peeled. He never had any problems with heart palpitations or other rheumatic complications. In other words, although antibiotics may be considered in the case of scarlatina, they are not mandatory, and Chinese medicine can be used to treat this disease. However, if there is a persistent high fever, vomiting, convulsions, dark red rashes or static spots, or local abscesses, the child should be referred to a Western MD. Otherwise, this condition could turn lethal if not adequately treated in time.

44. Mumps

Mumps are technically referred to as epidemic parotitis which simply means an epidemic inflammation of the parotid glands in the throat. Mumps are a type of viral infection which can attack a person at any age but which are usually far less serious and uncomfortable as a child than as a grown-up. Like many other viral contagions, once one has had mumps, one usually has a lifetime immunity, though it is possible for some few people to develop them a second time. Winter and spring are again the most likely seasons to contract this disease. In Chinese medicine, inflamed, painful swellings are often associated with the concept of toxins. Toxins are usually warm or hot, although not always. Toxins tend to cause very painful, swollen, red, and often times pussy, purulent conditions. Therefore, TCM divides mumps into two main patterns — warm toxins in the exterior and heat toxins in the interior.

Treatment based on pattern discrimination:

1. Warm toxins in the exterior

Main symptoms: Mild fever, mild aversion to chill, swelling and pain of the parotid region on one or both sides of the throat under the jaw, difficulty swallowing, a red, sore throat, a red tongue with thin, white or slightly yellow fur, a floating, bluish green finger vein, a floating, rapid pulse

Treatment principles: Dispel wind and clear heat, scatter nodulation and disperse swelling

Guiding formulas:
Yin Qiao San (Lonicera & Forsythia Powder)
Jin Yin Hua (Flos Lonicerae)
Lian Qiao (Fructus Forsythiae)
Jie Geng (Radix Platycodi)
Bo He (Herba Menthae Haplocalycis)
Dan Dou Chi (Semen Praeparatus Sojae)
Jing Jie Sui (Herba Schizonepetae)
Dan Zhu Ye (Herba Lophateri)
Lu Gen (Rhizoma Phragmitis)
Gan Cao (Radix Glycyrrhizae)

If heat is severe, add *Long Dan Cao* (Radix Gentianae), *Ban Lan Gen* (Radix Isatidis/Baphicacanthi), and *Shi Gao* (Gypsum Fibrosum). If swelling is severe, add *Xia Ku Cao* (Spica Prunellae).

Yin Qiao San Jia Jian (Lonicera & Forsythia Powder with Additions & Subtractions)
Jin Yin Hua (Flos Lonicerae)

Ban Lan Gen (Radix Isatidis/Baphicacanthi)
Jie Geng (Radix Platycodi)
Xia Ku Cao (Spica Prunellae)
Bo He (Herba Menthae Haplocalycis)
Niu Bang Zi (Fructus Arctii)
Gan Cao (Radix Glycyrrhizae)
Lu Gen (Rhizoma Phragmitis)
Ma Bo (Lasiosphaera/Calvatia)

Yin Qiao San Jia Jian (Lonicera & Forsythia Powder with Additions & Subtractions)
Jin Yin Hua (Flos Lonicerae)
Lian Qiao (Fructus Forsythiae)
Jie Geng (Radix Platycodi)
Niu Bang Zi (Fructus Arctii)
Ban Lan Gen (Radix Isatidis/Baphicacanthi)
Xia Ku Cao (Spica Prunellae)
Pu Gong Ying (Herba Taraxaci)
Bo He (Herba Menthae Haplocalycis)
Gan Cao (Radix Glycyrrhizae)

Yin Qiao San Jia Jian (Lonicera & Forsythia Powder with Additions & Subtractions)
Jin Yin Hua (Flos Lonicerae)
Lian Qiao (Fructus Forsythiae)
Bo He (Herba Menthae Haplocalycis)
Niu Bang Zi (Fructus Arctii)
Ban Lan Gen (Radix Isatidis/Baphicacanthi)
Xia Ku Cao (Spica Prunellae)
Jiang Can (Bombyx Batryticatus)

Unnamed formula
Jing Jie Sui (Herba Schizonepetae)
Fang Feng (Radix Saposhnikoviae)
Jie Geng (Radix Platycodi)
Gan Cao (Radix Glycyrrhizae)
Fu Ling (Sclerotium Poriae Coco)
Zhi Ke (Fructus Aurantii)
Qian Hu (Radix Peucedani)
Chai Hu (Radix Bupleuri)
Ban Lan Gen (Radix Isatidis/Baphicacanthi)
Zhe Bei Mu (Bulbus Fritillariae Thunbergii)
Xia Ku Cao (Spica Prunellae)
Jiang Can (Bombyx Batryticatus)

If the tongue fur is yellow, add *Huang Qin* (Radix Scutellariae) and *Long Dan Cao* (Radix Gentianae).

2. Heat toxins in the interior

Main symptoms: High fever, vexation and agitation, headache, oral thirst with a desire to drink, devitalized eating and drinking, possible vomiting, swelling and distention of the parotid glands which feel hard to the touch and painful when pressed, red, swollen, sore throat, difficulty swallowing, a red tongue with yellow fur, a slippery, rapid pulse

Treatment principles: Clear heat and resolve toxins, soften the hard and disperse swelling

Guiding formulas:
Pu Ji Xiao Du Yin (Universal Relief Disperse Toxins Beverage)

Huang Lian (Rhizoma Coptidis)
Huang Qin (Radix Scutellariae)
Lian Qiao (Fructus Forsythiae)
Ban Lan Gen (Radix Isatidis/Baphicacanthi)
Niu Bang Zi (Fructus Arctii)
Bo He (Herba Menthae Haplocalycis)
Jiang Can (Bombyx Batryticatus)
Xuan Shen (Radix Scrophulariae)
Ma Bo (Lasiosphaera/Calvatia)
Gan Cao (Radix Glycyrrhizae)
Jie Geng (Radix Platycodi)
Sheng Ma (Rhizoma Cimicifugae)
Chai Hu (Radix Bupleuri)

If the glands are especially swollen, hard, and do not scatter, add *Xia Ku Cao* (Spica Prunellae), *Kun Bu* (Thallus Algae), and *Hai Zao* (Sargassum). If heat toxins are congesting and exuberant and the stools are bound and constipated, add *Da Huang* (Radix Et Rhizoma Rhei) and *Mang Xiao* (Natri Sulfas).

Pu Ji Xiao Du Yin Jia Jian (Universal Relief Disperse Toxins Beverage with Additions & Subtractions)

Huang Qin (Radix Scutellariae)
Lian Qiao (Fructus Forsythiae)
Ban Lan Gen (Radix Isatidis/Baphicacanthi)
Xuan Shen (Radix Scrophulariae)
Ma Bo (Lasiosphaera/Calvatia)
Jiang Can (Bombyx Batryticatus)
Xia Ku Cao (Spica Prunellae)

If the swollen glands are hard to the touch and do not scatter, add *Kun Bu* (Thallus Algae) and *Hai Zao* (Sargassum).

Pu Ji Xiao Du Yin Jia Jian (Universal Relief Disperse Toxins Beverage with Additions & Subtractions)
Huang Qin (Radix Scutellariae)
Lian Qiao (Fructus Forsythiae)
Xuan Shen (Radix Scrophulariae)
Ban Lan Gen (Radix Isatidis/Baphicacanthi)
Jiang Can (Bombyx Batryticatus)
Jie Geng (Radix Platycodi)
Bo He (Herba Menthae Haplocalycis)
Xia Ku Cao (Spica Prunellae)
Pu Gong Ying (Herba Taraxaci)
Qing Dai (Pulvis Indigonis)

If there is a high fever, add uncooked *Shi Gao* (Gypsum Fibrosum), *Da Qing Ye* (Folium Daqingye), and *Zhi Zi* (Fructus Gardeniae). If the glands are swollen and hard, add *Kun Bu* (Thallus Algae) and *Hai Zao* (Sargassum). If the stools are constipated, add uncooked *Da Huang* (Radix Et Rhizoma Rhei) and/or *Mang Xiao* (Natri Sulfas). If the testes are swollen and painful, add *Long Dan Cao* (Radix Gentianae), *Li Zhi He* (Semen Litchi), *Yan Hu Suo* (Rhizoma Corydalis), and *Mu Tong* (Caulis Akebiae). If there is encephalitis, add *Da Qing Ye* (Folium Daqingye), *Zi Hua Di Ding* (Herba Violae), and ginger-processed *Zhu Ru* (Caulis Bambusae In Taeniis).

Unnamed formula
Zi Hua Di Ding (Herba Violae)
Niu Bang Zi (Fructus Arctii)
Zhe Bei Mu (Bulbus Fritillariae Thunbergii)
Dan Pi (Cortex Moutan)
Chi Shao (Radix Paeoniae Rubrae)
Hai Ge Ke (Concha Cyclinae/Meretricis)
Bo He (Herba Menthae Haplocalycis)
Chai Hu (Radix Bupleuri)
Kun Bu (Thallus Algae)
Jin Yin Hua (Flos Lonicerae)
Lian Qiao (Fructus Forsythiae)
Shan Ci Gu (Bulbus Shancigu)
Xia Ku Cao (Spica Prunellae)

If glandular swelling and pain are severe, delete the *Ge Fen* and add *Ban Lan Gen* (Radix Isatidis/Baphicacanthi), *Xuan Shen* (Radix Scrophulariae), uncooked *Mu Li* (Concha Ostreae), and *Qing Dai* (Pulvis Indigonis). If damp phlegm is heavy, add *Ban Xia* (Rhizoma Pinelliae) and *Chen Pi* (Pericarpium Citri Reticulatae).

Qing Jie Tang (Clearing & Resolving Decoction)
Long Dan Cao (Radix Gentianae)

Huang Qin (Radix Scutellariae)
Lian Qiao (Fructus Forsythiae)
Ban Lan Gen (Radix Isatidis/Baphicacanthi)
Pu Gong Ying (Herba Taraxaci)
Zhi Zi (Fructus Gardeniae)
Xia Ku Cao (Spica Prunellae)
Gan Cao (Radix Glycyrrhizae)

Acupuncture & moxibustion

Needle *He Gu* (LI 4), *Yi Feng* (TB 17), *Jia Che* (St 6), and *Tian Rong* (SI 17). If there is fever, add *Qu Chi* (LI 11) and *Da Zhui* (GV 14). If there is testicular swelling and pain, add *San Yin Jiao* (Sp 6) and *Xue Hai* (Sp 10). If there is sore throat, bleed *Shao Shang* (Lu 11) and/or *Shang Yang* (LI 1). In addition, the center of the swollen gland may be needled up to a depth of 2.5 inches, or the swollen gland may be pricked to bleed at the upper, middle, and lower parts of the swelling. If the latter method is used and the child will permit it, cup over these last three bled points to increase treatment efficacy.

Adjunctive treatments

Because both these patterns are heat patterns, the patient should avoid eating anything greasy or fatty or hot and spicy. Chinese folk remedies for mumps include boiling 20 grams of dried lily flowers and drinking this as a soup after adding some salt to taste. As for external applications, there are a number of these in Chinese medicine. One is to crush 10 grams of peeled garlic in 10ml of rice vinegar and then apply this externally to the swollen gland(s). Another is to crush a potato and squeeze out the juice. Mix this juice with vinegar and apply this locally. One can also grind 50-70 aduki beans into a powder. Mix this with warm water and egg white or with honey to make into a paste. Apply this paste over the affected glands and cover with a gauze bandage. Further, one can pound either fresh hibiscus leaves or fresh portulaca into a paste and apply this over the swollen glands. The portulaca (Herba Portulacae, *Ma Chi Xian*) that is used is the common purslane that grows as a weed in gardens and in sidewalk cracks. Or infuse some *Pu Gong Ying* (Herba Taraxaci) and *Ye Ju Hua* (Flos Chrysanthemi Indici) in boiling water. Then mash and mix with vinegar and apply to the affected area. And finally, one can mix three grams of *Mang Xiao* (Natri Sulfas) and six grams of *Qing Dai* (Pulvis Indigonis) with vinegar and spread this paste over the affected area.

To reduce the pain and swelling of swollen glands (from mumps and other sources), one can also use alternating hot and cold compresses. Begin by thoroughly wetting a towel with hot water. Wring out the towel so that it does not drip and wrap this around the child's throat being sure that it covers the swollen glands. Cover this wet towel with a dry one to both keep in the heat and prevent dripping. Be sure that the rest of the child's body is covered by a blanket in order to prevent chilling. Leave this warm compress in place for 15 minutes. Then remove and replace with a towel that has been run under very cold water. Leave this in place for five minutes, covered the same way as the hot compress. Again replace this cold compress with a hot compress and leave in place for 15 minutes. This can be repeated one, two, or three times each day to provide relief from pain and to help speed up the course of recovery.

Comments

Once glands get swollen and hard, they do not go down that quickly. Therefore, parents should not get worried if the glands are still relatively large and hard after all the other symptoms have disappeared. In adults, mumps can involve the testes in men and the breasts in women, but these complications rarely occur in children.

45. Diphtheria

Diphtheria is an acute, bacterial, upper respiratory tract infection. It is characterized by the formation of greyish white membranes over the mucus membranes of the pharynx, larynx, and nose. This is accompanied by fever, sore throat, and cough with noisy inhalation. Although this disease may occur in any season of the year, it is most prevalent in the fall and winter, and children under 10 years of age are most susceptible. Furthermore, the younger the child, the more severe this disease tends to be. Even though this disease is not a common one in the West, because a growing number of parents are choosing not to immunize their children against it, I have chosen to say something about its Chinese treatment in this book. Nonetheless, any child suspected of having diphtheria should be under the care of a Western MD as well as any care by a practitioner of Chinese medicine. Diphtheria is a life-threatening disease.

In Chinese medicine, diphtheria is categorized as a seasonal, pestilential disease due to invasion by a particularly virulent hot pathogenic qi. Because the throat is associated with both the lungs and stomach in Chinese medicine and because infants and young children often have stomach heat due to food depression, heat evils assailing the lungs may easily give rise to mutual exacerbation of stomach heat with this heat harassing the throat above. The treatment of diphtheria in Chinese medicine is based on the discrimination of five basic patterns.

Treatment based on pattern discrimination:

1. Wind heat pestilential toxins

Main symptoms: Mild fever, inflamed, swollen, sore throat, greyish white spot-like membranes covering the back of the throat which are difficult to scrape off, difficulty swallowing, a red-tipped tongue with thin, white fur, a bluish green, purplish finger vein, a floating, rapid pulse

Treatment principles: Dispel wind, clear heat, and resolve toxins

Guiding formulas:
Yin Qiao San Jia Jian (Lonicera & Forsythia Powder with Additions & Subtractions)

Jin Yin Hua (Flos Lonicerae)
Lian Qiao (Fructus Forsythiae)
Bo He (Herba Menthae Haplocalycis)
Niu Bang Zi (Fructus Arctii)
Chan Tui (Periostracum Cicadae)
Gan Cao (Radix Glycyrrhizae)
Zhi Zi (Fructus Gardeniae)
Xuan Shen (Radix Scrophulariae)
Shan Dou Gen (Radix Sophorae Subprostratae)
Lu Gen (Rhizoma Phragmitis)
Tu Niu Xi (Radix Achyranthis Bidentatae)

If swelling and pain of the throat is pronounced, add *Ban Lan Gen* (Radix Isatidis/ Baphicacanthi) and *Jin Guo Lan* (Radix Tinosporae). If the mouth and throat are dry and the tongue is red, add *Sheng Di* (uncooked Radix Rehmanniae) and *Mai Men Dong* (Tuber Ophiopogonis).

Unnamed formula

Sang Ye (Folium Mori)
Dan Zhu Ye (Herba Lophateri)
Pi Pa Ye (Folium Eriobotryae)
Bo He (Herba Menthae Haplocalycis)
Chuan Bei Mu (Bulbus Fritillariae Cirrhosae)
Sheng Di (uncooked Radix Rehmnniae)
Mu Tong (Caulis Akebiae)
Jin Yin Hua (Flos Lonicerae)
Gan Cao (Radix Glycyrrhizae)

If the tongue coating is yellow and heat is severe, add *Huang Qin* (Radix Scutellariae). If there are diminished mouth fluids, delete the Akebia and add *Tian Men Dong* (Tuber Asparagi) and *Mai Men Dong* (Tuber Ophiopogonis).

2. Interior heat blazing & exuberant (a.k.a. pestilential toxins attacking the throat)

Main symptoms: High fever with sweating which does not abate the fever, a red, swollen, painful throat, greyish, white or greenish membranes over the back of the throat, heart vexation, rapid dyspneic breathing, oral thirst, bad breath, short, diminished urination, a red face and red eyes, swollen and distended neck region, cyanotic lips, a red tongue with thick, yellow fur, a bluish green, purplish finger vein, a surging, rapid or slippery, rapid pulse

Treatment principles: Clear heat and drain fire, resolve toxins and flush phlegm

Guiding formulas:
Xian Fang Huo Ming Yin Jia Jian (Immortal Formula for Quickening the Destiny Beverage with Additions & Subtractions)
  Huang Lian (Rhizoma Coptidis)
  Huang Bai (Cortex Phellodendri)
  Shi Gao (Gypsum Fibrosum)
  Zhi Zi (Fructus Gardeniae)
  Ban Lan Gen (Radix Isatidis/Baphicacanthi)
  Jin Yin Hua (Flos Lonicerae)
  Xuan Shen (Radix Scrophulariae)
  Sheng Di (uncooked Radix Rehmanniae)
  Gan Cao (Radix Glycyrrhizae)
  Jiang Can (Bombyx Batryticatus)
  Tu Niu Xi (Radix Achyranthis Bidentatae)

If there is constipation with coarse, yellow tongue fur, which is due to heat binding in the intestines and stomach, add uncooked *Da Huang* (Radix Et Rhizoma Rhei), *Zhi Shi* (Fructus Immaturus Aurantii), and *Gua Lou Ren* (Semen Trichosanthis). If there is simultaneous epistaxis or bleeding gums, which is due to fire toxins damaging the network vessels, add *Dan Pi* (Cortex Moutan) and *Chi Shao* (Radix Paeoniae Rubrae).

Huang Lian Jie Du Tang (Coptis Resolve Toxins Decoction)
  Huang Lian (Rhizoma Coptidis)
  Huang Qin (Radix Scutellariae)
  Huang Bai (Cortex Phellodendri)
  Zhi Zi (Fructus Gardeniae)

If there is simultaneous yin damage and fire effulgence, add *Shi Gao* (Gypsum Fibrosum) and *Sheng Di* (uncooked Radix Rehmanniae) to clear heat and foster yin, and uncooked *Da Huang* (Radix Et Rhizoma Rhei), *Mang Xiao* (Natri Sulfas), *Meng Shi* (Lapis Chloriti/Mica), and *Zhu Li* (Succus Bambusae) to drain fire and flush phlegm.

Unnamed formula
  Long Dan Cao (Radix Gentianae)
  Xuan Shen (Radix Scrophulariae)
  Ma Dou Ling (Radix Aristolochiae)
  Ban Lan Gen (Radix Isatidis/Baphicacanthi)
  uncooked Shi Gao (Gypsum Fibrosum)
  Bai Shao (Radix Paeoniae Albae)
  Huang Bai (Cortex Phellodendri)
  Sheng Di (uncooked Radix Rehmanniae)
  Gua Lou (Fructus Trichosanthis)
  Zhi Zi (Fructus Gardeniae)
  Gan Cao (Radix Glycyrrhizae)
  Mai Men Dong (Tuber Ophiopogonis)

Lian Qiao (Fructus Forsythiae)
Niu Xi (Radix Achyranthis Bidentatae)

If the throat is severely swollen and red, add *She Gan* (Rhizoma Belamcandae) and *Niu Bang Zi* (Fructus Arctii). If the stools are dry and knotted, subtract the *Bai Shao* and *Ma Dou Ling* and double the amounts of *Mai Men Dong*, *Xuan Shen*, and *Sheng Di*. If the tongue is scarlet red and heat is in the blood division, replace *Bai Shao* with *Chi Shao* (Radix Paeoniae Rubrae) and add *Dan Pi* (Cortex Moutan).

3. Yin vacuity

Main symptoms: An inflamed, swollen throat with greyish yellow, stripe-like membranes spreading over the uvula and upper palate, only slight pain in the throat, a dry mouth and throat, dry lips, dry nose, lassitude of the spirit, lack of strength, low-grade fever after having had a high fever, cough, a hoarse voice, bad breath, a dark red tongue with diminished fluids and diminished, yellow fur, a purple, stagnant finger vein, a fine, rapid pulse

Treatment principles: Nourish yin, clear heat, and resolve toxins

Guiding formulas:
Yang Yin Qing Fei Tang Jia Wei (Nourish Yin & Clear the Lungs Decoction with Added Flavors)

Sheng Di (uncooked Radix Rehmanniae)
Xuan Shen (Radix Scrophulariae)
Mai Men Dong (Tuber Ophiopogonis)
Dan Pi (Cortex Moutan)
Bai Shao (Radix Paeoniae Albae)
Chuan Bei Mu (Bulbus Fritillariae Cirrhosae)
Gan Cao (Radix Glycyrrhizae)
Bo He (Herba Menthae Haplocalycis)
Jin Yin Hua (Flos Lonicerae)
Tu Niu Xi (Radix Achyranthis Bidentatae)

If there is a recurrence of high fever, add uncooked *Shi Gao* (Gypsum Fibrosum) and *Zhi Mu* (Rhizoma Anemarrhenae). If the throat is markedly painful, add *Huang Lian* (Rhizoma Coptidis) and *Shan Dou Gen* (Radix Sophorae Subprostratae). If it is red, swollen, and painful, add *Zi Hua Di Ding* (Herba Violae) and *Lian Qiao* (Fructus Forsythiae). If there is constipation, add whole *Quan Gua Lou* (Fructus Trichosanthis) and *Huo Ma Ren* (Semen Cannabis) and sometimes it is necessary to add *Mang Xiao* (Natri Sulfas).

Yang Yin Qing Fei Tang Jia Jian (Nourish Yin & Clear the Lungs Decoction with Additions & Subtractions)

Sheng Di (uncooked Radix Rehmanniae)
Xuan Shen (Radix Scrophulariae)

Mai Men Dong (Tuber Ophiopogonis)
Dan Pi (Cortex Moutan)
Bai Shao (Radix Paeoniae Albae)
Chuan Bei Mu (Bulbus Fritillariae Cirrhosae)
Bo He (Herba Menthae Haplocalycis)
Gan Cao (Radix Glycyrrhizae)

If vacuity is severe, add *Shu Di* (cooked Radix Rehmanniae). If heat is severe, delete *Bo He* and add *Lian Qiao* (Fructus Forsythiae) and *Tu Niu Xi* (Radix Achyranthis Bidentatae). If dryness is severe, add *Tian Men Dong* (Tuber Asparagi). If there is constipation, double the amounts of *Mai Men Dong*, *Shu Di*, and *Xuan Shen* or add a small amount of *Mang Xiao* (Natri Sulfas).

4. Phlegm turbidity congesting & obstructing

Main symptoms: The sound of phlegm in the throat, difficult, encumbered breathing, cough sounding like a dog's bark, a hoarse voice, vexation and agitation, sweating, a false membrane spreading from the lower to upper throat, a somber, white facial complexion, bluish green, purplish lips, thick, turbid tongue fur, a slippery pulse

Note: This is an emergency condition which may arise suddenly.

Treatment principles: Dispel phlegm and transform turbidity, diffuse congestion and resolve toxins

Guiding formulas:
Unnamed formula
Da Huang (Radix Et Rhizoma Rhei)
Ting Li Zi (Semen Lepidii/Descurainiae)
Meng Shi (Lapis Chloriti/Mica)
Tu Niu Xi (Radix Achyranthis Bidentatae)
Zhu Li (Succus Bambusae)
Ma Huang (Herba Ephedrae)

Unnamed formula
Zao Jiao (Fructus Gleditschiae), 30g
Mi Cu (Rice vinegar), 500g

Decoct for 20 minutes and administer warm in one dose.

5. Yang qi vacuity & debility
A. Heart qi vacuity weakness

Main symptoms: The white patches in the throat spread into plaques. There is sweating from the head and face, lassitude of the spirit, lack of strength, a somber white facial complexion, a pale tongue, and a vacuous, weak, skipping pulse.

Treatment principles: Boost the qi and nourish the heart

Guiding formulas:
Sheng Mai San Jia Wei (Engender the Pulse Powder with Added Flavors)
Ren Shen (Radix Ginseng)
Mai Men Dong (Tuber Ophiopogonis)
Wu Wei Zi (Fructus Schisandrae)
Gan Cao (Radix Glycyrrhizae)
Dan Shen (Radix Salviae Miltiorrhizae)

If there is sweating from the entire body, add calcined *Long Gu* (Os Draconis) and calcined *Mu Li* (Concha Ostreae).

Sheng Mai San Jia Jian (Engender the Pulse Powder with Additions & Subtractions)
Dang Shen (Radix Codonopsitis)
Mai Men Dong (Tuber Ophiopogonis)
Wu Wei Zi (Fructus Schisandrae)
mix-fried *Gan Cao* (Radix Glycyrrhizae)
Yuan Zhi (Radix Polygalae)
Long Gu (Os Draconis)
Mu Li (Concha Ostreae)

If there is inversion counterflow chilling of the limbs, add *Fu Zi* (Radix Lateralis Praeparatus Aconiti Carmichaeli) and *Huang Qi* (Radix Astragali). If the tongue is scarlet red with diminished fluids, add *Bai Shao* (Radix Paeoniae Albae), *Sheng Di* (uncooked Radix Rehmanniae), and *Yu Zhu* (Rhizoma Polygonati Odorati).

B. Devitalized heart yang

Main symptoms: The white membranes in the throat do not recede. There is essence spirit listlessness, fatigue and a desire to lie down, chilling of the four limbs, exiting of chilly sweat, diminished spirit in both eyes, a bright white facial complexion, a faint, fine pulse, an indistinct finger vein.

Treatment principles: Rescue yang and stem counterflow, support the righteous and secure desertion

Guiding formula:
Shen Fu Long Mu Jiu Ni Tang Jia Jian (Ginseng, Aconite, Dragon Bone & Oyster Shell Stem Counterflow Decoction with Additions & Subtractions)
Ren Shen (Radix Ginseng)
Fu Zi (Radix Lateralis Praeparatus Aconiti Carmichaeli)
Gan Jiang (dry Rhizoma Zingiberis)

calcined *Long Gu* (Os Draconis)
calcined *Mu Li* (Concha Ostreae)
Gan Cao (Radix Glycyrrhizae)

Acupuncture & moxibustion

Bleed *Shao Shang* (Lu 11) and needle *He Gu* (LI 4) or bleed both *Shao Shang* and *Shang Yang* (LI 1). If there is profuse phlegm, needle *Feng Long* (St 40). To disinhibit the throat and disperse swelling, needle *Tian Tu* (CV 22) and *Lian Quan* (CV 23). If there is shortness of breath, add *Shan Zhong* (CV 17). For yin vacuity, needle *San Yin Jiao* (Sp 6), and for yang vacuity, moxa *Shen Que* (CV 8) and *Guan Yuan* (CV 4).

Adjunctive treatments

A clear, bland, easily digestible but nutritious diet is important. This usually includes eating less salt. A simple Chinese herbal home remedy for diphtheria is to drink a tea made out of carrot tops. However, one should not think that this is a sufficient treatment for such a potentially serious and life-threatening disease. It is merely offered here as an adjunctive or supporting treatment when drunk as a background beverage or tea. Other beverage teas can be made from *Da Qing Ye* (Folium Daqingye) and *Ban Lan Gen* (Radix Isatidis/Baphicacanthi) or from *Tu Niu Xi* (Radix Achyranthis Bidentatae). *Xi Gua Shuang* (Water Melon Frost) or *Xi Lei San* (Black Tin Powder), both Chinese ready-made medicines, can be sprayed into the mouth. For the first two patterns, one can also take *Liu Shen Wan* (Six Spirits Pills, another Chinese ready-made medicine) along with the medicinal decoctions.

Comments

Diphtheria is a very dangerous disease and may present with various, complicated patterns. Correct and immediate treatment are essential. Even in China, this disease is usually treated with a combination of modern Western and traditional Chinese medicines.

46. Traumatic Injuries

Kids will be kids, and that means a certain amount of cuts and bruises, and burns and stings are part of the process of growing up. Children's coordination is not mature, nor is their assessment of what is safe. Therefore, although Chinese pediatric texts do not say anything about traumatic injuries, I have included a short selection of simple Chinese home remedies which practitioners can teach to their patients' parents. For more serious or complex traumatic injuries, practitioners are referred to Chinese traumatology texts, such as *Shaolin Secret Formulas for the Treatment of External Injuries* by De Chan, Blue Poppy Press.

Burns

There are a number of very simple Chinese herbal home remedies for burns. These include putting either fresh carrot juice, fresh cucumber juice, fresh potato juice, fresh aloe juice, fresh ginger juice, or honey to the burn itself. One can also apply roasted sesame oil or ground sesame seeds, *i.e.*, *tahini*.

There are a number of safe and effective Chinese ready-made medicines for external and first aid use in the case of traumatic injuries. One such Chinese ready-made medicine for burns is Ching Wan Burn Ointment. This is the single best burn ointment I know. It is available at Chinese apothecaries in Chinatowns in major Western cities.

Bruises

A bruise or contusion is a closed wound typically due to being struck or in a fall. Bruises cause a black and blue mark which, in Chinese medicine, is static blood which has pooled outside the blood vessels due to the strike or fall causing the local blood vessels to break or rupture. The Chinese medical treatment principles for dealing with bruises are, therefore, to move the blood and dispel stasis. Two effective Chinese ready-made medicines for external application to bruises and contusions are Tieh Ta Yao Gin and Wan Hua Oil.

Cuts

In order to stop bleeding, one can sprinkle *Xue Yu Tan* (Crinis Carbonisatus) into the wound. Another possibility is to sprinkle *Bai Fan* (Alumen) into a cut or dry ginger powder. There is also the Chinese ready-made medicine, Yunnan Bai Yao. This powder can be sprinkled into a cut to stop bleeding. It also comes as capsules which can be taken internally to stop more serious bleeding. Yet another possibility is to sprinkle powdered *Wu Zei Gu* (Endoconcha Sepiae) into the cut.

If a cut becomes infected, as they sometimes do with children who have a propensity for playing in the dirt and for picking at scabs, then one can make a poultice of crushed burdock roots applied warm to the affected area. Burdock is a common weed growing widely throughout North America and it is also available as a food (sometimes under the Japanese name, *gobo*) at health food stores. Another possibility is to make a compress out of raw, crushed garlic. At the same time, drink 1 teacup of warm, boiled water mixed with 1 teacup of freshly squeezed *daikon* radish juice. Or powder some *Da Huang* (Radix Et Rhizoma Rhei), mix with honey to form a thin paste, and apply locally.

Sprains & strains

When running and playing, it is not uncommon for children to twist their ankle or to strain a joint. Typically, our first response in the West is to ice such injuries. In Chinese medicine, ice may be applied for the first 24 hours, but after that, because the intense cold further restricts the flow of blood and since such injuries already involve blood stasis, we do not recommend using ice after that. If the joint is still swollen, red, and inflamed, then one can make a poultice or plaster out of grated potato or grated taro root mixed with a little white flour to hold it together. This will help clear heat and thus eliminate inflammation as well as eliminate the dampness associated with the swelling and edema. Another possibility during the swollen, inflamed stage is to make a poultice out of crushed tofu and a little white flour. Such poultices are applied to the affected area, which should be kept raised and immobile, and replaced every couple of hours.

If the sprain or strain is no longer hot to the touch or red to the sight but is still markedly swollen, then one can cook some buckwheat and mix that with white flour to make a poultice. Apply this to the swollen area in order to help eliminate the dampness and edema.

There are also so-called "hit pills" (*Die Da Wan* or *Tieh Ta Wan* depending on whether they are manufactured in the People's Republic of China or Hong Kong/Taiwan). These are large pills made from powdered herbs mixed with honey. They contain a number of ingredients in order to move the qi and blood, dispel stasis and stop pain. One pill or a part of a pill may be taken 1-2 times per day for serious strains, sprains, contusions, and even dislocations and broken bones *as long as there is no marked bleeding*. In addition, there are a number of commercially available Chinese herbal liniments, plasters, soaks, and compresses. Parents of active children may find it useful to keep a selection of these kinds of ready-made medicines in a Chinese herbal first aid kit. A simple home liniment for external application can be made by boiling some safflowers in some vinegar. Then straining out the safflowers and bottling this for later use.

Imbedded foreign objects

If one gets a thorn or splinter or some other, *small* foreign object imbedded in the skin, one can draw this out by taking a half of onion and roasting it in an oven until soft. This is then applied over the object while still warm and kept in place for some time. Such a poultice of roasted onion can help pull a foreign object from the skin.

Insect stings

A simple Chinese herbal home remedy for bee and other insect stings is to rub garlic juice into the site of injury. Another simple herbal remedy is to chew some tea leaves into a mash and then place this poultice on the site of the sting. And a third herbal home remedy is to make a taro root plaster with a pinch of salt and apply to the affected area.

47. Developmental & Constitutional Problems

The more traditional a Chinese pediatric text is, the more likely it will include a series of diseases prefaced by the word five. There are three sets of five describing developmental or constitutional problems in infants and young children. These three sets of five are the five slows, the five softs, and the five hards. To these three groups of five, some Chinese books add the categories of chicken breast, turtle back, and split skull. While no Western parent is likely to bring in their child complaining of the five slows or the five softs, it is important for the TCM pediatric specialist to understand these conditions nonetheless. In fact, they may be useful for diagnosing and treating some children even if their parents or Western physicians might scoff at these seemingly unsophisticated but very descriptive Chinese disease names.

The Five Slows

The five slows refer to slower than normal standing, slower than normal movement, slower than normal hair growth, slower than normal growth of teeth, and slower than normal speaking. In modern TCM pediatrics, these are treated based on the discrimination of two basic patterns: Liver-kidney insufficiency and heart blood insufficiency.

Treatment based on pattern discrimination:

1. Liver-kidney insufficiency (a.k.a. Liver-kidney depletion & vacuity)

Main symptoms: Sinews and bones atonic and weak, obviously abnormally slow development in sitting up, standing, and moving erect, slow development of the teeth

Treatment principles: Supplement the kidneys and nourish the liver

Guiding formulas:
Jia Wei Liu Wei Di Huang Wan (Added Flavors Six Flavors Rehmannia Pills)
Shu Di (cooked Radix Rehmanniae)
Shan Yao (Radix Dioscoreae)
Fu Ling (Poria)
Shan Zhu Yu (Fructus Corni)
Ze Xie (Rhizoma Alismatis)
Dan Pi (Cortex Moutan)
Lu Rong (Cornu Parvum Cervi)
Wu Jia Pi (Cortex Acanthopanacis)

If movement and arising are retarded and slow, one can use **Hu Gu San Jia Jian (Tiger Bone Powder with Additions & Subtractions):**
Zhu Gu (Os Porci)
Niu Xi (Radix Achyranthis Bidentatae)
Dang Gui (Radix Angelicae Sinensis)
Chuan Xiong (Rhizoma Chuanxiong)
Sheng Di (uncooked Radix Rehmanniae)
Rou Gui (Cortex Cinnamomi)
Suan Zao Ren (Semen Zizyphi Spinosae)
Fu Ling (Poria)
Fang Feng (Radix Saposhnikoviae)

If the teeth are particularly slow in growing, one can use **Tang Shi Xiong Huang San (Master Tang's Ligusticum Powder)**:

  Chuan Xiong (Rhizoma Chuanxiong)
  Dang Gui (Radix Angelicae Sinensis)
  Sheng Di (uncooked Radix Rehmanniae)
  Shan Yao (Radix Dioscoreae)
  Gan Cao (Radix Glycyrrhizae)

If growth and development are particularly slow, one can use **Cong Rong Wan (Cistanches Pills)**:

  Rou Cong Rong (Herba Cistanchis)
  Sheng Di (uncooked Radix Rehmanniae)
  Hei Dou (black Semen Glycinis)
  Dang Gui (Radix Angelicae Sinensis)
  Bai Shao (Radix Paeoniae Albae)

2. Heart blood insufficiency (heart/spleen insufficiency)

Main symptoms: Intelligence not complete, listlessness of the essence spirit, no speech after several years, speech not clear and intelligible, skin color a somber white, sparse, withered, yellowish hair, reduced food intake, constipation, a glossy tongue with no fur

Treatment principles: Supplement the heart and nourish the blood

Guiding formulas:
Chang Pu Wan (Acorus Pills)

  Dang Shen (Radix Codonopsitis)
  Dang Gui (Radix Angelicae Sinensis)
  Chuan Xiong (Rhizoma Chuanxiong)
  Yuan Zhi (Radix Polygalae)
  Shi Chang Pu (Rhizoma Acori Tatarinowii)

Chang Pu Wan Jia Wei (Acorus Pills with Added Flavors)

  Ren Shen (Radix Ginseng)
  Dang Gui (Radix Angelicae Sinensis)
  Chuan Xiong (Rhizoma Chuanxiong)
  Yuan Zhi (Radix Polygalae)
  Shi Chang Pu (Rhizoma Acori Tatarinowii)
  Ru Xiang (Olibanum)
  Mai Men Dong (Tuber Ophiopogonis)
  Wu Wei Zi (Fructus Schisandrae)
  Bai Zi Ren (Semen Platycladi)

Acupuncture & moxibustion

For slow speech, moxa the ankles of both feet and *Xin Shu* (Bl 15) with three cones each time, one time each day.

The Five Softs (and/or Weaks)

The five softs or weaks refer to a soft head and weak neck, a weak mouth, soft hair, weak feet, and soft muscles and flesh. The treatment of these various pediatric insufficiencies is based on discriminating two basic patterns: Spleen-kidney dual vacuity and qi and blood vacuity weakness.

Treatment based on pattern discrimination:

1. Spleen-kidney dual vacuity

Main symptoms: Head and neck soft and weak, the neck not able to hold the head upright, soft mouth and weak gums not able to suckle, flowing drool, soft hair which easily falls out, soft, weak feet and inability to stand up, no strength in movement, pale lips, diminished tongue fur

Treatment principles: Fortify the spleen and supplement the kidneys

Guiding formula:
Bu Shen Di Huang Wan (Supplement the Kidneys Rehmannia Pills) plus Bu Zhong Yi Qi Tang (Supplement the Center & Boost the Qi Decoction) with additions and subtractions

Shu Di (cooked Radix Rehmanniae)
Shan Zhu Yu (Fructus Corni)
Fu Ling (Poria)
Ren Shen (Radix Ginseng)
Huang Qi (Radix Astragali)
Bai Zhu (Rhizoma Atractylodis Macrocephalae)
Sheng Ma (Rhizoma Cimicifugae)
Bu Gu Zhi (Fructus Psoraleae)
Niu Xi (Radix Achyranthis Bidentatae)
Lu Rong (Cornu Parvum Cervi)
Dang Gui (Radix Angelicae Sinensis)
Shi Chang Pu (Rhizoma Acori Tatarinowii)

2. Qi & blood vacuity weakness

Main symptoms: Soft, weak body and limbs, soft joints of the four limbs, listlessness of the essence spirit, slow intelligence, a somber white facial complexion, lack of warmth in the four limbs, the opening of the mouth does not meet and the tongue lolls out, diminished eating, lack of transformation (*i.e.*, poor digestion), white lips, a glossy tongue

Treatment principles: Boost the qi and nourish the blood

Guiding formula:
Ba Zhen Tang (Eight Pearls Decoction)
    Ren Shen (Radix Ginseng)
    Fu Ling (Poria)
    Bai Zhu (Rhizoma Atractylodis Macrocephalae)
    Gan Cao (Radix Glycyrrhizae)
    Dang Gui (Radix Angelicae Sinensis)
    Chuan Xiong (Rhizoma Chuanxiong)
    Shu Di (cooked Radix Rehmanniae)
    Bai Shao (Radix Paeoniae Albae)

Acupuncture & moxibustion

Choose from among *Bai Hui* (GV 20), *Da Zhui* (GV 14), *An Mian* (N-HN-22b), *Ya Men* (GV 15), *Nei Guan* (Per 6), *He Gu* (LI 4), and *Zu San Li* (St 36) and needle one time each day.

The Five Hards

The five hards refer to a hard head and neck, a hard mouth, hard hair, hard feet, and hard muscles and flesh. Although the above two series of fives can cover a variety of Western diseases, the five hards specifically correspond to scleroderma neonatorum. This typically occurs in premature infants and infants with other disorders who are abnormally vacuous and weak 7-10 days after birth. It is characterized by sclerosis and edema of the subcutaneous fat and occurs more often in cold seasons. If not treated promptly, this can be a life-threatening condition. In severe cases, this condition is complicated by lung bleeding. Modern TCM pediatrics divides the five hards into two basic patterns: Yang qi vacuity and debility and cold congelation with astringing and stagnancy of the blood.

Treatment based on pattern discrimination:

1. Yang qi vacuity & debility

Main symptoms: The child's body is vacuous and weak. The whole body feels frozen and chilled. There is diminished movements during sleep, sleep is excessive, and breathing is faint and weak. The sound of crying lacks strength, the joints are inhibited, and the head and body have difficulty moving. The skin is hard like wood and is a somber white color and puffy. There is pitting of the skin when pressed. The lips and tongue are pale white.

Treatment principles: Boost the qi and warm yang

Guiding formula: *Shen Fu Tang Jia Wei* (Ginseng & Aconite Decoction with Added Flavors)
    Ren Shen (Radix Ginseng)
    Fu Zi (Radix Lateralis Praeparatus Aconiti Carmichaeli)
    Gui Zhi (Ramulus Cinnamomi)
    Huang Qi (Radix Astragali)
    Dang Gui (Radix Angelicae Sinensis)
    Hong Hua (Flos Carthami)

2. Cold congelation, stagnant blood

Main symptoms: The four limbs emit coolness, and the whole body lacks warmth. The skin lacks suppleness and softness and cannot be pinched up. This begins in the legs and then spreads to the upper limbs and cheeks. The skin color is dull purplish or red and swollen as if damaged by frostbite. There is a dark, dull facial complexion and a dark red tongue and lips.

Treatment principles: Warm the channels and open the network vessels

Guiding formulas:
Dang Gui Si Ni Tang Jia Wei (Dang Gui Four Counterflows Decoction with Added Flavors)
    Dang Gui (Radix Angelicae Sinensis)
    Chi Shao (Radix Paeoniae Rubrae)
    Bai Shao (Radix Paeoniae Albae)
    Xi Xin (Herba Asari)
    Gui Zhi (Ramulus Cinnamomi)
    Dang Shen (Radix Codonopsitis)
    Huang Qi (Radix Astragali)
    Mu Tong (Caulis Akebiae)
    Sheng Jiang (uncooked Rhizoma Zingiberis)
    Gan Cao (Radix Glycyrrhizae)

Dang Gui Si Ni Tang Jia Jian (Dang Gui Four Counterflows Decoction with Additions & Subtractions)
    Dang Gui (Radix Angelicae Sinensis)
    Gui Zhi (Ramulus Cinnamomi)
    Huang Qi (Radix Astragali)
    Ji Xue Teng (Caulis Spatholobi)
    Bai Shao (Radix Paeoniae Albae)
    Gan Cao (Radix Glycyrrhizae)

If the limbs are very cold, add *Wu Zhu Yu* (Fructus Evodiae). If the skin is dark purple due to more severe blood stasis, add *Hong Hua* (Flos Carthami) and *Dan Shen* (Radix Salviae Miltiorrhizae).

Acupuncture & moxibustion

The affected areas can be slowly and gently warmed with indirect moxibustion.

Adjunctive treatments

The baby should be kept warm by wrapping them in a blanket or quilt. A hot water bottle may also be used. However, it is important that the temperature be raised slowly to prevent bleeding. The baby's temperature should be measured every one to two hours until it is 35 C or higher, at which time the quilt or blanket can be removed.

Comments

This condition is a very dangerous one. It needs to be treated by both internally administered decoctions and external warming therapies. In most cases, the child should be treated in a hospital where they will probably be placed in an incubator. Hospitalization is important in case there is hemorrhaging. Since this condition is mostly seen in premature babies and since most premature babies will be hospitalized, it is unlikely that many Western TCM practitioners will be called on to treat this condition.

Chicken Breast

Chicken breast or chest is also called turtle breast in the Chinese medical literature. In this case, the child's breastbone or sternum protrudes abnormally outward, thus appearing like a chicken's breast. In Chinese medicine, this condition is due to a former heaven or prenatal insufficiency and is treated by mainly supplementing the kidneys. However, because of the interrelationship between the former and latter heavens or pre- and postnatal, in clinical practice, both the spleen and kidneys are usually addressed.

> **Main symptoms:** An abnormally shaped sternum which protrudes ventrally too much, either a thin body or a vacuous fat body, listlessness of the essence spirit, shortness of breath, lack of strength in movement, a somber white facial complexion, a pale red finger vein
>
> **Treatment principles:** Enrich yin and fortify the spleen, supplement and boost the qi and blood
>
> ### Guiding formula:
> **Bu Tian Da Zao Wan Jia Jian (Supplement Heaven Great Creation Pills with Additions & Subtractions)**
> *Zi He Che* (Placenta Hominis)
> *Lu Jiao* (Cornu Cervi)
> *Gui Ban* (Plastrum Testudinis)

Tu Si Zi (Semen Cuscutae)
Du Zhong (Cortex Eucommiae)
Niu Xi (Radix Achyranthis Bidentatae)
Shan Yao (Radix Dioscoreae)
Ren Shen (Radix Ginseng)
Bai Zhu (Rhizoma Atractylodis Macrocephalae)
Shu Di (cooked Radix Rehmanniae)
Mai Men Dong (Tuber Ophiopogonis)
Wu Wei Zi (Fructus Schisandrae)
Dang Gui (Radix Angelicae Sinensis)
Gou Qi Zi (Fructus Lycii)
Fu Ling (Poria)

Turtle Back

Turtle back is also called bulging upper back. It is a type of abnormal development of the child's bones in which case the spine in the upper back protrudes dorsally abnormally. As in the preceding condition, in Chinese medicine, turtle back is seen as a combination of former heaven insufficiency affecting the marrow and latter heaven insufficiency failing to nourish and moisten the sinews with the governing vessel left vacuous and debilitated. Thus treatment is directed mainly towards supplementing the kidneys while boosting the spleen at the same time.

Main symptoms: A crooked and outwardly protruding upper back like a turtle's back, a thin body with flabby, slack muscles and flesh, a lusterless facial complexion, a pale colored finger vein

Treatment principles: Supplement the kidneys and boost the spleen

Guiding formula:
Bu Tian Da Zao Wan Jia Jian (Supplement Heaven Great Creation Pills with Additions & Subtractions)
Zi He Che (Placenta Hominis)
Lu Jiao (Cornu Cervi)
Gui Ban (Plastrum Testudinis)
Shu Di (cooked Radix Rehmanniae)
Shan Yao (Radix Dioscoreae)
Gou Qi Zi (Fructus Lycii)
Dang Gui (Radix Angelicae Sinensis)
Du Zhong (Cortex Eucommiae)
Niu Xi (Radix Achyranthis Bidentatae)
Rou Cong Rong (Herba Cistanchis)
Tian Men Dong (Tuber Asparagi)
Fu Ling (Poria)
Gan Cao (Radix Glycyrrhizae)

If there is profuse sweating, add *Long Gu* (Os Draconis) and *Mu Li* (Concha Ostreae).

Acupuncture & moxibustion

Choose from among and moxa *Da Zhu* (Bl 11), *Feng Chi* (GB 20), *Jue Gu* (GB 39), *Hou Xi* (SI 3), *Fei Shu* (Bl 13), and *Xin Shu* (Bl 15).

Split Skull

Split skull refers to the child's fontanelles being too large and the bones of the skull not closing and joining properly. Although some Chinese pediatric books regard this as simply due to kidney insufficiency *vis a vis* the bones and marrow, others divide this condition and its treatment into four patterns.

Treatment based on pattern discrimination:

1. Kidney qi depletion & detriment

Main symptoms: Non-closure of the fontanelles after birth or gradual reopening of the fontanelles after they had closed, an obviously enlarged skull, the skin on the head bare and tight, blue-green sinews (*i.e.*, veins) sticking out and revealed, the pupils of the eyes contracted and small, smaller than normal and blackish eye whites, a large head but fine neck, a thin body, delayed development, a torpid spirit

Treatment principles: Supplement the kidneys and boost the marrow

Guiding formula:
Bu Shen Di Huang Wan (Supplement the Kidneys Rehmannia Pills)
    Shu Di (cooked Radix Rehmanniae)
    Shan Zhu Yu (Fructus Corni)
    Fu Ling (Poria)
    Shan Yao (Radix Dioscoreae)
    Niu Xi (Radix Achyranthis Bidentatae)

If the sinews and bones are soft and weak, add *Du Zhong* (Cortex Eucommiae) and *Xu Duan* (Radix Dipsaci). If the qi and blood are vacuous and weak, add *Dang Shen* (Radix Codonopsitis) and *Huang Qi* (Radix Astragali). If there is heat in the hands, feet, and heart with a dry mouth and red tongue, vexation and agitation, and restlessness, add *Mu Li* (Concha Ostreae), *Sheng Di* (uncooked Radix Rehmanniae), and *Shi Hu* (Herba Dendrobii).

2. Kidney vacuity with liver hyperactivity

Main symptoms: The fontanelles are open and the forebrain is enlarged. There are visible blue-green sinews (*i.e.*, veins) on the forehead. The whites of the eyes are especially obvious. There is no spirit in the eyes but there is vexation of the spirit and restlessness with heat in the hands, feet, and heart. There may be occasional tremors and spasms, and the mouth is dry and the tongue is red.

Treatment principles: Boost the kidneys and disinhibit water, level the liver and extinguish wind

Guiding formula:
Zhi Bai Di Huang Tang (Anemarrhena & Phellodendron Rehmannia Decoction) plus San Jia Fu Mai Tang (Three Shells Restore the Pulse Decoction)

Zhi Mu (Rhizoma Anemarrhenae)
Huang Bai (Cortex Phellodendri)
Bie Jia (Carapax Trionycis)
Mu Li (Concha Ostreae)
Gui Ban (Plastrum Testudinis)
Shu Di (cooked Radix Rehmanniae)
Shan Yao (Radix Dioscoreae)
Shan Zhu Yu (Fructus Corni)
Fu Ling (Poria)
Ze Xie (Rhizoma Alismatis)
Dan Pi (Cortex Moutan)

If there is vexation, agitation, and restlessness, add *Dan Zhu Ye* (Herba Lophateri), *Mu Tong* (Caulis Akebiae), and *Zhi Zi* (Fructus Gardeniae). If there is fright, paranoia, lack of tranquility, and, if severe, tremors and spasms, add *Shi Jue Ming* (Concha Haliotidis) and *Gou Teng* (Ramulus Uncariae Cum Uncis).

3. Spleen vacuity, water flooding

Main symptoms: A bright white facial complexion, lack of spirit in the eyes, fontanelles of the head open and not joining, shiny skin on the head, tapping it presents a broken kettle sound, a thin body, devitalized eating and drinking, loose stools, torpid and stagnant essence affect, inhibited urination, thin, white tongue fur, and a pale tongue

Treatment principles: Support the spleen and disinhibit water

Guiding formula:
Fu Zi Li Zhong Tang (Aconite Rectify the Center Decoction) plus Wu Ling San (Five [Ingredients] Poria Powder)

Ren Shen (Radix Ginseng)
Bai Zhu (Rhizoma Atractylodis Macrocephalae)
Gan Jiang (dry Rhizoma Zingiberis)
Fu Zi (Radix Lateralis Praeparatus Aconiti Carmichaeli)
Zhu Ling (Polyporus)

Fu Ling (Poria)
Ze Xie (Rhizoma Alismatis)
Gui Zhi (Ramulus Cinnamomi)

If qi and blood are both depleted, add *Huang Qi* (Radix Astragali) and *Dang Gui* (Radix Angelicae Sinensis). If there is abdominal distention and loose stools, add *Mu Xiang* (Radix Auklandiae) and *Sha Ren* (Fructus Amomi).

4. Heat toxins blockage & stagnation

Main symptoms: The fontanelles joined but then reopened. When pressed, there is a floating, soft feeling. The skin on the head is shiny and tight. There are visible purplish sinews (*i.e.*, veins) which appear angry and distended. Both eyes droop downward. There is headache, a dry mouth, fever, rapid dyspneic breathing, a red face and red lips, short, reddish urination, and dry, constipated stools.

Treatment principles: Clear heat and open the network vessels

Guiding formula:
Xi Di Qing Luo Yin (Rhinoceros & Rehmannia Clear the Network Vessels Beverage) plus *Hua Du Dan* (Transform Toxins Elixir) with additions and subtractions
Shui Niu Jiao (Cornu Bubali)
Sheng Di (uncooked Radix Rehmanniae)
Dan Pi (Cortex Moutan)
Chi Shao (Radix Paeoniae Rubrae)

If there is agitation, stirring and restlessness, spirit vexation, and insomnia, add *Shan Yang Jiao* (Cornu Caprae) and *Gou Teng* (Ramulus Uncariae Cum Uncis).

Acupuncture & moxibustion

Choose from among the following groups of points depending upon the presenting pattern. In all cases, needle *Bai Hui* (GV 20) through to *Si Shen Cong* (M-HN-1). If there is liver hyperactivity or heat toxins, needle *Feng Fu* (GV 16) through to *Ya Men* (GV 15), and *Feng Chi* (GB 20) through to *Da Zhu* (Bl 11) and *Da Zhui* (GV 14). If there is inhibited urination, needle *San Jiao Shu* (Bl 22) through to *Shen Shu* (Bl 23) and *Shui Fen* (CV 9) through to *Zhong Ji* (CV 3). If there is spleen vacuity, needle *Zu San Li* (St 36) through to *Yin Ling Quan* (Sp 9). If there is liver hyperactivity, needle *Yin Ling Quan* (Sp 9) through to *Yang Ling Quan* (GB 34). And if there is kidney vacuity, needle *San Yin Jiao* (Sp 6) through to *Fu Liu* (Ki 7).

Comments

Obviously, the above acupuncture protocol requires expert needle technique and is not for the fainthearted. Extreme care must be taken when needling *Bai Hui* (GV 20) through to *Si Shen Cong* (M-HN-1).

48. Premature Sexual Development

Sexual development is considered premature in girls 8 years old or younger and in boys 10 years old or younger. In TCM, sexual development is a function of the exuberance of the life-gate fire, while premature sexual development is mostly related to kidney yin insufficiency. In that case, yin is vacuous and fire is, therefore, prematurely effulgent. Thus vacuity fire stirs frenetically. This means that, typically, most cases of premature sexual development are treated based on the principles of enriching yin and downbearing fire. However, if premature development of breast buds is the main symptom, this may also be treated as liver depression transforming heat with yin vacuity. Parenthetically, the mental/emotional agitation experienced by adolescents is likewise due to stirring of life-gate or ministerial fire.

Treatment based on pattern discrimination:

1. Yin vacuity, fire effulgence

Main symptoms: Breast development, increased vaginal discharge, tension, agitation, easy anger, oral thirst, constipation, vexatious heat in the five hearts, a red tongue with dry or diminished fur, a fine, rapid pulse

Treatment principles: Enrich yin and drain fire

Guiding formulas:
Zi Yin Xie Huo Fang (Enrich Yin & Drain Fire Formula)
Sheng Di (uncooked Radix Rehmanniae)
Zhi Mu (Rhizoma Anemarrhenae)
Xuan Shen (Radix Scrophulariae)
Xia Ku Cao (Spica Prunellae)
Huang Bai (Cortex Phellodendri)
Ze Xie (Rhizoma Alismatis)
Chi Shao (Radix Paeoniae Rubrae)
San Leng (Rhizoma Sparganii)
mix-fried Chuan Shan Jia (Squama Manitis)
Long Dan Cao (Radix Gentianae)
Mai Ya (Fructus Germinatus Hordei)
Gan Cao (Radix Glycyrrhizae)

Zi Yin An Shen Tang (Enrich Yin & Quiet the Spirit Decoction)
Ye Jiao Teng (Caulis Polygoni Multiflori)
Suan Zao Ren (Semen Zizyphi Spinosae)
Huang Bai (Cortex Phellodendri)
Zhi Mu (Rhizoma Anemarrhenae)
Shu Di (cooked Radix Rehmanniae)
Gou Qi Zi (Fructus Lycii)
Shan Yao (Radix Dioscoreae)

Dan Pi (Cortex Moutan)
Ze Xie (Rhizoma Alismatis)

2. Liver depression transforming heat

Main symptoms: Premature breast development, increased vaginal discharge, sexual and emotional tension and agitation, thin, yellow tongue fur, a wiry, rapid pulse

Treatment principles: Soothe the liver and scatter nodulation, clear heat and disinhibit dampness

Guiding formula:
Shu Gan Qing Re Tang (Soothe the Liver & Clear Heat Decoction)
Chai Hu (Radix Bupleuri)
Huang Qin (Radix Scutellariae)
Ze Xie (Rhizoma Alismatis)
Zhi Ke (Fructus Aurantii)
Bai Shao (Radix Paeoniae Albae)
Xuan Shen (Radix Scrophulariae)
Dang Gui (Radix Angelicae Sinensis)
Sheng Di (uncooked Radix Rehmanniae)
Zhe Bei Mu (Bulbus Fritillariae Thunbergii)
Xia Ku Cao (Spica Prunellae)
Fu Ling (Poria)
Chi Shao (Radix Paeoniae Rubrae)
Dan Pi (Cortex Moutan)
Gan Cao (Radix Glycyrrhizae

Comments

Because this condition is primarily related to the disease mechanisms of insufficient yin, liver depression, and damp heat in the liver channel, a clear, bland diet is important in all cases involving damp heat. Improving stress-coping skills and solving emotional or familial problems as best as one can is important in liver depression. And adequate rest and a nourishing diet are important in yin vacuity patterns. In my experience, this condition is more common in young girls than in young boys. Since growth in girls slows and then stops within a year or so after menarche, premature sexual development in girls may lead to an extremely short stature.

2
Emergency Formulas

The formulas in this section are meant for emergency use only. They each include only one or a very few ingredients and do not require an elaborate pattern discrimination. However, when possible, more balanced formulas should be used based on a more complete pattern discrimination. These formulas are only meant as a first aid response until more complete professional treatment can be administered.

High fever

1. *Shi Gao* (Gypsum Fibrosum), 50g

Decoct in water and administer for high fever *with sweating*.

2. *Bai Luo Bu Zhi* (Daikon radish juice)

Administer orally for high fever *with sweating*.

Convulsions & seizures

uncooked *Ban Xia* (Rhizoma Pinelliae), 3g
Zao Jiao (Fructus Gleditschiae), 1.5g

Grind into powder and blow a small amount into the nostrils for acute and chronic convulsions and spirit clouding, *i.e.*, loss of consciousness.

Reversal (i.e., fainting or shock)

Heat reversal
Ren Shen (Radix Ginseng), 9g
Shi Gao (Gypsum Fibrosum), 20g
Gan Cao (Radix Glycyrrhizae), 6g
Zhi Mu (Rhizoma Anemarrhenae), 9g
Mai Men Dong (Tuber Ophiopogonis), 9g

Wu Wei Zi (Fructus Schisandrae), 6g
Geng Mi (Semen Oryzae), 20g

Decoct in water and administer 1-2 packets per day at 6 hour intervals.

Cold reversal

1. *Ren Shen* (Radix Ginseng), 10g
Fu Zi (Radix Lateralis Praeparatus Aconiti Carmichaeli), 6g
Gan Jiang (dry Rhizoma Zingiberis), 6g
mix-fried *Gan Cao* (Radix Glycyrrhizae), 3g

Decoct in water and administer 1-2 packets per day at 6 hour intervals.

2. *Gan Jiang* (dry Rhizoma Zingiberis), 20g

Decoct in water and administer frequently.

3. *Ren Shen* (Radix Ginseng), 10g
Gan Jiang (dry Rhizoma Zingiberis), 5g

Decoct in water and administer frequently.

Block & repulsion

Block and repulsion refers to a combination of vomiting, constipation, and anuria.

1. *Da Huang* (Radix Et Rhizoma Rhei), 24-30g

Decoct in 200ml of water and administer as an enema.

2. *Ren Shen* (Radix Ginseng), 9g
Mai Men Dong (Tuber Ophiopogonis), 9g
Wu Wei Zi (Fructus Schisandrae), 6g
Yu Zhu (Rhizoma Polygonati Odorati), 9g
Xing Ren (Semen Armeniacae), 9g

Decoct in water and administer in 3 doses for block and repulsion with a red tongue and a fine, rapid pulse.

3. *Ren Shen* (Radix Ginseng), 9g
Mai Men Dong (Tuber Ophiopogonis), 9g
E Jiao (Gelatinum Corii Asini), 6g
Shu Di (cooked Radix Rehmanniae), 9g
Bai Shao (Radix Paeoniae Albae), 6g
Niu Xi (Radix Achyranthis Bidentatae), 6g
Wu Mei (Fructus Mume), 6g

Decoct in water and administer in 3 doses for block and repulsion with a red tongue with diminished fur and a fine, rapid pulse.

4. *Zhi Zi* (Fructus Gardeniae), 6g
   Huang Lian (Rhizoma Coptidis), 3g
   Zhu Ru (Caulis Bambusae In Taeniis), 9g
   Lu Gen (Rhizoma Phragmitis), 9g
   Shui Niu Jiao (Cornu Bubali), 10g

Decoct in water and administer in 3 doses for block and repulsion with fire exuberance and a surging, large pulse.

5. *Chen Pi* (Pericarpium Citri Reticulatae), 3g
   Ban Xia (Rhizoma Pinelliae), 6g
   Fu Ling (Poria), 6g
   mix-fried *Gan Cao* (Radix Glycyrrhizae), 3g
   Zhi Shi (Fructus Immaturus Aurantii), 6g
   Bing Lang (Semen Arecae), 6g
   Hou Po (Cortex Magnoliae), 3g
   Mu Tong (Caulis Akebiae), 6g
   Ze Xie (Rhizoma Alismatis), 5g

Decoct in water and administer in 3 doses for block and repulsion with a deep, slippery pulse.

6. *Shu Di* (cooked Radix Rehmanniae), 9g
   Mai Men Dong (Tuber Ophiopogonis), 9g
   Zhi Ke (Fructus Aurantii), 6g
   Gan Cao (Radix Glycyrrhizae), 3g
   Pi Pa Ye (Folium Eriobotryae), 5g
   Shi Hu (Herba Dendrobii), 6g
   Sheng Di (uncooked Radix Rehmanniae), 6g
   Tian Men Dong (Tuber Asparagi), 6g

Decoct in water and administer in 3 doses for block and repulsion with a vacuous, wiry pulse.

7. uncooked *Da Huang* (Radix Et Rhizoma Rhei)
   Jie Geng (Radix Platycodi)
   Huai Hua Mi (Flos Immaturus Sophorae), 30g each

Decoct in water and administer as an enema for block and repulsion.

8. *Qu Mai* (Herba Dianthi), 10g
   Che Qian Cao (Herba Plantaginis), 15g

Bai Ji Guan Hua (Flos Celosiae Cristatae), 10g

Decoct in water and administer 1 packet per day for block and repulsion with anuria or scanty urination.

Acute abdominal pain

1. *Wu Mei* (Fructus Mume)
Yan Hu Suo (Rhizoma Corydalis)
Ru Xiang (Olibanum)
Mo Yao (Myrrha)
Gou Teng (Ramulus Uncariae Cum Uncis), 7.5g each

Grind into powder and use 6g each time, decocted in boiling water for chilly pain below the umbilicus.

2. *Yan Hu Suo* (Rhizoma Corydalis)
Xiao Hui Xiang (Fructus Foeniculi), equal amounts

Grind into powder and use 1-3 grams each time drunk down with rice soup for an acute suppurative inflammation of the intestines that ruptures through the umbilical wall at the umbilicus.

Sudden vomiting, sudden diarrhea

1. *Huang Lian* (Rhizoma Coptidis), 3g
Zi Su Ye (Folium Perillae), 3g
Sheng Jiang (uncooked Rhizoma Zingiberis), 3 slices

Use 60g of *Fu Long Gan* (Terra Flava Usta) and dissolve in clear water. Use this water to decoct the above medicinals. Administer the resulting decoction for the treatment of sudden vomiting.

2. *Sheng Jiang Zhi* (ginger juice)

Rub this on the tip of the tongue or administer internally for sudden vomiting.

3. *Er Cha* (Catechu), 25-50mg per kilo of body weight

Divide this into 3-4 doses and administer orally for sudden diarrhea.

4. Powder some *Chuan Jiao* (Fructus Zanthoxyli) and fill the baby's navel. Cover with an adhesive plaster and leave in place for 24 hours for sudden diarrhea.

5. *Han Shui Shi* (Calcitum), 60g

Ku Fan (Alumen), 30g

Grind into powder and mix with flour and water to make into pills the size of mung beans. Give one pill each time washed down with rice soup for the treatment of watery diarrhea.

6. *Cang Zhu* (Rhizoma Atractylis), 6g
Chen Pi (Pericarpium Citri Reticulatae), 3g
Hou Po (Cortex Magnoliae), 6g
Ze Xie (Rhizoma Alismatis), 6g
Fu Ling (Poria), 6g
Huo Xiang (Herba Pogostemonis), 6g
Shen Qu (Massa Medica Fermentata), 5g
Che Qian Cao (Herba Plantaginis), 6g

Decoct in water and divide into 3 doses for oral administration for watery diarrhea.

7. *Ge Gen* (Radix Puerariae), 9g
Huang Lian (Rhizoma Coptidis), 3g
Huang Qin (Radix Scutellariae), 5g
Gan Cao (Radix Glycyrrhizae), 3g
Bai Shao (Radix Paeoniae Albae), 6g

Decoct in water and divide into 3 doses for oral administration for fire diarrhea.

8. *Huang Qin* (Radix Scutellariae), 9g
Huang Bai (Cortex Phellodendri), 9g
Bai Tou Weng (Radix Pulsatillae), 20g
Ge Gen (Radix Puerariae), 9g
Mu Xiang (Radix Auklandiae), 5g
Bai Shao (Radix Paeoniae Albae), 6g
Chi Shao (Radix Paeoniae Rubrae), 6g
Feng Wei Cao (Herba Pteridis), 20g

Decoct in water and administer orally in three doses for heat diarrhea.

Acute poisoning

1. *Bai Fan* (Alumen), 6g

Dissolve in boiling water and administer to hasten vomiting and, therefore, expel the poison.

2. *Mang Xiao* (Natri Sulfas), 15-30g

Dissolve in water and administer to clear the intestines and expel the poison.

3. powdered *Da Huang* (Radix Et Rhizoma Rhei), 9-15g

Stir into boiling water and administer to clear the intestines and expel the poison.

4. *Dang Gui* (Radix Angelicae Sinensis), 10g
   Da Huang (Radix Et Rhizoma Rhei), 30g
   Bai Fan (Alumen), 30g
   Gan Cao (Radix Glycyrrhizae), 15g

Decoct in water and divide into several doses for oral administration in order to clear the intestines and expel the poison.

5. *Che Qian Cao* (Herba Plantaginis)
   Bai Mao Gen (Rhizoma Imperatae), 30g each

Decoct in water and administer to disinhibit urination and resolve toxins.

6. *Lu Dou* (Semen Phaseoli Munginis), 60g
   Huang Lian (Rhizoma Coptidis), 6g
   Gan Cao (Radix Glycyrrhizae), 15g

Decoct in water, add brown sugar, and administer to treat Aconite poisoning.

7. *Sheng Jiang* (uncooked Rhizoma Zingiberis), several slices
   Shi Tang (Sugar), 60g

Decoct in water and administer for Arisaema poisoning.

8. *Gan Cao* (Radix Glycyrrhizae), 20g
   Lu Dou (Semen Phaseoli Munginis), 60g

Decoct in water and administer for Xanthium poisoning.

Nosebleed & hematemesis

1. *Bai Cao Shuang* (Pulvis Fumi Carbonisati), 6g

Mix with glutinous rice soup and administer for nosebleeding.

2. *Sheng Di* (uncooked Radix Rehmanniae)
   Xuan Shen (Radix Scrophulariae)
   Tian Men Dong (Tuber Asparagi), 20g each

Decoct in water and administer for nosebleeding.

3. *Zhi Zi* (Fructus Gardeniae)

Grind some of this medicinal into a fine powder and snuff into the nose for nosebleeding.

4. *Bai Ji* (Rhizoma Bletillae), 6g
Da Huang (Radix Et Rhizoma Rhei), 6g

Grind into a powder, stir into boiling water, and administer to treat hematemesis.

5. *Ren Shen* (Radix Ginseng), 6-9g
Sheng Di (uncooked Radix Rehmanniae), 30g

Decoct in water, chill, and administer for the treatment of massive hematemesis.

6. *Ce Bai Ye* (Cacumen Platycladi), 30g
Xue Yu Tan (Crinis Carbonisatus), 3g

Decoct the Biota in water, mix in the powdered carbonized hair, and administer to treat hematemesis.

7. *Wu Wei Zi* (Fructus Schisandraepensae), 10 pieces
Mai Men Dong (Tuber Ophiopogonis), 30g
Huang Qi (Radix Astragali), 30g

Decoct in water and administer to treat hematemesis which has lasted for days without healing.

Hematuria & hemafecia

1. *Bai Mao Gen* (Rhizoma Imperatae), 30g
Sheng Di (uncooked Radix Rehmanniae), 30g
Xiao Ji (Herba Cephanoploris), 12g

Decoct in water and administer for hematuria.

2. *Bai Mao Gen* (Rhizoma Imperatae), 30g
powdered *San Qi* (Radix Notoginseng), 6g

Decoct the *Bai Mao Gen* in water, mix in the *San Qi*, and administer to treat hematuria.

3. powdered *Da Huang* (Radix Et Rhizoma Rhei), 5-10g

Mix this powder into warm, boiled water and administer to treat hemafecia.

4. powdered *San Qi* (Radix Notoginseng), 3g
powdered *Bai Ji* (Rhizoma Bletillae), 3-9g

Mix into water and administer to treat hemafecia.

5. *Di Yu* (Radix Sanguisorbae)
blackened *Shan Zha* (Fructus Crataegi)
Huai Hua Mi (Flos Immaturus Sophorae), 5-15g each

Decoct in water and adiminster to treat hemafecia.

Subdermal bleeding & hemoptysis

1. *Huai Hua Mi* (Flos Immaturus Sophorae), 12g
Ce Bai Ye (Cacumen Platycladi), 10g
Da Zao (Fructus Jujubae), 60g

Decoct in water and administer to treat subdermal bleeding or purpura.

2. *Wu Mei* (Fructus Mume)
Dan Pi (Cortex Moutan)
Chi Shao (Radix Paeoniae Rubrae), 9g each
Fang Feng (Radix Saposhnikoviae), 6g
Da Zao (Fructus Jujubae), 7 pieces
Gan Cao (Radix Glycyrrhizae), 3g

Decoct in water and administer to treat subdermal bleeding.

3. *Jin Yin Hua* (Flos Lonicerae)
Lian Qiao (Fructus Forsythiae)
Dang Gui (Radix Angelicae Sinensis)
Sheng Di (uncooked Radix Rehmanniae)
Xuan Shen (Radix Scrophulariae)
Dan Pi (Cortex Moutan), 9g each
Sang Zhi (Ramulus Mori), 15g

Decoct in water and administer warm to treat subdermal bleeding.

4. powdered *San Qi* (Radix Notoginseng), 6g
Xue Yu Tan (Crinis Carbonisatus), 6g
Hua Rui Shi (Ophicalcitum), 24g

Grind into powder, divide into four doses, and administer to treat hemoptysis.

5. *Da Huang* (Radix Et Rhizoma Rhei)

Xue Yu Tan (Crinis Carbonisatus), 15g each
Qing Dai (Pulvis Indigonis)
Huai Hua Mi (Flos Immaturus Sophorae), 30g each

Grind into powder and take nine grams each time washed down with a decoction made from *Zhi Zi* (Fructus Gardeniae) and *Dan Pi* (Cortex Moutan) to treat hemoptysis.

6. *Bai Ji* (Rhizoma Bletillae), 15g
Ce Bai Ye (Cacumen Platycladi)
Xian He Cao (Herba Agrimoniae), 30g each

Decoct in water and administer to treat hemoptysis.

7. *E Jiao* (Gelatinum Corii Asini), 15g
Sheng Di (uncooked Radix Rehmanniae), 30g
stir-fried *Pu Huang* (Pollen Typhae), 15g

Decoct in water and administer to treat hemoptysis.

3
Case Histories

The following case histories give some idea how I treat infants and young children.

Cough

Case 1: The patient was a 9 1/2 month-old little girl. Her main complaint was a wet cough. She had green mucus coming from her nose. She was waking a lot at night and was having trouble breathing at night. For some time she had been having only one bowel movement every three days which was typically hard and dry. However, the day of the visit the child's stools were loose and contained mucus. Her mother also said that she had begun teething two days before.

The wet cough meant that there was excessive phlegm in the lungs. The fact that the visible mucus was green meant that there was pathological heat in the lungs. The constipation and dry stools likewise suggested that she was overheated, thus drying out the stools. However, the presently loose stools with mucus suggested spleen vacuity with excessive phlegm and dampness. Therefore, my diagnosis was lung heat with spleen dampness. In this case, the appropriate treatment principles were to clear heat from the lungs while fortifying the spleen and to transform phlegm and eliminate dampness. I wrote the child a Chinese herbal prescription which contained:

Zhi Mu (Rhizoma Anemarrhenae)
Bei Mu (Bulbus Fritillariae)
Ban Xia (Rhizoma Pinelliae)
Fu Ling (Poria)
Chen Pi (Pericarpium Citri Reticulatae)
Huang Qin (Radix Scutellariae)
Sang Bai Pi (Cortex Mori)
Zi Su Zi (Fructus Perillae)
Bai Zhi (Radix Angelicae Dahuricae)

In this formula, the *Zhi Mu*, *Huang Qin*, and *Sang Bai Pi* all clear heat from the lungs and upper part of the body. *Fu Ling*, *Chen Pi*, and *Ban Xia* all strengthen the spleen and eliminate dampness, while *Ban Xia*, *Chen Pi*, and *Bei Mu* transform phlegm. *Zi Su Zi* downbears the lung qi and thus helps stop cough, and *Bai Zhi* is a specific empirical remedy for green mucus coming from the nose. Thus each ingredient in this formula was chosen because its functions fulfilled one or more of the treatment principles or it relieved a specific symptom.

The mother was given one packet of the above and was instructed to boil these in two cups of water down to one cup. She was then to give the child two droppers of this "tea" 4-6 times each day. I also counselled the mother on eliminating dairy products and sugars and sweets, including fruit juices, from the child's diet. Three days later, the mother called back to say that the herbs had been "perfect." The phlegm was now 90% gone and the cough was almost nonexistent. At that point, I told the mother to discontinue the herbs and the child was completely better in a day or two.

Case 2: The patient was an eight month-old little girl. She had had a runny nose with yellow mucus for a couple of days. Recently she had developed a wet cough. Her mother said that she may be teething. There was no fever. The little girl was sleeping more than usual, her eyes were somewhat listless, and she had no appetite. Her extremities felt cold to the touch which her mother said were always that way since she had been born. There was a visible blue vein at the root of her nose between her two eyes. Thus my diagnosis was spleen vacuity and heat and phlegm in the lungs. The phlegm was shown by the wet cough, the heat by the yellow mucus, and the spleen vacuity by the cold extremities, fatigue, lack of appetite, and listless eyes. Therefore, the treatment principles were to fortify the spleen and supplement the qi, clear heat and transform phlegm. Although the diagnosis was similar in some regards to the previous patient's, in this case, spleen vacuity was more evident. The prescription I wrote contained:

Fu Ling (Poria)
Ban Xia (Rhizoma Pinelliae)
Chen Pi (Pericarpium Citri Reticulatae)
Dang Shen (Radix Codonopsitis)
Bai Zhu (Rhizoma Atractylodis Macrocephalae)
Huang Qin (Radix Scutellariae)
Xing Ren (Semen Armeniacae)
Zi Su Zi (Fructus Perillae)
Gu Ya (Fructus Germinatus Oryzae)
Ji Nei Jin (Corneum Endothelium Gigeriae Galli)

In this formula, *Dang Shen*, *Bai Zhu*, and *Fu Ling* all fortify the spleen and supplement the qi. *Ban Xia*, *Xing Ren*, *Zi Su Zi*, and *Chen Pi* transform phlegm and stop coughing. *Huang Qin* clears heat from the lungs. And *Gu Ya* and *Ji Nei Jin* help improve the appetite by eliminating any stagnant food in the stomach.

The patient's mother was instructed to make and administer this formula the same as for the preceding patient. I also instructed her on the importance of a clear, bland diet, no sugar or dairy, no fruit juices and raw foods. Two days later the mother called back to say that the child was no longer fatigued, her hands and feet were warmer, her appetite had returned, and her cough and runny nose had cleared up.

Vomiting

Case: The child was a two month-old little boy. He had been vomiting thick, white mucus ever since he was born one time every 2-3 or five days. For the past three weeks, he had been sounding very mucusy when he breathed. He was not colicky, but his stools were loose and watery. His mother said his urine was very pale, "amazingly clear." His appetite was reduced and he seemed fatigued. My diagnosis was vomiting due to a cold stomach. The white mucus, clear urine, fatigue, lack of appetite, and loose stools all pointed to a spleen vacuity cold type of vomiting with phlegm and dampness. Therefore, the treatment principles were to supplement the spleen and warm the center, transform phlegm and stop vomiting. The formula I wrote consisted of:

Ren Shen (Radix Ginseng)
Bai Zhu (Rhizoma Atractylodis Macrocephalae)
Ban Xia (Rhizoma Pinelliae)
mix-fried *Gan Cao* (Radix Glycyrrhizae)
Gan Jiang (dry Rhizoma Zingiberis)
Ding Xiang (Flos Caryophylli)
Wu Zhu Yu (Fructus Evodiae)
Rou Gui (Cortex Cinnamomi)

These were prescribed and administered the same as above. Four days later the mother reported that the child was much better. He had stopped vomiting, his stools were more formed, and he seemed much more energetic. In this formula, *Ren Shen*, *Bai Zhu*, and *Gan Cao* all fortify the spleen and supplement the qi. *Ban Xia* transforms phlegm and eliminates dampness. It also downbears the qi and vomiting is a symptom of erroneously upward counterflowing qi. *Gan Jiang*, *Ding Xiang*, *Wu Zhu Yu*, and *Rou Gui* all warm the center or stomach and also direct upwardly counterflowing qi downward.

Earache

Case 1: The child was a six year-old boy. He had had a bad cough for the preceding three days and now he had a bad earache. His stools were on the hard side and he had bad breath. His appetite was poor and he was fatigued. His tongue was red with a yellow coating and his pulse was slippery, full, and rapid. I diagnosed the earache as heat in the stomach and intestines counterflowing upward to accumulate in the ear. The treatment principles were, therefore, to clear heat from the lungs and stomach while supplementing the spleen. The formula I prescribed was a version of *Xiao Chai Hu Tang* (Minor Bupleurum Decoction):

Chai Hu (Radix Bupleuri)
Huang Qin (Radix Scutellariae)
Shi Gao (Gypsum Fibrosum)
Ban Xia (Rhizoma Pinelliae)

Dang Shen (Radix Codonopsitis)
mix-fried *Gan Cao* (Radix Glycyrrhizae)
Da Zao (Fructus Jujubae)
Sheng Jiang (uncooked Rhizoma Zingiberis)

At the same time I gave the mother some eardrops made from water, *Bai Fan* (Alumen), *Peng Sha* (Borax), and *Bing Pian* (Borneol). In addition, I needled *Pian Li* (LI 6). This is the point which controls the network vessel linking the stomach and intestines to the inner ear. For even more pain relief, I explained how to do alternating hot and cold compresses on the ear. The next day the earache was gone and the cough cleared up in another two days, at which time the child was back to normal.

Case 2: The child was a 16 month-old little boy. Nine months previously he had gotten his first ear infection. His pediatrician put him on antibiotics. Since then he had been on five different antibiotics. He would get an ear infection, take antibiotics, the ear infection would clear up, and it would come back again in five days to a week. At this point, the MD was recommending tubes in the ears. At the time I saw the child, his stools fluctuated between loose and normal. Sometimes he had asthmatic wheezing at night which was accompanied by cough and runny nose with the mucus ranging between being clear to yellow. He seemed paler than normal, a little puffy looking, and he had cold hands and feet. The day before seeing me, he had vomited a white, mucusy material. The vein at the base of his index finger was larger and more prominent than normal and was purple in color.

My diagnosis was spleen qi vacuity weakness with stagnant food and phlegm which periodically would transform into pathological heat. Because he did not have an earache at the time I saw this child, I prescribed a simple modification of *Xiao Chai Hu Tang* (Minor Bupleurum Decoction):

Chai Hu (Radix Bupleuri)
Dang Shen (Radix Codonopsitis)
Ban Xia (Rhizoma Pinelliae)
Huang Qi (Radix Scutellariae)
mix-fried *Gan Cao* (Radix Glycyrrhizae)
Da Zao (Fructus Jujubae)
Sheng Jiang (uncooked Rhizoma Zingiberis)
Shen Qu (Massa Medica Fermentata)

I told the mother to administer this formula to the child continuously for several months. I also gave her a long talk on proper diet. The child had been eating raw fruits and vegetables, cold fruit juices, cold milk, lots of bread, peanut butter, cheese, sugars and sweets, including ice cream and frozen yogurt — in other words, the full catastrophe. The mother said that it would be hard to change the child's diet so radically at this point, but she also said she would try. I told her that she could expect an earache as soon as the present course of antibiotics was finished and, when that happened, she should not run to the MD but rather call me.

Several days later, she did call me as predicted. The child had started batting at his ears as soon as the antibiotics were finished. His stools were very loose and an orangy-yellow color. There was the sound of mucus in his throat when he breathed. I prescribed a different version of *Xiao Chai Hu Tang*:

Chai Hu (Radix Bupleuri)
Ren Shen (Radix Ginseng)
Huang Qin (Radix Scutellariae)
Ban Xia (Rhizoma Pinellia)
mix-fried *Gan Cao* (Radix Glycyrrhizae)
Da Zao (Fructus Jujubae)
Sheng Jiang (uncooked Rhizoma Zingiberis)
Chen Pi (Pericarpium Citri Reticulatae)
Shi Chang Pu (Rhizoma Acori Tatarinowii)
Chuan Xiong (Rhizoma Chuanxiong)
Bai Zhi (Radix Angelicae Dahuricae)

The addition of *Chen Pi* was to eliminate dampness and transform phlegm. The *Shi Chang Pu* was to transform phlegm and open the portals of the ear. *Chuan Xiong* was meant to guide the other herbs up to the side of the head and to help stop pain. While *Bai Zhi* was meant to stop pain in the head and to clear heat and eliminate dampness in the head. In addition, I gave the child the same eardrops described in the previous case. Within a day the earache got better and the child went back to the original formula. Six months later, the child has not had another earache. His facial color is rosier, his hands and feet are warmer, and he does not look so pale and puffy. His breathing is clear and he seems to have more energy.

Diarrhea

Case: The child was a 2 1/2 month-old little boy. His mother brought him in to see me because he had explosive diarrhea which was greenish in color and which contained mucus. In addition, he drooled constantly, had hiccups two times a day for 15 minutes to an hour each time, and was real fussy due to gas pains. Sometimes he would scream and, when he screamed, his face would become very red and he would sweat. Otherwise he had cool hands and feet. My diagnosis of this case was spleen vacuity contracting fright. This meant that there was spleen vacuity and dampness but that this was aggravated by fright affecting the relationship between his spleen and liver. The treatment principles were, therefore, to fortify the spleen, relax the liver, and calm fright wind. The formula I wrote consisted of:

Dang Shen (Radix Codonopsitis)
Bai Zhu (Rhizoma Atractylodis Macrocephalae)
Fu Ling (Poria)
Ge Gen (Radix Puerariae)
Huo Xiang (Herba Pogostemonis)
Bian Dou (Semen Dolichoris)
Mu Xiang (Radix Auklandiae)
dry *Gan Jiang* (Rhizoma Zingiberis)

Bai Shao (Radix Paeoniae Albae)
Gou Teng (Ramulus Uncariae Cum Uncis)

This formula was made and administered the same as the others above. In this formula, *Dang Shen*, *Bai Zhu*, *Bian Dou*, *Fu Ling* and *Gan Jiang* fortify the spleen. *Huo Xiang* eliminates dampness. *Ge Gen* is empirically known to stop diarrhea. *Mu Xiang* harmonizes the liver and spleen. *Bai Shao* relaxes the liver and *Gou Teng* settles liver wind and calms fright. One week later, the mother called to say that the stools were now normal, the child had less colic, and that he was much happier ove all.

Thrush

Case: The patient was a six week-old little girl. She had thrush, gas, and cold hands and feet. Her nails were pale and the vein at the base of the index finger was fine and hardly visible. Although thrush is often due to dampness and heat, it may also be due to spleen vacuity. This is called vacuity pattern thrush and that is what this child's TCM pattern was. The treatment principles were to fortify the spleen and eliminate dampness. The formula consisted of:

Ren Shen (Radix Ginseng)
Bai Zhu (Rhizoma Atractylodis Macrocephalae)
Fu Ling (Poria)
Ge Gen (Radix Puerariae)
Mu Xiang (Radix Auklandiae)
Huo Xiang (Herba Pogostemonis)
Gan Cao (Radix Glycyrrhizae)

These herbs were prepared and administered the same as above. In this formula, *Ren Shen*, *Bai Zhu*, *Fu Ling*, and *Gan Cao* fortify the spleen. *Ge Gen* gets rid of heat due to spleen vacuity. *Huo Xiang* eliminates dampness. And *Mu Xiang* helps to regulate the qi, thus helping to eliminate gas. I also counselled the mother on sticking to a clear, bland diet. Incidentally, the mother had a long history of chronic candidiasis which had eventually developed into multiple sclerosis. After four days, this child's mother reported that she still had lots of gas but that her thrush was getting better. "The white stuff was coming loose." I represcribed the same formula but added *Bai Shao* (Radix Paeoniae Albae) to relieve the stomach cramps due to gas. After another two days, again the mother reported the thrush was still getting better. There was still some gas, but it did not seem to be so painful. We continued with this same formula for a total of 17 days after which there was no further thrush and no further colic.

Appendix 1
Developmental Mileposts

Although not strictly a part of traditional Chinese pediatrics, many parents, and especially those who do not have a Western medical pediatrician, will ask if their child's development is normal. Below are some general guidelines for practitioners to help answer parents' questions.

Height

Linear growth is measured with the child lying down on thier back if the child is under two years of age. If the child is over two, then they are measured standing up. Typically, infants height increases by 30% by five months and by more than 50% by one year. After that, height doubles by five years of age. From then to puberty, growth slows down, and then at puberty speeds back up again.

Weight

Growth in weight roughly parallels that of growth in height. The infant doubles their weight by five months and triples it by their first birthday. They then quadruple their weight by two years old. Between two and five years of age, the annual increments of weight are fairly similar. After five years, weight gain slows down until puberty when it increases again along with the height.

Teething

As the reader most likely already knows, the baby's first set of teeth are not their permanent teeth. These baby teeth are shed like leaves and are, therefore, called deciduous teeth similar to deciduous leaves shed in the fall. In terms of when these baby or deciduous teeth come in, the lower incisors should come in somewhere between 5-9 months. From 8-12 months, the upper central incisors come in. From 10-12 months, the upper lateral incisors break through, and from 12-15 months the lower lateral incisors come out. The first molars come in at between 10-16 months, the canines come in between 16 and 20 months, and the second molars break through somewhere between 20-30 months. These deciduous teeth are smaller than the permanent teeth which will replace them.

The second or permanent teeth begin to erupt somewhere after five years of age. For instance, the first molars come in between 5-7 years, the incisors erupt between 6-8 years, and the bicuspids break through between 9-12 years. Then the canines come in between 10-13 years, the second molars between 11-13 years, and the third molars between 17-25 years. These third molars are what are also called the wisdom teeth. Although both boys and girls develop their baby teeth at the same time, girls tend to get their permanent teeth earlier than boys.

Major developmental events

These are only rough guidelines. Individual children will do some of these things a bit earlier or later than others. When learning a new skill, it is common for the child to try something over and over without success, eventually becoming frustrated. Then they will not try that activity or skill for awhile. A bit later, they will suddenly be able to do that activity or skill as if from nowhere. Thus, often children will look like their development is going backwards when they are on the verge of making a new leap forward.

Birth

Newborns sleep most of the time. They can eat, clear their airway, and respond with crying to pain and displeasure.

Six weeks

By this time the child can look at objects in their line of sight. They can usually smile when spoken to and they can lie flat on their stomachs. If pulled into a sitting position, they cannot hold up their head, however.

Three months

By three months the child can smile spontaneously. They are vocalizing and they can follow a moving object with their eyes. They are capable of holding up their head themselves when sitting up and they can grasp objects placed in their hands.

Six months

By six months most children will be able to sit with support and to roll over. They can support themselves in a standing position, transfer objects from one hand to the other, and babble to toys.

Nine months

At nine months the child sits well, crawls, and pulls themself to a standing position. They usually say dada or mama, play pat-a-cake, and wave goodbye. They can also hold their own bottle.

One year

Most children this age can walk if held by their hand. They can speak several words and they can help to dress themselves.

Eighteen months

At this age the child walks well, can climb stairs holding on, turns several book pages at a time, speaks about 10 words, pulls toys on a string, and partially feeds itself.

Two years

By now most children run well, climb up and down stairs by themselves, turn single pages of a book at a time, can put on simple clothing, make simple 2-3 word sentences, and verbalize toilet needs. At this age, children are learning to be more independent, and necessarily so. Therefore, they often say no. For this reason, the age from 2-3 years is often called "the terrible twos."

Three years

The child can ride a tricycle, dresses well except for buttons and laces, counts to 10, uses plurals, questions constantly, and feeds itself well.

Four years

The child now alternates feet going up and down stairs, can throw a ball overhand, and can hop on one foot. They can copy a cross, they know at least one color, and can wash their hands and face. They also take care of their own toilet needs.

Five years

At this age, children can skip, catch a bounced ball, copy a triangle, know four colors, and dress and undress without assistance.

Appendix 2
Resources for Going Further

For more information on Chinese dietary therapy, see:

The Book of Jook: Chinese Medicinal Porridges, A Healthy Alternative to the Typical Western Breakfast by Bob Flaws, Blue Poppy Press, Inc., Boulder, CO, 1995. This book is specifically about Chinese medicinal porridges made with very simple combinations of Chinese medicinal herbs.

Chinese System of Food Cures: Prevention & Remedies by Henry C. Lu, Sterling Publishing Co., Inc., NY, 1986

Eating Your Way to Health — Dietotherapy in Traditional Chinese Medicine by Cai Jing-feng, Foreign Languages Press, Beijing, 1988

Harmony Rules: The Chinese Way of Health Through Food by Gary Butt & Frena Bloomfield, Samuel Weiser, Inc., York Beach, ME, 1985

A Practical English-Chinese Library of Traditional Chinese Medicine: Chinese Medicated Diet ed. by Zhang En-qin, Shanghai College of Traditional Chinese Medicine Publishing House, Shanghai, 1990

Prince Wen Hui's Cook: Chinese Dietary Therapy by Bob Flaws & Honora Lee Wolfe, Paradigm Publications, Brookline, MA, 1983. This book is an introduction to Chinese dietary therapy. Although some of the information it contains is dated, it does give the Chinese medicinal descriptions of most foods commonly eaten in the West.

The Tao of Healthy Eating: A Simple Guide to Healthy Eating According to Traditional Chinese Medicine by Bob Flaws, Blue Poppy Press, Inc., Boulder, CO, 1991. This book is a layperson's primer on Chinese dietary therapy. It includes detailed sections on the clear, bland diet as well as sections on chronic candidiasis and allergies.

The Tao of Nutrition by Maoshing Ni, Union of Tao and Man, Los Angeles, 1989

For more information on Chinese pediatric massage, see:

Chinese Pediatric Massage by Kyle Cline, Dharma Productions #301, Institute for Traditional Medicine, Portland, OR. This is a video tape.

Chinese Pediatric Massage: Parent's Reference Video by Kyle Cline, Dharma Productions #303, Institute for Traditional Medicine, Portland, OR. This is a video tape.

Chinese Pediatric Massage, Practitioner's Reference Manual by Kyle Cline, Institute for Traditional Medicine, Portland, OR, 1993

Chinese Pediatric Massage Therapy: A Parent's & Practitioner's Guide of the Treatment and Prevention of Childhood Disease by Fan Ya-li, Blue Poppy Press, Inc., Boulder, CO, 1994

Infantile Tuina Therapy by Luan Chang-ye, Foreign Languages Press, Beijing, 1989

Introduction to Chinese Pediatric Massage by Kyle Cline, Dharma Productions #302, Institute for Traditional Medicine, Portland, OR. This is a video tape.

A Parent's Guide to Chinese Pediatric Massage by Kyle Cline, Institute for Traditional Medicine, Portland, OR, 1993

For more information on the relationship of chronic candidiasis, allergies, and autoimmune diseases, see:

Allergies and Candida by Steven Roschlitz, Human Ecology Balancing Sciences, 1991

The Candidacans Yeast-free Cookbook by Pat Connolly, Keats Publishing, New Canaan, CT, 1985

The Candida Control Cookbook by Gail Burton, Aslan Publishing, Lower Lake, CA, 1993

Candida: The Symptoms, the Causes, the Cure by Luc de Schepper, self-published, Santa Monica, CA, 1990

Healthy at Last: Solutions to Chronic Ill Health by Cynthia Clinkscales, CEOM Publishing, Homer, AS, 1990

How to Prevent Yeast Infections, Yeast Consulting Services, P.O. Box 11157, Torrance, CA 90510

Solving the Puzzle of Your Hard-to-Raise Child by William G. Crook & Laura Stevens, Random House, NY, 1987

The Yeast Connection, A Medical Breakthrough by William G. Crook, Vintage Books, NY, 1986. Although this book was first written in 1986, it is still the standard for lay readers on chronic candidiasis in English.

The Yeast Connection Cookbook, William G. Crook & Marjorie Hunt Jones, Professional Books, 1989

The Yeast Connection & Women by William G. Crook, Professional Books, 1995. Although the title says this book is for women, in fact, it contains all the updated materials Dr. Crook has learned about candidiasis since writing the above-mentioned book in the 1980s.

The Yeast Syndrome by John Parks Trowbridge & Martin Walker, Bantam Books, NY, 1988

For more information on the possible side effects of immunizations, see:

DPT: A Shot in the Dark by Harris L. Coulter & Barbara Joe Fisher, Avery Publishing Group, NY

Epidemiology and Prevention of Vaccine Preventable Diseases by William Atkinson *et al.*, Department of Health and Human Services and Centers for Disease Control and Prevention, 1995, 2nd edition; 1-800-223-SHOT

Immunization: The Reality Behind the Myth by Walene James, Bergin & Garvey, MA, 1995, revised edition

The Immunization Resource Guide by Diane Rozario, Patter Publications, Burlington, IA, 1995, revised edition

Immunization: The Terrible Risks Your Children Face That Your Doctor Won't Reveal by Robert S. Mendelsohn, Second Opinion, 1993

Medicine: What Works & What Doesn't by the editors of *What Doctors Don't Tell You*, The Wallace Press, 1995

Vaccination and Immunization: Danger, Delusion and Alternatives by Leon Chaitow, C.W. Daniel Company Ltd., London, 2004

Vaccination: 100 Years of Orthodox Research Shows That Vaccines Represent a Medical Assault on the Immune System by Viera Scheibner, The Australia Print group, Maryborough, Victoria, 1993

Vaccinations: The Rest of the Story, *Mothering* (magazine), Santa Fe, NM, 1996, 2nd revised and expanded edition

Vaccination, Social Violence & Criminality: The Medical Assault on the American Brain by Harris L. Coulter, North Atlantic Books, Berkeley, CA, 1990

The Vaccine Guide by Randall Neustaedter, North Atlantic Books, Berkeley, CA, 1996

Vaccines: Are they Really Safe and Effective? A Parents Guide to Childhood Shots by Neil Z. Miller, New Atlantean Press, Santa Fe, NM, 1996

Vaccines by Stanley Plotkin & Edward Mortimer, W.B. Saunders, Philadelphia, 1994, 2nd edition

What About Immunization? Exposing the Vaccine Philosophy by Cynthia Cournoyer, Clear Communications, Grants Pass, OR, 1995

Organizations providing information on vaccinations

Vaccine Research Institute
P.O. Box 4182
Northbrook, IL 60065
Tel. 847-564-1403

National Vaccine Information Center (NVIC), Dissatisfied Parents Together (DPT)
512 W. Maple Ave. #206
Vienna, VA 22180
1-800-909-SHOT; Fax: 703-938-5768

Determined Parents to Stop Hurting Our Tots
915 S. University Ave.
Beaverdam, WI 53916
Tel. 414-887-1133

Parents for Freedom of Choice
7009 Caldwell Ln.
Plano, TX 75025
Tel. 214-517-4282

Citizens for Vaccination Liberation
2101 Pallets Ct.
Virginia Beach, VA 23454
Tel. 804-486-3129

Partenership for Individual Freedom
P.O. Box 685
Boonton, NJ 07005
Tel. 201-316-8142

Natural Immunity Information Network
209 E. 7th St.
NY, NY 10009
Tel. 212-979-7622

Vaccination Alternatives: The Right to Know,
the Freedom to Abstain
P.O. Box 346
NY, NY 10023
Tel. 212-873-5051

National Vaccine Injury Compensation Program
Health Resources & Services Administration
Parklawn Bldg., Room 8A-35
5600 Fishers Ln.
Rockville, MD 20857
1-800-338-2382

State exemptions

All states in the United States provide certain exemptions to otherwise compulsory pediatric immunizations. These exemptions fall into three categories: religious, medical, and philosophical. A religious exemption means that the parents of the child are members of a religious organization or hold religious beliefs that prevent them from immunizing their children. A medical exemption means that an MD has stated in writing that, in their professional reason, to immunize a particular child would place that child in some sort of medical risk. In other words, to obtain a medical exemption, an MD must be willing to say for the record that immunizations are contraindicated for a medical reason in a particular child. Philosophical exemptions mean that the parents simply hold a philosophical belief, for whatever reason, that immunizations are wrong for their child. This is the most lenient and liberal of these three types of immunization exemptions.

States with medical exemptions only

Mississippi   West Virginia

States with medical & religious exemptions

Alaska	Montana
Arkansas	Nevada
Connecticut	New Jersey
Delaware	New York
Florida	North Carolina
Georgia	Oregon
Illinois	Rhode Island
Indiana	South Carolina
Iowa	Tennessee
Kansas	Texas
Kentucky	Virginia
Maryland	Washington, DC
Missouri	Wyoming

States with medical, religious & philosophical exemptions

Alabama	New Hampshire
Arizona	New Mexico
California	North Dakota
Colorado	Ohio
Hawaii	Oklahoma
Idaho	Pennsylvania
Louisiana	South Dakota
Maine	Utah
Michigan	Vermont
Minnesota	Washington
Nebraska	Wisconsin

For more information on antibiotics, see:

The Antibiotic Paradox: How Miracle Drugs are Destroying the Miracle by Stuart B. Levy, Plenum Press, 1992

Beyond Antibiotics by Micheal Schmidt, Lenden H. Smith & Keith W. Sehnert, North Atlantic Books, 1993

How to Raise a Healthy Child, In Spite of Your Doctor by Robert S. Mendelsohn, Contemporary Books, 1984

The Plague Makers: How We Are Creating Catastrophe by Jeffrey Fisher, Simon & Schuster

Bibliography

Chinese language bibliography:

Er Ke Bing Liang Fang (Fine Formulas for Pediatric Diseases) by He Yuan-lin *et al.*, Yunnan University Press, Kunming, 1991

Er Ke Zheng Zhi (Pediatric Proven Treatments) by Cao Xu, Shanxi Science & Technology Press, Xian, 1980

Er Ke Zheng Zhi Xin Fa (Heart Methods of Proven Treatments in Pediatrics) by Cheng Shao-en *et al.*, Beijing Science & Technology Press, Beijing, 1990

Jian Ming Xiao Er Tui Na (Simple, Clear Pediatric Tuina) by Zhang Shi-da *et al.*, Shanxi People's Press, Xian, 1983

Xiao Er Bing Zheng Wai Zhi Fa (External Treatment Methods in Pediatric Diseases & Conditions) by Zhang Qi-wen, Shandong Science & Technology Press, Jinan, 1991

Xiao Er Tui Na (Pediatric Tuina) by Jin Yi-cheng, Shanghai Science & Technology Press, Shanghai, 1981

Xiao Er Xiao Hua Bu Liang (Pediatric Indigestion) by Zhou Run-zhi *et al.*, People's Health & Hygiene Press, Beijing, 1985

You Ke Tie Jing (The Iron Mirror of Pediatrics) by Xia Jiang, Qing dynasty, Chinese National Press, Beijing, 1987

You You Ji Cheng (Comprehensive Pediatrics) by Chen Fu-zheng, Yuan dynasty, People's Army Press, Beijing, 1988

Zhi You Xin Shu (The Heart Book of Treating Children) by Ceng Shi-rong, Yuan dynasty, Beijing Municipal Chinese National Book Store, Beijing, 1985

Zhong Yi Er Ke Lin Chuang Shou Ce (A Clinical Handbook of Chinese Medicine Pediatrics) by the Shanghai College of Chinese Medicine, Shanghai Science & Technology Press, Shanghai, 1983

Zhong Yi Er Ke Xue (A Study of Chinese Medicine Pediatrics) by the Guangdong College of Chinese Medicine, Shanghai Science & Technology Press, Shanghai, 1981

Zhong Yi Er Ke Xue (A Study of Chinese Medicine Pediatrics) by Guo Zhen-qiu, Shanghai Science & Technology Press, Shanghai, 1983

Zhong Yi Er Ke Xue (A Study of Chinese Medicine Pediatrics) by Jiang You-ren *et al.*, Shanghai Science & Technology Press, Shanghai, 1991

Zhong Yi Er Ke Xue (A Study of Chinese Medicine Pediatrics) by the Shanghai College of Chinese Medicine & the Shanghai Municipal Department of Health, People's Health & Hygiene Press, Beijing, 1983

Zhong Yi Zi Xue Cong Shu (Chinese Medicine Self-study Collection of Books): Er Ke (Pediatrics) by Yang Yi-ya, Hebei Science & Technology Press, Shijiazhuang, 1987

Zhong Yi Er Ke Zheng Zhi (Chinese Medicine Pediatrics Proven Treatments) by Zhou Tian-xin, Guangdong Science & Technology Press, Guangzhou, 1990

English language bibliography:

Acupuncture in the Treatment of Children, Revised Edition by Julian Scott, Eastland Press, Seattle, WA, 1992

A Barefoot Doctor's Manual, Revised & Enlarged Edition prepared by the Revolutionary Health Committee of Hunan Province, Cloudburst Press, Mayne Isle & Seattle, 1977

The English-Chinese Encyclopedia of Practical Traditional Chinese Medicine: Paediatrics ed. by Xu Xiang-cai, Higher Education Press, Beijing, 1991

Essentials of Traditional Chinese Pediatrics by Cao Ji-ming *et al.*, Foreign Languages Press, Beijing, 1990

The Merck Manual, 15th Edition ed. by Robert Berkow, Merck Sharp & Dohme Research Laboratories, Rahway, NJ, 1987

Pediatric Bronchitis: Its TCM Cause, Diagnosis, Treatment & Prevention by Xiao Shu-qin *et al.*, Blue Poppy Press, Inc., Boulder, CO, 1991

General Index

A
A Collection of Pediatric Cases, 3
A Study of Chinese Medicine Pediatrics, 8, 332
abdomen, full feeling in the upper, 172
abdomen, rubbing the, 77
abdominal distention, 14, 53, 63, 65-66, 70-71, 77, 80-82, 116-117, 137, 153, 159, 168, 173, 184, 198, 203, 218, 229, 233, 302
abdominal distention after eating, 53, 153, 233
abdominal distention, lower, 71
abdominal pain, acute, 308
abdominal pain and distention, 88-89
abdominal pain desiring pressure and warmth, 82
abdominal pain is relatively severe, 90
abdominal, lower, sagging and distention, 216
acid eructation, 81, 88
acupuncture, laser, 50
Aging & Blood Stasis, 9
air, fresh, 4
allergies, 8, 13, 15, 20, 33, 38, 41, 53, 96, 106, 130, 176, 181, 195-197, 206, 213, 226-227, 325-326
allergies, upper respiratory, 196
American Medical Association, 54
An Exposition on Pediatrics, 4
anal prolapse, 94
anaphylactic shock, 54, 56, 58
anger, easy, 86, 238, 241-242, 303

antibiotics, 51-55, 57, 59, 112, 121, 128-131, 166, 176-177, 180-181, 195, 278, 318-319, 330
antinuclear antibodies, 223
anuria, 306, 308
anus, dampness and itching of the, 21
appetite, poor, 110, 141, 238
arched neck rigidity, 164
arthritis, rheumatoid, 53, 112, 223, 226
asthma, 8, 13, 15, 30, 53, 130, 155, 164, 166-170, 175-176, 195-196, 204, 250, 259
asthma, chronic, 175
attention deficit disorder, 57, 237
auditory duct of the ear, swelling and pain of the, 21
autoimmune diseases, 53, 326
aversion to cold, 72, 90, 108, 113-115, 121, 127, 147-149, 155-157, 213, 218
aversion to wind, 114, 209, 261

B
Bao Ying Cuo Yao, 3
bed-wetting at night, 173, 239
Bei Ji Qian Jin Yao Fang, 3
bilirubin lights, 63
birth trauma, history of, 242
bleeding, subdermal, 312
block & repulsion, 306
blood, ejection of, 66, 151
blue vein at the bridge of the nose, 78, 82
body aches, 177
body and limbs, endless twitching move-

ment of the, 234
body, cold, 94, 169, 173, 225
body, weak, 67, 103, 295
Bordetella parapertussis, 147
Bordetella pertussis, 147
bowel movements, irregular, 226
brain damage, 56, 67
breast-feeding, 26, 33-34, 67, 77, 87, 100, 106
breast milk, substitutes for human, 33, 35
bad breath, 30, 81, 88, 101, 182, 198, 210, 229, 285, 287, 317
breath, shortness of, 142, 144, 155, 157-158, 160, 162, 167, 169, 171, 189, 205, 226, 238, 244, 256, 290, 298
breathing, difficulty, 167
breathing, exertion causing heart palpitations and rapid, 173
breathing, heavy, 141
breathing, obstructed, 159
breathing, rapid dyspneic, 68, 117, 169, 262, 285, 302
breathing, rough, 138
bronchitis, 8, 30, 41, 131, 155, 332
bruises, 290-291
burns, 290-291
burping and belching, 15, 86

C

candidiasis, 97, 101, 105-106, 176, 320, 325-327
candidiasis, polysystemic chronic, 106
canker sores, 20, 30, 211-212
case histories, 57, 315, 317, 319
Chao Yuan-fang, 3, 7
cheeks, red, redder than normal, 18, 85, 103, 141, 153, 169
lateral costal pain, 218
chest glomus, 159, 168
chest, fullness and oppression, 141, 145, 183, 241
chest, tight or heavy feeling in the, 110
chicken breast, 293, 298
chicken pox, 3, 11, 21, 57-58, 265, 267, 271
Chinese Pediatric Massage Therapy, 77
aversion to cold draft and chill 72, 90, 108, 113-115, 121, 127, 147-149, 155-157, 213, 218
cold, fear of, 144, 188, 221-222
cold hands and feet, 53, 78, 144, 318, 320
cold limbs, 18, 22, 65, 244, 246
cold limbs and a chilly sweat, 18
cold reversal, 306
cold sores, 186
colic, 13, 15, 33-35, 37, 41, 76-81, 320
common cold, 20, 38, 90, 131
cold, easily catches, 142-143, 225
conjunctivitis, 213-215
consciousness, loss of, 49, 120, 227, 230-231, 253, 305
constipation, 14, 37, 63-67, 73, 81-85, 102-103, 105, 112, 116-117, 122, 136, 138, 159, 167-168, 178, 180, 185, 187, 198, 210-212, 214, 220, 225, 229, 249, 255, 263-264, 269-270, 275-276, 286-288, 294, 303, 306, 315
convulsions, 19-20, 24, 49, 56-57, 81, 95, 113, 115, 117-118, 120, 122, 131, 155, 164, 247, 251, 260, 274, 277-278, 305
convulsions & seizures, 305
convulsions due to high fever, 122, 164, 247, 251
corneal opacity, slight, 20
cough, 13, 15, 24, 39, 41, 55, 58, 108, 110, 114, 131-132, 134-139, 141-147, 149-155, 157-162, 167, 169-170, 172-173, 177, 209, 244-245, 247-248, 250, 256-257, 259, 261-262, 265, 271, 276, 284, 287-288, 315-318
cough, dry, 24, 110, 160, 248, 276
cough, enduring, with little or no phlegm, 141
cough, heavy sounding, which is worse at night, 149
cough, severe, 158, 161, 244, 247, 250
cough, severe paroxysmal, 138
cough, spasmodic, with thicker, pastier phlegm, 150
cough, spasmodic, with thin, watery phlegm, 147
cough, strong, 24
cough, weak but enduring, 142
cough, weak, 24, 161
cough, wet, 24, 39, 315-316
cough, whooping, 55, 58, 147, 154-155

cough with thin, white or clear mucus, 132
cough with clear, watery, white-colored phlegm, 169
cough, with copious, white, watery phlegm, 175
cough with little or no phlegm, 136, 141
cough with profuse phlegm, 137, 170, 172, 245
cough with sticky, yellow phlegm, 157
Coulter, Harris L., 56, 327-328
cradle cap, 99-100
cry, forceless, 78
cry, loud energetic, 77
cry low weak, 67
cry, obstructed sound to their, 68
crying and restlessness, 76, 122
crying and shouting, 230-231
crying, excessive, 86, 101
crying, red face when, 77
cupping, 175, 180, 197, 206
cursing, incessant, 234
cuts, 195, 290-291

D

Dan Xi Xin Fa (Dan-xi's Heart Methods), 9
deafness, 121
decoctions, 31, 43, 49, 87, 208, 290, 298
defecation, neonate, non free-flowing, 69
delirium, 24-25, 247
dental caries, 20, 211
dermatitis, allergic, 196
development, abnormally slow, 293
developmental mileposts, 321, 323
diabetes, 53, 57
diaper rash, 21, 24, 96-97, 99
diarrhea, 9, 14-15, 24, 39, 41, 50, 53, 81, 88-96, 117-119, 214, 224, 229, 238, 245, 308-309, 319-320
diarrhea, enduring, 92, 94-95
diarrhea after eating, 92, 94
diarrhea, pain relieved by, 88
diarrhea, sudden, 308
diarrhea, watery, with reduced urination, 90
diarrhea which is sour or foul-smelling, 81

diarrhea of yellow water, 95
digestion, 8, 13-16, 19, 29, 35-38, 52-53, 77, 195, 296
digestion, poor, 15, 29, 296
diphtheria, 21, 55, 284, 290
Dissatisfied Parents Together, 57, 328
Dou Zhen Liang Fang, 4
Dou Zhen Shi Yi Xin Fa, 4
DPT, 55-57, 327-328
DPT: A Shot in the Dark, 56, 327
drink, desire to, 83, 102, 150, 167, 224, 247, 262, 273, 281
drink a lot yet no desire to eat food, 184
drinks, desire for cold, 141, 178, 206, 212, 214
drool, clear, running from the mouth, 103
drooling, excessive, 101, 107

E

ear blockage, 121
ear, greenish yellow, purulent discharge from the, 21
ear infections, 121, 127, 129-131
ear, pain in the, 122
ear, sounds inside the, 121
ear, swelling and pain of the auditory duct of the, 21
earache, 13, 16, 39, 107, 121, 130-131, 317-319
earaches, recurrent, 53, 124, 128, 130
earwax, increased, 124
eat, no desire to, 63, 262
eat or drink, refusal to, 101, 182, 184
eating and drinking, diminished, 122, 232
eczema, 13, 53, 141, 195-197, 199
eyelids, edema of the, 152, 221
electroacupuncture, 50
emaciated, thin muscles and flesh, 92
emaciation, 103, 119, 172, 257
emotional restlessness, 79
emotional tension and agitation, 190, 236, 304
encephalitis, 56, 58, 120, 131, 282
endangered species, 47
epilepsy, 113, 120, 227-234, 237
epilepsy, chronic and enduring, 232
Er Ke Zheng Zhi Xin Fa, 76, 331
eructation, acid, 81, 88

essence spirit depression and oppression, 86
essence spirit, extreme listlessness of the, 118
Essentials for the Care & Protection of Infants, 3
Essentials of the Golden Cabinet, 3
external genitalia are red and moist, 21
eyelids, edema of the, 152, 221
eyes and fontanel, sunken, 95
eyes, both staring upward, 116, 164
eyes, brightly colored yellow skin and, 63
eyes, dull yellow skin and, 65
eyes feel dry and rough, 258
eyes, frightened looking, when crying, 79

F

face flushed, in the late afternoon and evening, 141
face is bluish green, 117
face, pale, with flushed cheeks, 123
face, white, and pale lips, 71
face, white, edematous, 18
face, yellowish, and pale lips, 160
facial complexion, bluish grey, 250, 254
facial complexion, bright yellow, 18
facial complexion, darkish, dull, 144
facial complexion, dirty looking, 159
facial complexion, dull white or somber white, 171
facial complexion, flushed red, 119
facial complexion, green-blue, 18
facial complexion, greyish greenish, 79
facial complexion, lusterless, 111, 172, 182, 232, 299
facial complexion, pale, 18, 78, 139, 141-142, 161, 188, 205, 246
facial complexion, red, 18, 119
facial complexion, sallow yellow, 92, 118, 124, 184, 222, 226
facial complexion, somber or dull white, 173
facial complexion, yellow, 18, 92, 118, 124, 184, 222, 226, 236
facial complexion, yellow, lusterless, 172
fainting, 305
Family Secrets in Pediatrics, 4
Fan Ya-li, 77, 326

fatigue, 24, 53, 63, 65, 91, 111, 123, 125, 143-144, 153, 168, 171-172, 183-184, 205, 238, 246, 249, 289, 316-317
febrile seizures, 57
feeding, scheduled, 34-35
feeding, unregulated, 22, 24, 34
feet, and heart, heat in the hands, 85, 141, 153, 185, 236, 300-301
feet, heat in the centers of the hands and, 119
lack of warmth particularly in the feet, 173
feet, spasms and contractions of the hands and, 230
fetal toxins, 11, 57-58, 243-244
fever, and a red face, 101
fever blisters, 186
fever, high, 24, 49, 109, 111, 113-115, 120, 122, 126, 134-135, 138, 146, 158, 164, 178, 223, 244, 246-247, 250-251, 253, 260, 263-264, 266-267, 272-274, 276-278, 281-282, 285, 287, 305
fever, high, which does not abate, 109, 247
fever, low-grade, 111, 119, 160-161, 219, 224, 276, 287
fever, slight or mild, 24, 58, 132, 147, 155, 261, 279, 284
fever, slight, with no perspiration, 155
fever, tidal, 85, 110, 119, 142, 153, 224, 253, 257, 260
fever, tidal, in the afternoon, 85
Fine Formulas for Poxes & Rashes, 4
Fine Formulas in Pediatrics, 4
finger vein, pale purplish, 259
finger vein is purplish and stagnant, 117
finger vein, red, 219, 257, 298
Fisher, Barbara Loe, 56
five hards, 292, 296
five slows, 292-293
five softs, 292-293, 295
flatulence, 182, 198
flesh, withered and shrunken muscles and, 224
flesh, thin muscles and, 92
fontanel, sunken eyes and, 95
fontanelles, non-closure of the, 300
foods, introducing solid, 36, 39

foreign objects, imbedded, 292
fright tremors and spasms, 94

G
Gao Yu-li, 41
genitalia, external, are red and moist, 21
glands, swollen, 13, 39, 41, 176-177, 181, 281, 283
glomus and lumpiness, right-sided, 66
goat's milk, 35
gua sha, 112, 145, 165, 175, 180
Guillain-Barre syndrome, 57
gums, bleeding, 211, 255, 286
gums, red, swollen, 20
guts, leaky, 52

H
hair, withered and brittle or sparse, 19
hair, soft, which easily falls out, 295
Halloween, 39, 129, 146
hands and feet, hot, 137
hands and feet, spasms and contractions of the, 230
hands and feet, squirming movements of the, 118
hands, feet and heart, heat in the, 85, 141, 153, 185, 236, 300-301
He Meng-yao, 4
head, large, but fine neck, 300
headache, 24, 108, 113-115, 120, 132-133, 177, 209, 213, 216, 231, 265, 271, 281, 302
headache, severe, 115, 120
Heart Methods Handed Through the Generations for Poxes & Rashes, 4
Heart Methods of Proven Treatments in Pediatrics, 331
heart palpitations, 173, 238-239, 277-278
heart palpitations, exertion causing, 173
heart vexation, 102, 114-115, 135, 234, 248, 250, 254, 259-260, 268, 285
hemafecia, 74, 311-312
hematemesis, 74, 310-311
hematuria, 22, 311
hemoptysis, 151, 312-313
hemorrhage, intracranial, 242
Hempel, Velia, 56
Herpes simplex, 186

hiccup, 15
hives, 195-196, 200, 202, 204
How to Raise a Healthy Child In Spite of Your Doctor, 181, 330
hunger, frequent, 214
hypertonicity, bodily, 115

I
immune deficiencies, 53
immunizations, 51, 53-59, 327, 329
impetigo, 21-22, 192, 194-195, 199
inhalation, noisy, 284
injuries, traumatic, 41, 290-291
insect stings, 292
insomnia, 228, 231, 238-239, 302
Institute of Medicine, 55-56
intelligence, slow, 295
intestinal gas, 81
intestinal noises, 90
intestinal parasites, 18-20, 202
intracranial hemorrhage, 242
irritability, 137, 241, 247
irritability, pronounced, 241
itching, incessant, 263

J, K
jaundice, neonatal, 63, 67
Jin Gui Yao Lue, 3
joints, red, swollen painful, 223-224
joints, swollen, distended, abnormally formed, 226
Keeping Your Child Healthy with Chinese Medicine, 29

L
laser acupuncture, 50
lateral costal pain, 218
leaky guts, 52
legs, lack of strength in the lower, 173
legs, pumping of the, to the abdomen, 77
Li Dong-yuan, 10
Li Shi-zhen, 25-26
life bar, 23-24
limbs, chilled, 18, 90, 94, 173, 188, 225, 251
limbs, endless twitching movement of the body and, 234
limbs, icy chill of the four, 118

limbs, lack of strength in the four, 110
limbs, lack of warmth in the four, 67, 82-83, 162, 169, 171, 250
limbs, rigidity of the body and, 119
limbs, tremors of the four, 113, 119, 164, 228
Ling Shu, 7
lips, chapped, 136, 248
lips, cyanotic, 19, 158, 162, 250-251, 256, 285
lips, dark red, 66, 262
lips, dry, 110, 153, 158, 219, 263, 269, 276, 287
lips, dry red, 83
lips, pale, 67, 71, 111, 160, 238, 295
lips, recurrent blistery lesions on the, 187
listlessness, 66, 92, 96, 117-119, 221, 228, 230, 232, 256-257, 289, 294-295, 298
Liu Fang, 3
low back and knee soreness and weakness, 123
lymph nodes, submaxillary swollen, 179

M

Macrobiotics, 34
macules, static, 66, 231
Mai Jing, 3
massage, 4, 30, 49, 77, 100, 112, 120, 129, 155, 166, 176, 194, 326
massage, Chinese pediatric, 4, 30, 49, 77, 112, 326
Master Shen on the Importance of Preserving Life, 4
measles, 3, 20-21, 57-58, 155, 185, 243-244, 246, 250-251, 253-261, 265
memory, poor, 238
Mendelsohn, Robert S., 181, 327, 330
meningitis, 56, 120, 131
milk, soy, 35
Morris, Dr., 55
mouth and lips, dry, 63
mouth and nose, dry, 209
mouth and throat, dry, parched, 84
mouth, 18-20, 22, 31, 36, 48, 63, 67, 70-71, 84, 87, 95, 101-103, 105, 110, 122, 124, 136, 150, 160, 169, 178, 180, 184, 186-187, 209, 212, 218, 227, 234, 236, 242, 245, 248, 253, 267, 269-270, 285, 287, 290, 295-296, 300-302
mouth, bitter taste in the, 122, 178, 218
mouth, bland taste in the, 110
mouth, dry, 63, 71, 95, 102-103, 110, 124, 150, 160, 169, 184, 186, 209, 212, 253, 267, 269-270, 287, 300, 302
mouth, dry tongue and, 70
mouth, dry, but no thirst, 103
mouth, dry, but only scanty drinking, 110
mouth, white slimy coating or membrane over the, 101
movement and arising are retarded and slow, 293
moxibustion, 4, 33, 49, 69-70, 72, 80, 86, 95, 105, 111, 120, 126, 145, 154, 165, 175, 180, 185, 187, 191, 204, 206-207, 211, 215, 222, 226, 233, 237, 243, 260, 264, 270, 277, 283, 290, 295-296, 298, 300, 302
multiple sclerosis, 53, 320
mumps, 21, 58, 279, 283-284
muscles and flesh, withered and shrunken, 224
muscles, flaccid, 141
muscular aches and pain, 108

N

nasal congestion, 108, 121, 132, 204-205, 213, 265
nasal flaring, 158
nasal mucus, dry, yellow, 20
nasal obstruction, 91, 175
National Academy of Science, 55
nausea, 84, 89, 91, 110, 115, 183, 216, 218, 224, 241
nausea and vomiting, 89, 115, 216
nausea upon eating, 84
neck, large head but fine, 300
neck not able to hold the head upright, 295
neck, rigidity of the, 19
night sweats, 110, 119, 123, 142, 153, 160, 219, 224, 239, 257
night-crying, 76, 88
nose, crusting around the, 20
nose, itchy, 168, 204-205
nose, runny, 14, 20, 39, 108, 114, 121, q132, 141, 147, 175, 177, 204-205, 261,

265, 316-318
nose, sound of phlegm obstructing the, 24
nose, stuffy, 14, 20, 234
nose, turbid runny, 141
nose, visible blue vein at the bridge of the, 82
nose, wings of the, tremble, 20
nosebleed, 150, 209-212, 310

O

oral cavity, numerous sores and lesions in the, 101
oral mucosa, pale, 103
oral sores, 101
oral thrush, 101, 105

P

pain relieved by diarrhea, 88
panting, 167-168, 170, 250-251, 259
Pao Zhi: An Introduction to the Use of Processed Chinese Medicinals, 46
parapertussis, 147
glands, inflammation of the parotid, 279
parotid glands, swelling and distention of the, 281
parotitis, epidemic, 21, 279
pattern discrimination, ten different methods of, 26
Pediatric Bronchitis: Its TCM Cause Diagnosis Treatment & Prevention, 41, 332
perspiration, easy, 184
perspiration, slight, 108, 149, 177
perspiration, spontaneous, 111, 142, 153, 161, 171, 173, 189, 205, 224, 230
pertussis, 55-56, 112, 147, 155
phlegm, blood-streaked, 141-142, 150
phlegm, sound of, rattling in the throat, 139, 160, 169
Pi Wei Lun, 10
pink eye, 213
plantar warts, 206
pneumonia, 19-20, 44, 55, 58, 147, 155, 162, 165-166, 250
poison ivy, 207-208
poisoning, acute, 309
polio, 57

polysystemic chronic candidiasis, 106
prickly heat, 97-98
psoriasis, 196
Pulse Classic, 3
pupils, abnormally dilated or contracted, 20

Q, R

qi bar, 23-24, 116, 263
Qian Yi, 3, 7
Qian Zhong-yang, 3
Qin Bo-wei, 43
rash indistinct bright red,, 271
rash, moist, red, made up of water blisters, 265
rash, red maculopapular, starting first behind the ears, 247
rash, red, swollen, which is scaly and hard, 198
rash, with bright red macular eruptions, 22
rash, with fine, raised papules which then become water blisters, 21
rash, with pale-colored wheels, 200
rash, with red-colored wheels, 201
rash, with small, fine papular eruptions, 21
rash, with turbid pus-filled lesions with red bases, 22
respiration, weak, 67
restlessness, 76, 79, 86, 102, 105, 115, 119, 122, 126, 137, 158, 162, 214, 227, 230-231, 241, 244, 247, 251, 259-260, 263, 268, 277, 300-302
restlessness when lying down at night, 137
rheumatoid arthritis, 53, 112, 223, 226
rice soup, 35-37, 165, 308-310
rubella, 11, 21, 57-58, 261, 265
rubeola, 11, 243

S

sclera, black or dark bluish spots in the, 20
sclera, yellow, 20
scrotum is unusually flaccid, 21
seizures, febrile, 57
sexual development, premature, 303-304

shan gen, 19
Shang Han Lun, 10
Shen Shi Zan Sheng Su, 4
shock, 54, 56-58, 305
shonishin, 50
sinews and bones atonic and weak, 293
skin and eyes, brightly colored yellow, 63
skin and eyes, Dull yellow, 65
skin colored bluish green and purple, 231
skin dry, 185
skin feels hot to the touch, 98
skin itches incessantly, 259
skull, enlarged, 300
split skull, 293, 300
sleep, difficulty going to, at night, 259
sleep, restless, 86, 88, 153, 233
talking in their sleep, 190
sleeping habits, 19
sleeping, sudden jerking movements while, 86
sneezing, 8, 14, 132, 204
solid foods, introducing, 36, 39
soy milk, 35
spasms and contractions of the hands and feet, 230
spasms and tremors, forceless, indistinct, 117
spasms and tremors of the four limbs, 113, 164, 228
speak, disinclination to, 25, 111, 142, 153, 161, 171, 189, 205, 226
speech, delirious, 114, 164, 248, 251, 273, 277
spine in the upper back protrudes dorsally, 299
spirit clouding, 63, 117, 227, 251, 273, 277, 305
spirit, depressed, 184
spirit, lassitude of the, 66, 78, 90, 92, 103, 111, 119, 123, 139, 142, 144, 161, 169, 189, 229, 232, 287-288
Spiritual Pivot, 7
sprains & strains, 291
staring straight ahead, 20
startled reactions, 19
startle reflex, exaggerated, 113, 227
sternum protrudes abnormally outward, 298

Stewart, Gordon, 55
stomachache, 14-15
stools, blood and pus or mucus in the, 22
stools, dry, 22, 110, 119, 135, 167, 185-187, 273, 276, 315
stools, dry, constipated, 302
stools, foul-smelling, 83, 88, 101
stools, greenish, 94
stools, greyish white, 66
stools, incomplete, 172
stools, light colored, with no foul odor, 92
stools, loose, 22, 37, 39, 53, 64-66, 78-79, 82, 88, 92, 101, 103, 110-111, 118, 137, 141, 143, 153, 161, 168, 172-173, 184, 189-190, 205, 221-222, 224, 238, 256, 301-302, 315, 317
stools loose, containing white milk curds, 22
stools,, loose, foul-smelling, 101
stools, loose, which are greenish in color, 79
stools not crisp, 183
stools, small, hard, round, dry, 22
stools, tendency to loose, 238
stools, undigested food in the, 94, 184
stools, watery, loose, 173
strength, lack of, 63, 110, 119, 125, 142-143, 153, 171-173, 189, 205, 229, 232, 246, 287-288, 298
strep throat, 181, 271
Streptococcus pneumoniae, 155
subdermal bleeding, 312
sudden infant death syndrome, 57
Sun Si-miao, 17
swallowing, desire to eat but difficulty, 102
swallowing, difficulty, 102, 177, 279, 281, 284
sweating but no reduction in the fever, 134
sweating, excessive, 141, 143
sweating profuse, from the forehead, 118
sweating, no, 108, 113, 115, 148, 156, 244, 246, 274
sweating on slight exertion, 111
sweats, night, 110, 119, 123, 142, 153, 160, 219, 224, 239, 257
swollen glands, 13, 39, 41, 176-177, 181,

281, 283

T
Tao Xi-yu, Dr. (Eric) 15, 41, 50
teeth are particularly slow in growing, 294
teeth clenched tightly shut, 164
teething, 18, 106-107, 121, 127, 195, 315-316, 321
tetanus, 55-56
The Heart Book of Pediatrics, 3
The Merck Manual, 77, 80-81, 332
thirst and a preference for cold drinks, 210
thirst, annoying or upsetting, 109
thirst, oral, 72, 82-84, 91, 115, 135, 149, 156, 158, 178, 206, 216, 220, 224, 250, 262-263, 271, 273, 281, 285, 303
thirst with a desire for hot drinks, 169
thirst with a desire to drink, 150, 167, 224, 247, 273, 281
dry throat, 110, 122, 141, 153, 179, 219
dry, sore throat, 136
greyish white membrane covering the back wall of the throat, 21
red and inflamed throat*****
throat is red and inflamed, 20
throat, sore, 25, 121, 127, 134, 136, 149, 176-179, 245-246, 253, 270-271, 276, 279, 281, 283-284, 341
throat, greyish white membrane covering the back wall of the, 21
throat, red, 114, 134, 179
throat, red, painful, 108
throat, severe sore, 178
throat, slight sore, 179
throat, sound of phlegm rattling in the, 139, 160, 169
throat, strep, 181, 271
throat, swelling, pain, erosion, and ulceration of the, 273
thrush, oral, 101, 105
timidity, excessive, 227
tongue, moist glossy mouth and, 70
tongue sores, 103, 255
tongue, static spots on the, 66
tongue, ulcers and lesions on the tip or top of the, 102

tonsillitis, 21, 30, 38, 49, 53, 129-130, 176-177, 179-181, 271
tonsils are swollen and inflamed, 21
tonsils, red, swollen, 177
tonsils, swollen, 177-179
tonsillitis, recurrent, 53, 180
toothache, 212
torpid intake, 65-66, 78, 152, 184, 189, 218, 220, 224, 226
Tourette's syndrome, 234, 237
toxicity, 46
traumatic injuries, 41, 290-291
Treatise on Damage [Due to] Cold, 10
Treatise on the Origins of Pediatric Diseases & Their Treatments, 7
Treatise on the Spleen & Stomach, 10
tremors and spasms, fright, 94
tremors of the four limbs, 113, 119, 164, 228
turtle back, 293, 299

U
ulcers, 101-103, 105
umbilical bleeding, 74
umbilical dampness, 72
umbilical region, various conditions, 72
umbilical sore, 72
undigested water and grains, 92
upper respiratory allergies, 196
urinary tract, burning pain in the, 216
urination, copious clear, 144
urination, difficult, astringent, painful, 219
urination, frequent, 216, 220-221, 223
urination, frequent, urgent, short, red, 218
urination non free-flowing, in a neonate, 71
urination, short, reddish, 102, 110, 227, 263, 267, 302
urination, reddish, 102, 110, 227, 250, 263, 267, 302
urination, short scanty, 95
urine, reddish, 22, 250
urine, short, yellowish, 66
urine is dark yellow frequent and painful or burning, 22
urine, deep yellow, 63

urine, turbid, like rice-washing water, 219

V, W

Vaccine Advisory Committee, 55
Vaccine Injury Compensation Program, 54, 329
vacuity vexation and restlessness, 162
varicella, 265
vein, finger, is blue-green and purple, 116
vein, finger, is purplish and stagnant, 117
vein, pale purplish finger, 259
vein, purplish engorged, at the wind bar, 88
vein, red finger, 219, 257, 298
vein, visible blue, at the bridge of the nose, 82
vexation and agitation, 68, 70-72, 77, 82-83, 86, 95, 101, 114-115, 153, 156, 164, 186, 218, 263, 267, 270, 281, 288, 300
voice, hoarse, 254-255, 287-288
voice, weak, 25, 111, 153
voice, low, 171
voice, feeble, 70, 161, 236
vomiting, 9, 14-15, 24, 26, 37, 41, 50, 65-66, 68, 70, 78, 81-89, 95-96, 113, 115-118, 137, 148, 152, 169, 183, 216, 218, 227, 229-230, 245, 255, 271, 278, 281, 306, 308-309, 317
vomiting and diarrhea of sour putrid substances, 229
vomiting drool, 227, 230
vomiting is without force, 82
vomiting of milk, 26, 78, 81, 113
vomiting of sour water, 86
vomiting of sticky phlegm, 137
vomiting, projectile, 83, 87-88
vomitus looking just like the milk, 82
vomitus, sour, foul-smelling, 83
Wai Tai Mi Yao, 3
Wan Mi-zhai, 3
Wan Quan, 3-4
Wang Luan, 3
warts, 206-207
warts, plantar, 206
wheezing, 14, 24, 142-145, 157-160, 167, 171, 254, 318
wheezing and dyspnea, 159-160
wheezing provoked by movement, 144
whooping cough, 55, 58, 147, 154-155
wind, aversion to, 114, 209, 261
wind bar, 22-24, 88, 137

X

Xiao Er Bing Yuan Fang Lun, 7
Xiao er tui na, 4, 331
Xiao Er Yao Zheng Zhi, 3, 7
Xiao Er Yao Zheng Zhi Jue, 3, 7
Xiao Shu-qin et al., 41, 332
Xue Liang-wu, 3

Y

Yan De-xin, 9
You Ke Fa Hui, 4
You Ke Lei Cui, 3
You Ke Liang Fang, 4
You You Xin Shu, 3
Yu Ying Jia Mi, 4

Z

Zhen Jiu Da Cheng, 4
Zhong Yi Er Ke Xue, 8, 332
Zhou You-fan, 17
Zhu Bing Yuan Hou Lun, 3, 7
Zhu Dan-xi, 9

Formula Index

A, B

An Gong Niu Huang Wan, 73, 116, 165, 252-253, 274
Ba Zhen Tang, 125, 131, 226, 296
Ba Zhen Tang Jia Jian, 226
Ba Zhen Tang Jia Wei, 125
Ba Zheng San, 216
Bai Hu Cheng Qi Tang, 212
Bai Hu Tang, 122, 211-212
Bai Mao Gen Tang, 217
Bai Tou Weng Tang Jia Jian, 258
Bao He Wan, 30, 77, 81, 88, 117, 137, 229
Bao He Wan Jia Jian, 81, 88, 117, 137, 229
Bao Ying Wan, 30
Bei Xie Shen Shi Tang, 197
Bei Xie Shen Shi Tang Jia Jian, 197
Bi Yan Pian, 206
Bu Shen Di Huang Wan, 295, 300
Bu Shen Er Xian Tang, 241
Bu Shen Huo Xue Tang, 241
Bu Shen Yi Zhi Tang, 240
Bu Tian Da Zao Wan Jia Jian, 298-299
Bu Zhong Yi Qi Tang, 105-106, 111, 189-190, 205, 256, 295
Bu Zhong Yi Qi Tang Jia Jian, 190, 256
Bu Zhong Yi Qi Tang Jia Wei, 205

C, D

Cang Ling Tang, 91
Chang Pu Wan, 294
Chang Pu Wu Wei San, 241
Chang Zhi Long Mu Tang, 242
Chu Feng Xiao Zhen Fang, 201
Cong Rong Wan, 294
Da Bu Yuan Jian, 229
Da Cheng Qi Tang, 117
Da Ding Feng Zhu Jia Jian, 119
Da Huang Gan Cao Tang, 84
Da Qing Long Tang Jia Wei, 156
Dang Gui Hong Hua Yin, 247
Dang Gui Si Ni Tang Jia Jian, 297
Dang Gui Si Ni Tang Jia Wei, 297
Dao Chi San Jia Jian, 78
Dao Chi San Jia Wei, 71, 250
Di Gu Pi Yin Jia Jian, 257
Di Tan Tang, 231
Die Da Wan, 292
Ding Chen Si Jun Zi Tang, 83
Ding Chuan Er Hao, 164
Ding Chuan Tang, 167, 170
Ding Chuan Tang Jia Jian, 167, 170
Ding Jing Wan Jia Jian, 227
Ding Ming San, 117
Ding Po Wan Jia Jian, 228
Ding Shi Qing Luo Yin Jia Jian, 224
Ding Tu Wan, 86
Ding Xian Wan, 231
Ding Yu Li Zhong Tang Jia Wei, 83
Du Shen Tang, 68, 70-71

E

Er Chen Tang Jia Wei, 130, 140-141, 173
Er Dong Tang, 151
Er Huang Er Zi Tang, 168
Er Miao San, 72, 193, 198, 208
Er Miao San Jia Wei, 72, 193, 208
Er Zhi Zi Yin Yin, 220

F, G

Fang Feng Tong Shen San Jia Jian, 202
Fei Zi Fen, 98
Fu Tu Yi Mu Tang, 236
Fu Zi Li Zhong Tang, 94, 301
Gan Lu Xiao Du Dan, 64, 102, 183
Gan Lu Xiao Du Dan Jia Jian, 102, 183
Gan Lu Yin, 211-212
Gan Mai Da Zao Tang, 239
Ge Gen Qin Lian Tang, 91-92, 96, 258
Ge Gen Qin Lian Tang Jia Jian, 92
Ge Gen Qin Lian Tang Jia Wei, 91, 258
Ge Gen Sha Shen Tang, 220
Ge Gen Tang Jia Jian, 113
Gu Ben Pei Yuan Fen, 174
Gui Pi Tang, 74, 239
Gui Pi Tang Jia Jian, 74
Gui Pi Tang Jia Wei, 74
Gui Zhi Jia Huang Qi Tang Jia Jian, 172
Gui Zhi Shao Yao Zhi Mu Tang, 225
Gui Zhi Tang, 108, 114, 143, 171, 200, 238
Gui Zhi Tang Jia Jian, 200

H, I

Hang Xie Dan, 69
He Che Ba Wei Wan Jia Jian, 232
He Qi Yin, 90
Hu Gu San Jia Jian, 293
Hua Ban Tang, 254
Hua Du Dan, 302
Hua Gai San Jia Jian, 156
Hua Shi San, 218
Hua Tan Xi Feng Tang, 235
Huang Bai Shi Wei Tang, 217
Huang Lian Jie Du Tang, 122, 270, 286
Huang Lian Jie Du Tang Jia Wei, 270
Huang Lian Wen Dan Tang Jia Jian, 242
Huang Qi Jian Zhong Tang, 131
Huang Qin Hua Shi Tang, 218
Hui Yang Jiu Ji Tang Jia Jian, 256
Huo Lian Tang, 84
Huo Po Huang Lian Tang Jia Jian, 84
Huo Po Xia Ling Tang, 110
Huo Tan Xi Feng Tang, 234
Huo Xiang Zheng Qi San Jia Jian, 90

J

Ji Sheng Shen Qi Wan, 221-222
Jia Jian Sheng Jiang San, 248
Jia Wei Jie Geng Tang, 255
Jia Wei Liu Wei Di Huang Wan, 293
Jia Wei Wen Dan Tang, 84
Jia Wei Xiao Du Yin, 259, 262, 268
Jian Pi Bu Shen Tang, 184
Jian Pi Hua Tan Tang, 140
Jian Pi Wan Jia Jian, 78
Jian Pi Xiao Ji Tang, 183
Jiang Can Jing Gong Yin, 201
Jie Du Xie Re Yin, 270
Jie Gan Jian, 86
Jie Ji Tou Sha Tang, 273
Jie Xiao Tang, 171
Jin Fu Hua San Jia Jian, 148
Jin Gui Shen Qi Wan Jia Jian, 174
Jin Gui Shen Qi Wan Jia Wei, 173-174
Jin Huang San, 73, 187
Jin Sha San Jia Wei, 217
Jin Suo Gu Jing Wan, 188, 192
Jing Fang Bai Du San, 108, 200
Jing Fang Bai Du San Jia Jian, 200
Jing Jie Bai Du San Jia Jian, 132
Jing Jie Tou Zhen Tang, 247
Jing Ke Ling, 152
Ju Hua Tong Sheng San Jia Jian, 214
Ju Pi Zhu Ru Tang Jia Wei, 85

K, L

Ku Jiang Xin Kai Fang, 159
Ku Shen Tang, 194, 208
Kuan Dong Hua Tang, 152
Lai Mei Jie Du Tang, 268
Lai Mei Jie Du Tang Jia Jian, 268
Li Ma Tou Fa Tang, 246
Li Zhong Tang, 65-66, 68, 78, 83, 94, 118, 301
Li Zhong Tang Jia Jian, 65, 83, 118
Lian Mei Tang Jia Jian, 95
Liang Ge Lian Qiao San, 214
Liang Ge San, 101
Liang Ge San Jia Jian, 101
Liang Ying Qing Qi Tang Jia Jian, 274
Ling Jiao Gou Teng Tang, 164-165, 252
Ling Jiao Gou Teng Tang Jia Jian, 164-165, 252
Liu Jun Zi Tang, 144, 172, 184, 231
Liu Jun Zi Tang Jia Jian, 144

Liu Jun Zi Tang Jia Wei, 184, 231
Liu Shen Wan, 254-255, 290
Liu Wei Di Huang Wan, 43, 104, 293
Liu Wei Di Huang Wan Jia Wei, 104
Long Dan Xie Gan Tang Jia Jian, 122, 190-191, 218
Lu Dou Tang, 98

M, N, P

Ma Huang Yi Zhi Tang, 189
Ma Xing Shi Gan Tang, 44, 135, 150, 157-159, 168, 170, 250-251
Ma Xing Shi Gan Tang Jia Jian, 135, 170
Ma Xing Shi Gan Tang Jia Wei, 150, 157-158, 168, 250-251
Mai Men Dong Tang Jia Jian, 153
Mai Men Dong Yin, 220
Mai Wei Di Huang Wan, 145
Mu Xiang Bing Lang Wan, 80
Niao Beng Fang, 219
Niao Beng Ji Ben Fang Jia Jian, 219
Ning Gan Xi Feng Tang, 235
Ping Wei San, 144, 199, 203
Ping Wei San Jia Jian, 203
Pu Di Ren Tang, 98
Pu Ji Xiao Du Yin, 178, 281-282
Pu Ji Xiao Du Yin Jia Jian, 281-282

Q

Qi Ju Di Huang Wan Jia Jian, 258
Qi Wei Bai Zhu San Jia Wei, 92
Qian Gen Tang, 75
Qian Gen Tang Jia Jian, 75
Qian Jin Long Dan Tang, 230
Qiang Huo Sheng Feng Tang Jia Jian, 213
Qiao He Tang, 263
Qin Jiao Bie Jia San, 110
Qing Dai Gao, 106, 199
Qing Dai San, 194, 199, 209
Qing Fei Yin, 135, 186
Qing Jie Tang, 282
Qing Jie Tou Biao Tang, 247
Qing Li Jie Du Tang, 269
Qing Liang Zhi Nu Tang, 210
Qing Nao Yi Zhi Tang, 240
Qing Pi Chu Shi Yin, 193
Qing Re Jie Du Tang, 248
Qing Re Li Niao Fang, 217
Qing Re Li Shi Tang, 92
Qing Re Liang Xue Yin, 210
Qing Re Xie Huo Tang, 103
Qing Re Xie Pi San, 69, 103
Qing Re Xie Pi San Jia Jian, 103
Qing Shu Tang, 98, 193
Qing Shu Tang Jia Jian, 193
Qing Wei Jie Du Tang, 268
Qing Wen Bai Du Yin Jia Jian, 116, 274-275
Qing Yan Li Ge Tang, 178
Qing Yan Xia Tan Tang, 254-255
Qing Yan Xia Tan Tang Jia Jian, 255
Qing Ying Bai Du Yin, 252
Qing Ying Tang Jia Jian, 252, 269, 275
Qing Zao Jiu Fei Tang Jia Jian, 154
Qu Feng San Re Yin Zi Jia Jian, 215
Qu Mai Zhi Zhu Wan, 182

R, S

Ren Shen Wu Wei Zi Tang, 143, 153, 161, 173
Ren Shen Wu Wei Zi Tang Jia Jian, 153, 161
Ren Shen Wu Wei Zi Tang Jia Wei, 173
San Ao Tang Jia Wei, 148, 156
San Huang Xi Ji, 98, 194, 199, 209
San Jia Fu Mai Tang, 236, 301
San Ju Yin Jia Jian, 149
Sang Bai Pi Tang, 150
Sang Ju Yin, 108, 134
Sang Ju Yin Jia Jian, 134
Sang Piao Xiao San Jia Jian, 188
Sang Xing Tang Jia Wei, 136
Sha Shen Mai Dong Tang, 85, 110, 141, 161, 248-249, 276
Sha Shen Mai Dong Tang Jia Jian, 85, 141, 161, 249, 276
Shang Shi Fu Tong Zhi Xie Tang, 89
She Gan Xiao Du Yin, 255
Shen Fu Long Mu Jiu Ni Tang, 163, 289
Shen Fu Tang, 116, 162-163, 297
Shen Fu Tang Jia Wei, 162-163, 297
Shen Ling Bai Zhu San, 93, 162, 183, 222
Shen Ling Bai Zhu San Jia Jian, 162, 183
Shen Ling Bai Zhu San Jia Wei, 162
Shen Xiang Tang, 82
Shen Zhu Tang, 93
Sheng Ma Ge Gen Tang, 245

Sheng Mai San, 169, 289
Sheng Mai San Jia Jian, 289
Sheng Mai San Jia Wei, 289
Sheng Mai Yin, 240
Shi Gao Zhi Mu Tang, 109
Shi Wei Dao Chi San, 216
Shu Feng Qing Re Tang Jia Jian, 121
Shu Feng Qu Shi Tang, 198
Shu Gan Qing Re Tang, 304
Shu Jin Chu Bi Tang Jia Jian, 225
Shui Dou Fang, 267
Si Jun Zi Tang, 68, 83, 143, 172, 221
Si Jun Zi Tang Jia Wei, 143, 172
Si Ni Tang Jia Wei, 163, 297
Si Qi Tang, 86
Si Shen Wan, 94
Si Wu Tang, 199, 259
Su Ting Gun Tan Wan Jia Jian, 150
Su Zi Jiang Qi Tang, 140, 143
Suan Zao Ren Tang, 107
Suo Quan Wan, 189-190, 221

T, W

Tang Shi Xiong Huang San, 294
Ting Li Da Zao Xie Fei Tang, 159
Tong Ming San, 126
Tong Qiao Huo Xue Tang, 232
Tong Qiao Huo Xue Tang Jia Jian, 232
Tou Zhen Liang Jie Tang Jia Jian, 263
Tu Si Zi San, 188
Wei Jing Tang Jia Wei, 139
Wen Dan Tang, 84, 228, 242
Wen Fei Kang Min Tang, 171
Wen Fei Zhi Ke Yin, 145
Wen Fei Zhi Liu Dan Jia Jian, 205
Wu Lin San Jia Wei, 217
Wu Ling San, 71, 130, 301
Wu Ling San Jia Wei, 130
Wu Sheng Dan, 175
Wu Wei Xiao Du Yin, 208
Wu Yao San, 79

X

Xi Di Qing Luo Yin, 302
Xi Jiao Di Huang Tang, 253-254
Xi Jiao Di Huang Tang Jia Jian, 253
Xi Jiao San Jia Jian, 65
Xi Jiao Xiao Du Yin Jia Jian, 73

Xi Liang Tou Biao Tang, 246
Xian Fang Huo Ming Yin Jia Jian, 286
Xiang Ru Yin Jia Wei, 115
Xiang Sha Liu Jun Zi Tang Jia Wei, 184
Xiao Chai Hu Tang, 128-129, 180, 223, 317-319
Xiao Chai Hu Tang Jia Wei, 128
Xiao Du Yin Jia Jian, 73, 122, 281-282
Xiao E Tang, 177
Xiao Er Hui Chun Dan, 117
Xiao Feng San Jia Jian, 201
Xiao Ji Hua Zhi Tang, 182
Xiao Jian Zhong Tang, 78
Xiao Mi Qing Tang, 96
Xiao Qing Long Tang, 133, 148, 160, 169-170
Xiao Qing Long Tang Jia Jian, 133, 170
Xiao Qing Long Tang Jia Wei, 148
Xiao Ru Tang, 82
Xiao Ru Wan, 79, 89
Xiao Shi Hua Ji Yin, 89
Xie Bai San Jia Jian, 138
Xie Qing Wan Jia Jian, 230
Xie Xin Dao Chi Tang, 102
Xin Yi Qing Fei Yin, 186
Xing Su San, 133-134
Xing Su San Jia Jian, 133-134
Xuan Du Fa Biao Tang, 245-246
Xuan Du Fa Biao Tang Jia Jian, 246
Xue Fu Zhu Yu Tang, 67

Y

Yang Wei Zeng Jin Tang, 185
Yang Xin Tang, 228
Yang Yin Jie Du Tang, 249
Yang Yin Qing Fei Tang, 276, 287
Yang Yin Qing Fei Tang Jia Wei, 287
Ye Ju Niu Zi Tang Jia Wei, 99
Ye Shi Yang Wei Tang Jia Jian, 185
Yi Gan San, 238
Yi Gong San, 111
Yi Pi Zhen Jing San, 94
Yi Qi Bu Pi Tang, 93
Yi Qi Gu She Tang, 222
Yi Xin Hua Yu Tang, 163
Yin Chen Hao Tang, 64
Yin Chen Hao Tang Jia Jian, 64
Yin Chen Hao Tang Jia Wei, 64

Yin Chen Li Zhong Tang, 65-66
Yin Chen Li Zhong Tang Jia Jian, 65
Yin Chen Li Zhong Tang Jia Wei, 66
Yin Chen Si Ling Tang, 64
Yin Dai Tang, 159
Yin Guo San, 157
Yin Hua Zi Cao Tang, 262
Yin Qiao Er Ding Tang, 266
Yin Qiao Ma Bo She Gan Tang Jia Jian, 271-272
Yin Qiao San, 73, 109, 114, 158, 177, 246, 261, 265-266, 268, 273, 279-280, 285
Yin Qiao San Jia Jian, 73, 114, 177, 246, 261, 265-266, 268, 273, 279-280, 285
Yin Shi Tang, 267
You Yin Qian Yang Wan, 239
Yu Ping Feng San, 171
Yu Quan Wan, 220
Yu Shu Dan, 117

Yun Qi San, 68
Yun Qi San Jia Jian, 68

Z

Zhen Gan Xi Feng Tang, 235
Zhi Bai Di Huang Wan, 104, 124, 131, 191
Zhi Bai Di Huang Wan Jia Jian, 124
Zhi Bai Di Huang Wan Jia Wei, 104, 124
Zhi Jing Er Chen Tang, 152
Zhi Ke San Jia Wei, 149
Zhi Yi Xi Fang, 100
Zhi Zhu San Jia Jian, 203
Zhong Bai Zhu Ye Tang, 102
Zhu Ye Shi Gao Tang, 187
Zi Cao San, 201
Zi Yin An Shen Tang, 303
Zi Yin Xie Huo Fang, 303
Zuo Gui Wan Jia Jian, 240
Zuo Jin Wan, 86

OTHER BOOKS ON CHINESE MEDICINE AVAILABLE FROM:
BLUE POPPY PRESS

5441 Western, Suite 2, Boulder, CO 80301
For ordering 1-800-487-9296 PH. 303\447-8372 FAX 303\245-8362
Email: info@bluepoppy.com Website: www.bluepoppy.com

ACUPOINT POCKET REFERENCE
by Bob Flaws
ISBN 0-936185-93-7

ACUPUNCTURE & IVF
by Lifang Liang
ISBN 0-891845-24-1

ACUPUNCTURE AND MOXIBUSTION FORMULAS & TREATMENTS
by Cheng Dan-an, trans. by Wu Ming
ISBN 0-936185-68-6

ACUPUNCTURE PHYSICAL MEDICINE: An Acupuncture Touchpoint Approach to the Treatment of Chronic Pain, Fatigue, and Stress Disorders
by Mark Seem
ISBN 1-891845-13-6

AGING & BLOOD STASIS:
A New Approach to TCM Geriatrics
by Yan De-xin
ISBN 0-936185-63-5

A NEW AMERICAN ACUPUNTURE
By Mark Seem
ISBN 0-936185-44-9

BETTER BREAST HEALTH NATURALLY with CHINESE MEDICINE
by Honora Lee Wolfe & Bob Flaws
ISBN 0-936185-90-2

THE BOOK OF JOOK:
Chinese Medicinal Porridges
by B. Flaws
ISBN 0-936185-60-0

CHANNEL DIVERGENCES
Deeper Pathways of the Web
by Miki Shima and Charles Chase
ISBN 1-891845-15-2

CHINESE MEDICAL OBSTETRICS
by Bob Flaws
ISBN 1-891845-30-6

CHINESE MEDICAL PALMISTRY:
Your Health in Your Hand
by Zong Xiao-fan & Gary Liscum
ISBN 0-936185-64-3

CHINESE MEDICAL PSYCHIATRY
A Textbook and Clinical Manual
by Bob Flaws and James Lake, MD
ISBN 1-845891-17-9

CHINESE MEDICINAL TEAS:
Simple, Proven, Folk Formulas for Common Diseases & Promoting Health
by Zong Xiao-fan & Gary Liscum
ISBN 0-936185-76-7

CHINESE MEDICINAL WINES & ELIXIRS
by Bob Flaws
ISBN 0-936185-58-9

CHINESE PEDIATRIC MASSAGE THERAPY: A Parent's & Practitioner's Guide to the Prevention & Treatment of Childhood Illness
by Fan Ya-li
ISBN 0-936185-54-6

CHINESE SELF-MASSAGE THERAPY:
The Easy Way to Health
by Fan Ya-li
ISBN 0-936185-74-0

THE CLASSIC OF DIFFICULTIES:
A Translation of the Nan Jing
translation by Bob Flaws
ISBN 1-891845-07-1

CLINICAL NEPHROLOGY
IN CHINESE MEDICINE
by Wei Li & David Frierman,
with Ben Luna & Bob Flaws
ISBN 1-891845-23-3

CONTROLLING DIABETES NATURALLY WITH CHINESE MEDICINE
by Lynn Kuchinski
ISBN 0-936185-06-3

CURING ARTHRITIS NATURALLY WITH CHINESE MEDICINE
by Douglas Frank & Bob Flaws
ISBN 0-936185-87-2

CURING DEPRESSION NATURALLY WITH CHINESE MEDICINE
by Rosa Schnyer & Bob Flaws
ISBN 0-936185-94-5

CURING FIBROMYALGIA NATURALLY WITH
CHINESE MEDICINE
by Bob Flaws
ISBN 1-891845-09-8

CURING HAY FEVER NATURALLY WITH CHINESE MEDICINE
by Bob Flaws
ISBN 0-936185-91-0

CURING HEADACHES NATURALLY WITH
CHINESE MEDICINE
by Bob Flaws
ISBN 0-936185-95-3

CURING IBS NATURALLY WITH CHINESE
MEDICINE
by Jane Bean Oberski
ISBN 1-891845-11-X

CURING INSOMNIA NATURALLY WITH CHINESE MEDICINE
by Bob Flaws
ISBN 0-936185-86-4

CURING PMS NATURALLY WITH
CHINESE MEDICINE
by Bob Flaws
ISBN 0-936185-85-6

THE DIVINE FARMER'S MATERIA MEDICA A
Translation of the Shen Nong Ben Cao
translation by Yang Shouz-zhong
ISBN 0-936185-96-1

DUI YAO: THE ART OF COMBINING
CHINESE HERBAL MEDICINALS
by Philippe Sionneau
ISBN 0-936185-81-3

ENDOMETRIOSIS, INFERTILITY AND TRADITIONAL CHINESE MEDICINE:
A Laywoman's Guide
by Bob Flaws
ISBN 0-936185-14-7

THE ESSENCE OF LIU FENG-WU'S
GYNECOLOGY
by Liu Feng-wu, translated by Yang Shou-zhong
ISBN 0-936185-88-0

EXTRA TREATISES BASED ON
INVESTIGATION & INQUIRY:
A Translation of Zhu Dan-xi's Ge Zhi Yu Lun
translation by Yang Shou-zhong
ISBN 0-936185-53-8

FIRE IN THE VALLEY: TCM Diagnosis &
Treatment of Vaginal Diseases
by Bob Flaws
ISBN 0-936185-25-2

FU QING-ZHU'S GYNECOLOGY
trans. by Yang Shou-zhong and Liu Da-wei
ISBN 0-936185-35-X

FULFILLING THE ESSENCE:
A Handbook of Traditional & Contemporary
Treatments for Female Infertility
by Bob Flaws
ISBN 0-936185-48-1

GOLDEN NEEDLE WANG LE-TING: A 20th
Century Master's Approach to Acupuncture
by Yu Hui-chan and Han Fu-ru, trans. by Shuai Xue-zhong
ISBN 0-936185-789-3

A GUIDE TO GYNECOLOGY
by Ye Heng-yin,
trans. by Bob Flaws and Shuai Xue-zhong
ISBN 1-891845-19-5

A HANDBOOK OF TCM PATTERNS
& TREATMENTS
by Bob Flaws & Daniel Finney
ISBN 0-936185-70-8

A HANDBOOK OF TRADITIONAL
CHINESE DERMATOLOGY
by Liang Jian-hui, trans. by Zhang Ting-liang & Bob Flaws
ISBN 0-936185-07-4

A HANDBOOK OF TRADITIONAL
CHINESE GYNECOLOGY
by Zhejiang College of TCM, trans. by Zhang Ting-liang & Bob Flaws
ISBN 0-936185-06-6 (4th edit.)

A HANDBOOK OF CHINESE HEMATOLOGY
by Simon Becker
ISBN 1-891845-16-0

A HANDBOOK OF MENSTRUAL DISEASES IN
CHINESE MEDICINE
by Bob Flaws
ISBN 0-936185-82-1

A HANDBOOK of TCM PEDIATRICS
by Bob Flaws
ISBN 0-936185-72-4

THE HEART & ESSENCE OF DAN-XI'S METHODS OF TREATMENT
by Xu Dan-xi, trans. by Yang Shou-zhong
ISBN 0-926185-49-X

HERB TOXICITIES & DRUG INTERACTIONS:
A Formula Approach
by Fred Jennes with Bob Flaws
ISBN 1-891845-26-8

IMPERIAL SECRETS OF HEALTH
& LONGEVITY
by Bob Flaws
ISBN 0-936185-51-1

INSIGHTS OF A SENIOR ACUPUNCTURIST
by Miriam Lee
ISBN 0-936185-33-3

INTRODUCTION TO THE USE OF
PROCESSED CHINESE MEDICINALS
by Philippe Sionneau
ISBN 0-936185-62-7

KEEPING YOUR CHILD HEALTHY WITH
CHINESE MEDICINE
by Bob Flaws
ISBN 0-936185-71-6

THE LAKESIDE MASTER'S STUDY
OF THE PULSE
by Li Shi-zhen, trans. by Bob Flaws
ISBN 1-891845-01-2

MASTER HUA'S CLASSIC OF THE
CENTRAL VISCERA
by Hua Tuo, trans. by Yang Shou-zhong
ISBN 0-936185-43-0

MASTER TONG'S ACUPUNCTURE
by Miriam Lee
ISBN 0-926185-37-6

THE MEDICAL I CHING: Oracle of the Healer
Within
by Miki Shima
ISBN 0-936185-38-4

MANAGING MENOPAUSE NATURALLY with
Chinese Medicine
by Honora Lee Wolfe
ISBN 0-936185-98-8

NCCAOM BIO-MEDICINE TEST PREP BOOK:
EXAM PREPARATION & STUDY GUIDE
by Zhong Bai-song
ISBN 978-1-891845-34-9

POINTS FOR PROFIT: The Essential Guide to
Practice Success for Acupuncturists
by Honora Wolfe, Eric Strand & Marilyn Allen
ISBN 1-891845-25-X

THE PULSE CLASSIC:
A Translation of the Mai Jing
by Wang Shu-he, trans. by Yang Shou-zhong
ISBN 0-936185-75-9

SHAOLIN SECRET FORMULAS for Treatment of
External Injuries
by De Chan, trans. by Zhang Ting-liang &
Bob Flaws
ISBN 0-936185-08-2

STATEMENTS OF FACT IN TRADITIONAL
CHINESE MEDICINE
by Bob Flaws
ISBN 0-936185-52-X

STICKING TO THE POINT 1:
A Rational Methodology for the Step by
Step Formulation & Administration of
an Acupuncture Treatment
by Bob Flaws
ISBN 0-936185-17-1

STICKING TO THE POINT 2:
A Study of Acupuncture & Moxibustion
Formulas and Strategies
by Bob Flaws
ISBN 0-936185-97-X

A STUDY OF DAOIST ACUPUNCTURE &
MOXIBUSTION
by Liu Zheng-cai
ISBN 1-891845-08-X

THE SUCCESSFUL CHINESE HERBALIST
by Bob Flaws and Honora Lee Wolfe
ISBN 1-891845-29-2

THE SYSTEMATIC CLASSIC OF
ACUPUNCTURE & MOXIBUSTION
A translation of the Jia Yi Jing
by Huang-fu Mi, trans. by Yang Shou-zhong & Charles
Chace
ISBN 0-936185-29-5

THE TAO OF HEALTHY EATING
ACCORDING TO CHINESE MEDICINE
by Bob Flaws
ISBN 0-936185-92-9

TEACH YOURSELF TO READ MODERN
MEDICAL CHINESE
by Bob Flaws
ISBN 0-936185-99-6

TREATING PEDIATRIC BED-WETTING WITH
ACUPUNCTURE & CHINESE MEDICINE
by Robert Helmer
ISBN 978-1-891845-33-0

THE TREATMENT OF CARDIOVASCULAR
DISEASES WITH CHINESE MEDICINE
by Simon Becker, Bob Flaws &
Robert Casañas, MD
ISBN 978-1-891845-27-6

THE TREATMENT OF DIABETES
MELLITUS WITH CHINESE MEDICINE
by Bob Flaws, Lynn Kuchinski &
Robert Casañas, M.D.
ISBN 1-891845-21-7

THE TREATMENT OF DISEASE IN TCM, Vol. 1: Diseases of the Head & Face, Including Mental & Emotional Disorders
by Philippe Sionneau & Lü Gang
ISBN 0-936185-69-4

THE TREATMENT OF DISEASE IN TCM, Vol. II: Diseases of the Eyes, Ears, Nose, & Throat
by Sionneau & Lü
ISBN 0-936185-69-4

THE TREATMENT OF DISEASE, Vol. III: Diseases of the Mouth, Lips, Tongue, Teeth & Gums
by Sionneau & Lü
ISBN 0-936185-79-1

THE TREATMENT OF DISEASE, Vol IV: Diseases of the Neck, Shoulders, Back, & Limbs
by Philippe Sionneau & Lü Gang
ISBN 0-936185-89-9

THE TREATMENT OF DISEASE, Vol V: Diseases of the Chest & Abdomen
by Philippe Sionneau & Lü Gang
ISBN 1-891845-02-0

THE TREATMENT OF DISEASE, Vol VI: Diseases of the Urogential System & Proctology
by Philippe Sionneau & Lü Gang
ISBN 1-891845-05-5

THE TREATMENT OF DISEASE, Vol VII: General Symptoms
by Philippe Sionneau & Lü Gang
ISBN 1-891845-14-4

THE TREATMENT OF EXTERNAL DISEASES WITH ACUPUNCTURE & MOXIBUSTION
by Yan Cui-lan and Zhu Yun-long, trans. by Yang Shou-zhong
ISBN 0-936185-80-5

THE TREATMENT OF MODERN WESTERN MEDICAL DISEASES WITH CHINESE MEDICINE
by Bob Flaws & Philippe Sionneau
ISBN 1-891845-20-9

THE TREATMENT OF DIABETES MELLITUS WITH CHINESE MEDICINE
by Bob Flaws, Lynn Kuchinski & Robert Casañas, MD
ISBN 1-891845-21-7

UNDERSTANDING THE DIFFICULT PATIENT: A Guide for Practitioners of Oriental Medicine
by Nancy Bilello, RN, L.ac.
ISBN 1-891845-32-2

70 ESSENTIAL CHINESE HERBAL FORMULAS
by Bob Flaws
ISBN 0-936185-59-7

160 ESSENTIAL CHINESE HERBAL PATENT MEDICINES
by Bob Flaws
ISBN 1-891945-12-8

630 QUESTIONS & ANSWERS ABOUT CHINESE HERBAL MEDICINE: A Workbook & Study Guide
by Bob Flaws
ISBN 1-891845-04-7

230 ESSENTIAL CHINESE MEDICINALS
by Bob Flaws
ISBN 1-891845-03-9

750 QUESTIONS & ANSWERS ABOUT ACUPUNCTURE
Exam Preparation & Study Guide
by Fred Jennes
ISBN 1-891845-22-5